CW00486704

ISBN 978-0-260-11534-8
PIBN 10928871

FB &c Ltd, Dalton House, 60 Windsor Avenue, London, SW19 2RR.
Company number 08720141. Registered in England and Wales.

PAPERS TO BE PRESENTED
BEFORE THE SECTION ON

OPHTHALMOLOGY

OF THE

AMERICAN MEDICAL ASSOCIATION

Chicago, June 2-5, 1908

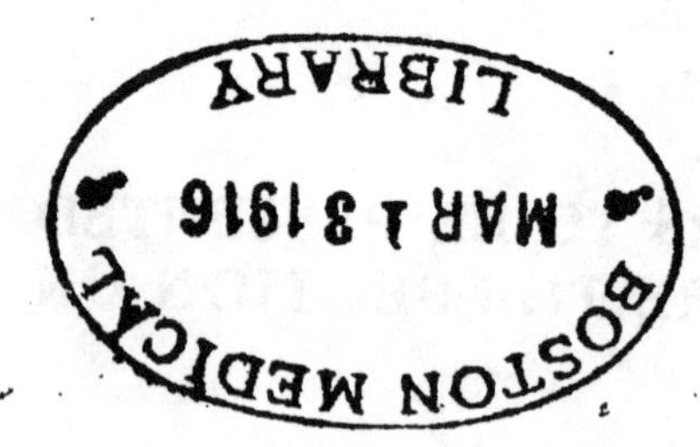

These papers, being the property of the American Medical Association, are not released for publication. They are here printed solely for the use of the members of the Section on Ophthalmology.

TO THE MEMBERS OF THE SECTION ON OPHTHALMOLOGY

OF THE

AMERICAN MEDICAL ASSOCIATION

In presenting to the members of the Section on Ophthalmology of the American Medical Association printed copies of the papers accepted for the Section program for the session that is to be held in Chicago, June 2-5, 1908, the officers and executive committee are continuing a progressive feature which proved so satisfactory the last two years.

Members are reminded that the following rules have been adopted:

1. No paper will be formally read at the session, though each essayist will be allowed not to exceed five minutes in which to close the discussion.

2. The member formally opening the discussion of a paper will be allowed not to exceed ten minutes, and subsequent speakers five minutes.

Members are, therefore, respectfully asked to read the papers carefully before going to Chicago, with a view not only of becoming familiar with the substance of the papers, but also for the purpose of preparation to take part in a more intelligent and comprehensive discussion which such a plan is certain to bring out.

Members are requested to take the printed papers to Chicago for reference during discussion.

The officers desire to express their appreciation of the co-operation of the essayists in carrying the plan to its present stage, and earnestly request the assistance of the members of the Section in an endeavor to make the Chicago session the best in our history.

Albert E. Bulson, Jr., Secretary.

William H. Wilder, Chairman.

CONTENTS

CONTENTS

AUTHORS' INDEX

AUTOINTOXICATION.

A FURTHER CONTRIBUTION TO THE POSSIBLE RELATIONSHIP OF AUTOINTOXICATION TO CERTAIN DISEASES OF THE CORNEA AND UVEAL TRACT.*

G. E. DE SCHWEINITZ, M.D.

WITH GENERAL AND LABORATORY EXAMINATIONS†

BY

CHARLES A. FIFE, M.D.

PHILADELPHIA.

At a meeting of the Section on Ophthalmology of the American Medical Association in Boston, 1906, I presented a paper on "Autointoxication in Relation to the Eye,"[1] and concluded this communication with the following summary: "Although we do not know the entity of a single autointoxication, except the acidosis of diabetic coma, and although we know that no known autointoxication is to be attributed to any known end product of any known metabolism, to quote Alonzo Taylor, we do know, from clinical analogy, at least, that autointoxications exist, even if their true nature is as yet a secret. We do know, too, that after food is swallowed, and before the end products of assimilation are eliminated, there may be processes arising under abnormal conditions which yield poisonous products foreign to normal metabolism, the reabsorption of which may be followed by definite symptoms. We have reason to believe, in the absence of other causes, that under these conditions ocular troubles may also arise largely in the corneo-scleral and uveal tracts, and probably, in

* This paper has been accepted by the Executive Committee of the Section on Ophthalmology of the American Medical Association, to be presented before the Section at the Chicago Session, June 2-5, 1908. Publication rights reserved by the American Medical Association.

† Laboratory examinations were made in the William Pepper Clinical Laboratory, Phœbe Hearst Foundation.

1. THE JOURNAL A. M. A., Feb. 9, 1907, p. 502.

so far as the nervous apparatus is concerned, in manifestations to which we apply the term acute or chronic retrobulbar neuritis. We do not know whether these toxins, whatever they may be, actually are the only and sole cause of these conditions, but such examinations as have been made by Elschnig, Kraus, Groyer, Edsall and myself, at least indicate that, to use Elschnig's term, they may be considered accessory causes. As Edsall and I have said, they may be able to play a certain part in the production of the symptoms, and at times are probably the direct cause of their continuance, even when other more commonly accepted etiologic factors have ceased to be active."

As the subject appears to have excited some interest among certain of my ophthalmic confreres, it seemed proper to continue these investigations and to record the results thus far obtained by the report of a series of cases which may be regarded as types of some of the ocular diseases in which, at least, the suspicion is justified that they may, perhaps, interpret one of the manifestations of the presence of endogenous intoxication. For the general and laboratory examinations in the study of the patients whose histories are reported, I am in largest measure indebted to Dr. Charles A. Fife.

It should distinctly be understood that if the detection and isolation of definite ptomains or toxins are necessary for the diagnosis of autointoxication, as is intimated by some authorities, then the cases which follow are not entitled to be regarded in any sense as ocular interpretations of nutritional or metabolic disorders. We are in entire accord with Alonzo Taylor that a loose interpretation of the facts of metabolism and their relation to disease should strongly be condemned, but believe, nevertheless, that presumptive clinical, laboratory and therapeutic testimony is worthy of consideration. Because the ocular conditions of the cases reported suggest a toxic state, because the constitutional symptoms in some of them are analogous to symptoms of chronic infections and gastro-intestinal diseases, and because the physical examinations of the patients were, in a measure, indicative of similar etiologic factors, there seems to be a certain justification for presenting them as worthy of consideration from the standpoint of autointoxication.

Before proceeding to a detailed statement of the study of these cases, it would seem proper to give a résumé[2] of those products detected by urinary analysis, examination of the feces and examination of the gastric contents, which permit one to indulge in the belief that autointoxication and its effects are worthy of consideration.

1. *Examination of Urine.*—The urine is usually scanty, of dark color, and albumin, cylindroids and casts may be detected. The presence of acetone, diacetic acid and oxybutyric acid suggests acidosis and derangement in fat metabolism. Indol and skatol, which are the result of bacterial action on an end product of tryptic digestion, unite chiefly with sulphuric acid, forming part of the so-called conjugated sulphates or ethereal sulphates. Phenol and cresol are formed from tyrosin by bacteria and are chiefly eliminated, as are indol and skatol, as conjugated sulphates. These aromatic bodies, that is, indol, skatol, phenol and cresol, but more especially their conjugated forms, are valuable indicators in the urine of protein decomposition products, that is, of intestinal putrefaction; but when considered alone they are not pathognomonic of autointoxication, even though tissue putrefaction is excluded, because the excretion of aromatic bodies may be much in excess of the average normal, and yet no other evidence of disease can be detected. This is especially true of any single type, such as indican.

Urobilin is probably formed from bile pigments in the intestines by the action of bacteria, and hence has been regarded as something of an index to bacterial activity in the intestinal tract. This, however, has not been proved. The volatile fatty acids (formic, acetic, butyric and propionic) have also been regarded, to a certain extent, as indications of carbohydrate fermentation in the intestinal tract. In this respect, however, the volatile fatty acids are uncertain guides, because under some conditions they are increased without the accompanying carbohydrate fermentation. Therefore, the degree of fatty acidity is not of value when considered alone, but in relation to the diet of the patient, to the presence or absence of acetone, aromatic bodies, urobilin, ammonia, nitrogen and conjugated sulphates, it is, at least, of interest and probably of value. The presence of cystin, leucin, tyrosin and hydrogen-sulphid is of no importance unless associated with other evidences of autointoxication.

The total nitrogen, urea, uric acid, ammonia nitrogen and albumin, when considered in connection with the character and amount of diet, furnish important data on the condition of nitrogen metabolism. The average output of these substances in twenty-four hours, on an average diet, of a

---

2. This résumé has been prepared by Dr. Fife.

healthy adult, is approximately: Urea, 20.0 gm.; uric acid, 0.2 gm.; ammonia nitrogen, 0.6 gm.; total nitrogen, 14.0 gm.

Inasmuch as ammonia nitrogen probably bears a reciprocal relation to urea, except where there is an increased formation of acids in the system, the increase of ammonia is an index, though not a perfectly trustworthy one, of acidosis to be confirmed by detection of excess of acetone, diacetic acid and oxybutyric acid. The sulphates are derived principally from the catabolism of protein material in the body. The largest amount unites with inorganic elements, forming the so-called preformed sulphates, approximately 1.5 to 2.5 gm., being the daily output of a normal adult on an average diet. The conjugated sulphates are the sulphates combined with the aromatic protein decomposition products, averaging from 0.1 to 0.25 gm. per day, the normal ratio to preformed sulphates being 1 to 10. An increase in amount of the conjugated sulphates is our most reliable evidence of intestinal putrefaction.

2. *Examination of Feces.*—Naturally, a diagnosis of intestinal autointoxication can not be made in the absence of thorough examination of the feces, and certainly not in the absence of inspection of the dejecta, in order to note their color, odor, reaction, consistency, state of digestion and the presence or absence of the signs of fermentation, etc.

3. *Examination of Gastric Contents.*—This also is important in order to ascertain the state of digestion of the test meal, the evidence of retention and decomposition, the presence of acid products of fermentation, the total gastric acidity and the amount of free hydrochloric acid, the presence of sarcenæ, yeast, etc.

It should be distinctly understood that the influence of syphilis and tuberculosis is definitely excluded as an etiologic factor in the cases which are utilized as types in this communication. The details of the laboratory and other examinations are purposely recorded, as in no other way can the character of the investigation to which the patients with these ocular disorders should be submitted be demonstrated satisfactorily.

REPORT OF CASES.

Case 1.—*Relapsing Sclero-Keratitis of Four Months' Duration; Clear Evidences of Gastrointestinal Decomposition and Faulty Nitrogen Metabolism.*—Mrs. A., aged 28, no children, no miscarriages, came for consultation on March 7, 1907.

Family History.—This is good in all respects, the patient coming from a long-lived family, the members of which have suffered from no heart, lung, liver, kidney, blood or nerve disease.

Personal History.—The patient has had measles, pertussis, tonsillitis once and influenza three times, but not in recent years, and none of the attacks was severe, and all were uncomplicated. Ten years ago she is said to have suffered from malaria, having been ill for two weeks. There is no history of typhoid fever or of scarlet fever, and none of diphtheria or rheumatism. Owing to a faulty position of the uterus, there is dysmenorrhea. During the past three years the patient has had six periods of unconsciousness, without convulsions, the symptoms indicating that the attacks were not epileptic in nature. They have usually been followed by the vomiting of large amounts of undigested food, which is said to have been very sour. These attacks are probably "fainting spells." Except for nausea, following indiscretions in diet, there are no dyspeptic symptoms. Constipation is moderate. The patient is of a nervous temperament, but leads a regular life; she drinks too much tea and coffee, and eats too much meat, taking insufficient exercise. Syphilis and tuberculosis are definitely eliminated.

Past Eye History.—Ten years prior to her examination there was an attack of inflammation of the right eye, which is said to have been phlyctenular keratitis, but which probably was of the same nature as her present trouble. Four months ago the right eye was again attacked with inflammation, and again the diagnosis of phlyctenular keratitis was made. She then consulted an oculist, who evidently recognized the true nature of the case, and for three months she was treated with the usual local remedies, and took internally iron, arsenic and quinin, as occasions seemed to demand, without, however, any relief from the constantly recurring inflammations. These were always confined to the right eye, the left remaining normal.

Examination.—Examination of the patient's face, neck and throat, except for the evidences of anemia, was negative. The tongue was slightly coated, the heart and lungs negative, the chest long and narrow, the liver normal in size and position, the spleen normal and the right kidney easily palpable and movable. There was slight gastroptosis. Otherwise the abdomen was negative. The station was good; the knee-jerks were exaggerated.

Examination of the Eyes.—Uncorrected vision of O. D. 6/30. There was a general scleral injection, a little more condensed in the region of the ciliary body, which gradually assumed a coarser character in a large, triangular patch, chiefly placed over the region of the insertion of the external rectus. This patch had a slightly violaceous hue. The outer and upper triangular segment of the cornea was occupied by a delicate punctate haze, which was coarser nearer the periphery, and which apparently was situated beneath Bowman's membrane. At the outer margin of the cornea there was thickening of the episcleral tissue, and in one spot a small scleral node. Adrenalin bleached the general surface of the sclera, but failed entirely to blanch the more coarsely enlarged vessels in the denser patch of scleritis over the external rectus. The pupil dilated readily with scopolamin, and there was no discoloration of the iris. Fluorescin did not stain either the epithelium or endothelium. On the inner side of the cornea there were some old superficial scars, evidently the remnants of the inflammation of ten years ago. Ophthalmoscopic examination of this eye was practically negative, in so far as pathologic conditions are concerned, the optic disc being a vertical oval, of good color, and the retinal circulation normal in appearance. A faint nystagmus was demonstrable.

After one week of treatment, practically negative in its results, in so far as any relief of the patient is concerned, she was admitted to the University Hospital, and Dr. Fife requested to make the usual examinations. On the day of her admission the scleral injection was especially marked, and the punctate haze or infiltrate in the cornea very clearly evident, in addition to which there were about fifteen scattered white dots in the deeper layers of the cornea, somewhat resembling those seen in punctate keratitis, but evidently not situated on Descemet's membrane.

V. of O. S. 6/5; amplitude of accommodation 9 D.; media clear; fundus healthy in all respects.

LABORATORY EXAMINATIONS.

GASTRIC CONTENTS.

Gastric Contents.—March 14, 1907. Total acidity, 20 (0.07 per cent.); free HCl, none; lactic acid, none; microscopic examination, negative.

March 17, 1907. Total acidity, 62 (0.22 per cent.); free HCl, 36 (0.3 per cent.); lactic acid, none; microscopic examination, little yeast; mucus; starch well digested.

Blood.—March 14, 1907. Hemoglobin, 90 per cent.; leucocytes, 10,900; red cells, 4,670,000; polymorphonuclears, 70 per cent.; lymphocytes, 19 per cent.; large mononuclears, 2 per cent.; eosinophiles, ½ per cent.; no granular degeneration.

Feces.—Liquid; brown; not offensive; neutral reaction; hydrobilirubin present; no occult blood; vegetable fiber and shells, large amount; small amount of mucus. Microscopically: much mucus; no leucocytes; no blood; no muscle; no fat.

Urine.—March 16, 1907. Diet, equivalent to about 9.25 gm. of nitrogen.

Quantity, 24 hours, 825 c.c.; acid; color, amber; cloudy; flocculent sediment; normal odor; sp. gr., 1010; serum-albumin, faint trace; indican, slight excess.

Quantitative determinations:

Total solids, 16.50 gm.; serum-albumin, very faint trace; serum-globulin, none; glucose, none; total nitrogen (Kjeldahl), 6.636 gm.; urea (Doremus), 10.8 gm.; uric acid (Folin-Hopkins' method), 0.247 gm.; ammonia nitrogen (Styer's apparatus), 0.218 gm.; volatile fatty acids (Blumenthal). 30 c.c., 1/10 N. solution; total chlorids, estimated as NaCl, 4.320 gm.; total phosphates, estimated as P_2O_5, 1.116 gm.; earthy phosphates, estimated as P_2O_5, 0.372 gm.; alkaline phosphates, estimated as P_2O_5, 0.744 gm.; total sulphates, estimated as H_2SO_4, 1.929 gm.; preformed sulphates, estimated as H_2SO_4, 1.663 gm.; conjugate sulphates, estimated as H_2SO_4, 0.266 gm.; purin nitrogen (Hall), 0.1632.

Microscopic examination, negative.

Urine.—March 17, 1907. Diet, equivalent to about 12 gm. nitrogen.

Quantity, 24 hours, 830 c.c.; amber; appearance, cloudy; flocculent sediment; normal odor; acid; sp. gr., 1014; serum-albumin, faint trace; no excess of indican.

Quantitative determinations:

Total solids, 23.24 gm.; serum-albumin, very faint trace; serum-globulin, none; glucose, none; total nitrogen (Kjeldahl), 7.12 gm.; urea (Doremus), 12.0 gm.; uric acid (Folin-Hopkins' method), 0.3096 gm.; ammonia nitrogen (Styer's apparatus), 0.168 gm.; volatile fatty acids (Blumenthal). 48 c.c.; 1/10 N. solution; total chlorids, estimated as NaCl, 5.52 gm.; total phosphates, estimated as P_2O_5, 1.55 gm.; earthy phosphates, estimated as P_2O_5, 0.42 gm.; alkaline phosphates, estimated as P_2O_4, 1.13 gm.; total sulphates, estimated as H_2SO_4, 1.747 gm.; preformed sulphates, estimated as H_2SO_4, 1.413 gm.; conjugate sulphates, estimated as H_2SO_4, 0.334 gm.; purin nitrogen (Hall), 0.210 gm.

Microscopic examination: No casts; few leucocytes.

Remarks.—The interesting symptoms from the general standpoint are the fainting attacks, accompanied by the vomiting of large amounts of undigested sour food, especially when these are considered in connection with the laboratory findings. The wide variation in the character of the gastric contents, the one being hypoacid and the other hyperacid, is probably due to nervous influences, and these and the anemia are in all likelihood, in large part, dependent on the gastrointestinal decomposition products. The evidences of intestinal decomposition are the large amount of ethereal (conjugate) sulphates as compared with the preformed sulphates and the increase of indican. The large proportion of uric acid and of purin nitrogen to the total nitrogen suggests deranged metabolism.

Treatment and Its Results.—After consultation with Dr. Fife, the following line of treatment was suggested: Exercise, hot baths, the withdrawal from the diet of foods rich in purins and of easily decomposing foods; the administration of plenty of water before meals. Locally, the following remedies were used: Scopolamin, sufficient to maintain mydriasis; dionin, occasional subconjunctival injections of saline solution, hot compresses at stated intervals, and the usual flushings with boric acid.

The improvement was prompt and rapid, and at the expiration of three weeks the eye was almost white, and the corneal haze, although still present, lessened in density and extent. Corrected vision was now 6/6 with + 1 ⌒ + 1 c. axis 105. This improvement continued unimpaired for another four weeks, when, after the patient had returned home, there was a sharp relapse on June 18. Whether this was due to any indiscretion in diet or any relaxation in the strict regimen which had been ordered, we are not able to say. It yielded promptly to a renewal of the treatment. The eye became white and quiet and the extensive corneal opacity disappeared, with the exception of a somewhat kidney-shaped area, almost central, 5 mm. in length and 3 mm. in width, which, however, was not of sufficient density to prevent normal visual acuity with suitable glasses. The only internal medication was one of the preparations of iron, and this was given only in occasional doses. At the last examination, seven months after the patient originally sought advice, there had been no renewal of the ocular difficulty. Moreover, we know there has been none up to the present time.

Case 2.—*Bilateral Parenchymatous Keratitis Apparently Dependent on or Associated with Serious Indiscretion in Diet and Obstinate Constipation.*—Miss X., aged 17, applied for treatment on March 6, 1907.

Family History.—The patient's parents are living and healthy, as are one brother and two sisters. One brother died of intestinal tuberculosis at the age of 11 and another in early infancy.

Past History.—The patient had the ordinary exanthemata of childhood, had never had diphtheria, but until recent years was a great sufferer from tonsillitis, but has not had rheumatism. Formerly the patient suffered from dysmenorrhea, but at the present time menstruation is normal. She has always suffered from constipation, it being, as her mother expressed it, one of the troubles of her life. She has been a most imprudent eater of all manner of sweet stuffs, particularly of candy, pastry, cakes and the like, and has exhibited a really shocking disregard of proper diet. Syphilis and tuberculosis, except as noted in the family history, were excluded.

Past Eye History.—The original examination of the patient's eyes took place on May 10, 1902, when she came for the relief of frontal headache. Ophthalmoscopic examination at that time revealed in the right eye a small patch of old chorioiditis on the outer side of the disc, but in other respects the fundus was normal, as was the fundus in the opposite eye. After the correction of a moderate hyperopic astigmatism, which yielded normal vision, the asthenopia disappeared. This returned two years later, when it was found necessary to increase the strength of the cylinder. The headaches disappeared and the patient led a comfortable eye life until March 6, 1907, when she reported with the statement that for a couple of weeks she had suffered with what appeared to be a cold in the head, associated with a great deal of headache and some watering of the eyes.

Examination.—The patient is a small but well-formed girl, weighing 98 pounds as compared with 114 pounds four months previously. At the right apex, immediately below the clavicle, there was some prolongation of expiration and impaired resonance on percussion, most marked on lying down. The examination of the neck and throat, of the heart and of the abdominal organs yielded negative results. There was no rhinopharyngeal disease and no evidence of sinus infection. The teeth are sound and there was no pyorrhea alveolaris.

Eye Examination.—The left eye and a few days later the right eye exhibited a marked ciliary flush, and at the outer margin of each cornea a few small infiltrates, together with one or two minute nodes in the episcleral tissue. Within a week, with deepening of the scleral flush, a decided central interstitial infiltrate developed in each cornea, through which were scattered numerous saturated spots, the whole associated with marked photophobia, but without any very definite involvement of the iris and certainly no synechia. Edema of the corneal epithelium was evident. The conditions exactly represented those in the early stage of a parenchymatous keratitis. She was admitted to the University Hospital for treatment.

LABORATORY EXAMINATIONS.

These were made in part by her physician, Dr. Hobart A. Hare, and in part in the laboratory of the University Hospital.

Blood.—Hemoglobin, 83 per cent.; erythrocytes, 5,600,000; leucocytes, 6,000; plaques, greatly diminished; color index, 0.74. There was moderate pallor of many of the red cells, but no deformities. A few microcytes were present, no megalocytes, no erythroblasts, and no parasites.

The differential leucocyte count was as follows: Small lymphocytes, 12.0 per cent.; large lymphocytes, 16.0 per cent.; polymorphonuclear cells, 68.0 per cent.; eosinophiles, 2.4 per cent.; mastcells, 1.6 per cent.; myelocytes, none.

Urine.—The urine was dilute; the urea 0.9 per cent., 4½ grains in a fluidounce, 256.5 grains in twenty-four hours; other solids barely 175 grains in twenty-four hours. Examinations for excess of uric acid, calcium oxylates, triple phosphates, amorphous urates and phosphates were negative. These examinations were repeated on three successive days, with practically identical results.

It is evident that the blood reveals moderate so-called chlorotic changes, while the urine reveals nothing, except that the urea is a little low. No definite examinations were made at that time for indican.

Treatment and Progress of Case.—The patient remained in the University Hospital from March 29 to May 7, and the treatment consisted of a light diet, easily assimilated, with absolute abstinence from sweets, tea, coffee and fresh bread. Fruit was permitted in moderation. For a week, inunctions of unguentum hydrargyrum were used, and citrate of potassium was exhibited until the elimination of the solids in the urine reached the normal proportion. Calomel was used as a laxative. Locally, dionin, atropin and hot compresses were ordered.

The improvement was prompt, and at the expiration of the time noted the corneas were entirely clear, with the exception of a small area, crescent-shaped, at the lower and outer side of each of them, and the vision was normal in each eye. The patient gained 17 pounds in weignt, and continued to maintain this weight until the beginning of the present year, when, after a relapse, in so far as diet is concerned, she having returned to the use of sweets, etc., the eyes flushed and there was a return of the photophobia. With the restoration of diet to normal and the regulation of the bowel action, which had previously been placed in a normal condition, there was a prompt disappearance of these symptoms. With a correction of the hyperopic astigmatism as follows:

O. D. + .50 ⊂⊃ + .60 c. axis 165.
O. S. + .75 ⊂⊃ + .25 c. axis 30, V. is 6/6 in each eye.

Remarks.—This case is inserted because it is an excellent example of one of the types of keratitis, associated, to use Mr. W. T. Holmes Spicer's phrase, with defective intestinal hygiene. It is true that the elaborate analyses recorded in connection with case 1 were not made, and therefore it is not possible to say from the laboratory standpoint that any of the indications of intestinal autointoxication were present. It can only be assumed that such a condition of affairs was possible, but it may be at least definitely stated that with the regulation of the diet and the elimination of the constipation, there was a more prompt disappearance of the corneal lesions, together with the restoration of absolutely normal vision, than one is accustomed to see in cases of this nature. To be sure, inunctions of mercury were used, but only for a comparatively short time, and while they may have had an influence, owing to their aplastic action, they do not appear to have been the largest contributing factor in the success of treatment. The treatment of this patient was, of course, that which any intelligent practitioner would institute, and, in a certain sense, the case does not belong to the series now under consideration, that is to say, in the absence of elaborate laboratory examinations to prove the presence of autointoxication. It is inserted because of the undoubted relationship of the development of the corneal lesions to dietetic imprudence and presumably to faulty metabolism, and because from the eye symptoms alone the lesions could perfectly well have been attributed to other well recognized causes. The importance of the administration of citrate of potassium in cases of this character, until the elimination of the solids in the urine reaches the normal standard, is worthy of mention.

CASE 3.—*Disseminated Exudative Chorioiditis, Right Eye; Cataract, Left Eye; Faulty Nitrogen Metabolism; Probable Moderate Intestinal Autointoxication.*—Miss N. R., aged 26, referred by Dr. Murphy of Chicago applied for treatment on June 18, 1907.

Family History.—The patient comes from a long-lived family, among the members of which there are no hereditary predispositions. Both her parents are living, and her mother has had attacks of inflammatory rheumatism in her feet and hands for about ten years. Two sisters and three brothers are living. The mother has had no miscarriages. One brother had eczema at birth, one sister eczema from the eighth to the tenth year, and one brother is "not strong," apparently being a sufferer from gastric hyperacidity. One sister has twice had muscular rheumatism.

Past History.—The patient had three attacks of "diphtheria" when quite young. During the years following she was prone to sore throat and frequent attacks of tonsillitis, from which for the past six years she has been free. The patient has never suffered from influenza, scarlet fever, rheumatism or nervous disease, and does not readily take cold. Her first attack of eczema occurred in her sixteenth year, and since this date she has always suffered more or less from this skin affection. If she exercises freely, and she has done much horseback riding, the eczema is better, as it is also when she lives on a meat-free diet. She stays in bed about eight hours during the night, but is not a good sleeper, and has sometimes taken tablets for insomnia. Her appetite is good, but she is a rapid eater, and for the last six years has omitted meat from her diet list.

Past Eye History.—When 14 years old she had an attack of inflammation of her eyes, of what character is not definitely known; again an attack (in all probability chorioiditis or uveitis) when she was 21, and finally a third attack one year prior to her present examination. These attacks appear to have chiefly concerned the left eye. During the three weeks before she came for treatment there had been a rapid increase in the faulty vision of the left eye and the appearance of a white mass in the pupil space. These attacks of ocular inflammation had not been accompanied with severe pain. Muscæ had appeared before the right eye and vision had been somewhat blurred.

Examination.—The patient is a well-formed girl, of good proportions, whose mucous membranes are a little pale. The chest was well developed, the clavicles slightly prominent, the lung expansion good, although not quite so good at the right apex as at the left; no bronchial breathing and no râles, but the expiratory murmur was slightly higher pitched at the right than at the left apex. The heart was a trifle enlarged, the left border being in the mid-clavicular line, the right border at the right border of the sternum, while the apex was at the fifth interspace in the mid-clavicular line. There were no murmurs. The liver was just palpable and slightly tender. The gall bladder was not palpable. The right kidney was palpable, but not very movable, and there was moderate gastroptosis. In other respects the abdomen was negative. The station and reflexes were normal, and there was no glandular involvement and no evidence of syphilis or tuberculosis. The teeth were sound; there was no active rhino-pharyngeal disease and no sign of sinus infection.

Examination of the Eyes.—O. D. V. = 6/5, accommodation 7 D. There were no spots on the posterior layer of the cornea. The disc was an irregular oval, of good color, and surrounded by thick masses of chorioidal pigment. Up and in from the disc there was a large patch of pigmented retino-chorioiditis, and throughout the eyeground smaller patches of disseminated exudative chorioiditis, none in an active stage. A few delicate vitreous opacities were demonstrable and very faint opacities in the periphery of the lens. V. of O. S. counts fingers at 25 cm.; white swollen cataract, showing the sectors of the lens plainly and still transmitting a faint reflex; no view of the eyeground. Marked contraction of the field in a circular manner.

LABORATORY EXAMINATIONS.

Blood.—June 20, 1907. Color, consistency and coagulability, normal; hemoglobin, 77 per cent.; erythrocytes, 4,610,000; leucocytes, 7,900.

Microscopic examination: Lymphocytes, 34 per cent.; large mononuclears, 1 per cent.; transitional, 2 per cent.; polymorphonuclears, 61 per cent.; eosinophiles, 2 per cent.; basophiles, none.

Gastric Contents.—June 19, 1907. Preliminary lavage; quantity removed, 92 c.c.; appearance, greenish; mucus, moderate amount; Congo test, present. Total acidity, 30 (0.10 per cent.); free HCl, 14 (0.05 per cent.); lactic acid, none; occult blood, none; bile, positive.

Microscopic examination: Mucus, present; starch, few whole; blood, none; pus, present; epithelium, gastric mucosa, fat and meat fiber, none; yeast, present; sarcinæ and Oppler-Boas bacilli, none.

June 25, 1907. Preliminary lavage, none; character of meal, Ewald; time meal taken, 8:30 a. m.; time meal removed, 9:25 a. m.; quantity removed, 40 c.c.; solid residue, 15 c.c.; appearance, well digested, yellowish; mucus, very little; Congo test, present. Total acidity, 56 (0.21 per cent.); free HCl, 24 (0.08 per cent.); combined HCl, 22 (0.08 per cent.); acid salts, 10 (0.03 per cent.); rennin, present; pepsin, present; lactic acid, none; occult blood, none; bile, present.

Microscopic examination: Mucus, very little; starch, well digested; blood, pus, epithelium, gastric mucosa, fat, meat fiber, yeast, none; sarcinæ and Oppler-Boas bacillus, absent.

Feces.—June 22, 1907. Hour stool passed 6 p. m., June 21, 1907. Period of passage, 57 hours then moved by a laxative. Consistency, liquid, some formed pieces; color, reddish brown; smell, somewhat offensive.

Macroscopic examination: Connective tissue, muscle fiber and fat, none; vegetable fiber and detritus, very little; mucus, few pieces; no blood, pus, occult blood, parasites, stones or other foreign bodies; reaction, alkaline; bile pigments, hydrobilirubin.

Microscopic examination: Mucus, present; no pus or blood; few epithelial cells; no muscle fiber or connective tissue; some vegetable fiber and starch cells; neutral fat present; fatty acids, present; soap, much; casein, none; crystals, few triple phosphates; parasites and bacteria, none.

June 24, 1907. Liquid, some formed pieces; reddish brown color; very offensive; odor ammoniacal.

Macroscopic examination: No connective tissue, muscle fiber, fat, detritus, blood, pus, parasites, stones or other foreign bodies; very little vegetable fiber, a few pieces of mucus; alkaline reaction; strong hydrobilirubin reaction.

Microscopic examination: Mucus, present; few epithelial cells; some vegetable fiber; no blood, muscle fiber, connective tissue or starch cells. No fat; many crystals; no soap; few triple phosphate crystals.

Urine.—June 21, 1907. Diet: (see diet list below).

Quantity, 24 hours, 1566 c.c.; straw-colored; cloudy; flocculent sediment; normal odor; faintly acid; sp. gr., 1004; serum-albumin, trace; acetic acid ppt., very slight; serum-globulin, very faint trace.

Quantitative determinations: Total solids, 12.8 gms; serum-albumin, faint trace; serum-globulin, very faint trace; glucose, none; total nitrogen (Kjeldahl), 8.064 gms.; urea (Doremus), 10.6 gm.; uric acid (Folin-Hopkins' method), 0.323 gm.; ammonia nitrogen (Styer's apparatus), 0.784 gm.; volatile fatty acids (Blumenthal), 126 c.c., 1/10 normal solution; total chlorids, estimated as NaCl, 6.240 gm.; total phosphates, estimated as P_2O_5, 1.250 gm.; earthy phosphates, estimated as P_2O_5, 0.264 gm.; alkaline phosphates, estimated as P_2O_5, 0.986 gm.; total sulphates, estimated as H_2SO_4, 2.612 gm.; preformed sulphates, estimated as H_2SO_4, 2.279 gm.; ratio of conjugate sulphates to preformed sulphates = 1 to 6.6; conjugate phosphates, estimated as H_2SO_4, 0.343 gm.; purin nitrogen (Hall), 0.2834 gm.; ammonia nitrogen coefficient, 9.72.

Microscopic examination: No casts; many amorphous phosphates; triple phosphates.

June 22, 1907. Diet: (see diet list below).

Quantity, 24 hours, 1260 c.c.; straw-colored; cloudy; flocculent sediment; normal odor; neutral reaction; sp. gr., 1002; serum albumin, faint trace.

Quantitative determinations: Total solids, 10.4 gms.; serum-albumin, very faint trace; no serum-globulin or glucose; total nitrogen (Kjeldahl), 5.46 gms.; urea (Doremus), 10.4 gms.; uric acid (Folin-Hopkins' method), 0.101 gm.; ammonia nitrogen (Styer's apparatus), 0.455 gm.; volatile fatty acids, ?; total chlorids, estimated as NaCl, 6.37 gms.; total phosphates, estimated as P_2O_5, 1.38 gm. Purin nitrogen (Hall) 0.304 gm.; ammonia nitrogen coefficient, 8.33.

Microscopic examination: Negative.

June 23, 1907. Diet: (see diet list below).

Quantity, 24 hours, 660 c.c.; pale amber; cloudy; flocculent sediment; normal odor; acid reaction; sp. gr., 1013; serum-albumin, nucleo-albumin. Serum-globulin, very faint traces.

Quantitative determinations: Total solids, 26.0 gms.; serum-albumin and serum-globulin, very faint trace; glucose, none; total nitrogen (Kjeldahl), 4.55 gms.; urea (Doremus), 8.00 gm.; uric acid (Folin-Hopkins' method), 0.348 gm.; ammonia nitrogen (Styer's apparatus), 0.574 gm.; volatile fatty acids (Blumenthal), 33 c.c., 1/10 normal solution; total chlorids, estimated as NaCl, 6.1 gms.; total phosphates, estimated as P_2O_5, 1,280 gms.; earthy phosphates, estimated as P_2O_5, 0.335 gm.; alkaline phosphates, estimated as P_2O_5, 0.945 gm.; total sulphates, estimated as H_2SO_4. 1.571 gm.; preformed sulphates, estimated as H_2SO_4, 1.388 gms.; conjugate sulphates, estimated as H_2SO_4, 0.183 gm.; ratio of conjugate to preformed sulphates = 1 to 7.6; purin nitrogen (Hall), 0.205 gm.; ammonia nitrogen coefficient, 12.6.

Microscopic examination: No casts; mucus moderate; few leucocytes.

June 24, 1907. Diet: (see diet list below).

Quantity, 24 hours, 1420 c.c.; straw colored; cloudy; flocculent sediment; normal odor; faintly acid; sp. gr., 1006; very faint trace of serum-albumin, nucleo-albumin, and serum globulin.

Quantitative determinations: Total solids, 18.0 gms.; very faint trace of serum-albumin and serum-globulin; no glucose; total nitrogen (Kjeldahl), 8.41 gms.; urea (Doremus), 9.75 gms.; uric acid (Folin-Hopkins' method), 1.168 gms.; ammonia nitrogen (Styer's apparatus), 0.408 gm.; volatile fatty acids (Blumenthal), = 30 c.c., 1/10 normal solution; total chlorids, estimated as NaCl, 4.65 gms.; total phosphates, estimated as P_2O_5, 1.23 gms; purin nitrogen (Hall), 0.2775 gm.; ammonia nitrogen coefficient, 5.2.

Microscopic examination: No casts; numerous epithelial cells; small amount of mucus; uric acid.

DIET LIST.

	June 20. Gms.	June 21. Gms.	June 22. Gms.	June 23. Gms.	Total. Gms.	Average.	Nitrogen equivalent.
Orange	100	95	95	100	390	97.5	0.0
Bread	150	145	145	195	605	151.0	1.91
Oatmeal	22	22	22	22	88	22.0	.49
Egg	52	57	55	54	218	54.0	1.08
Chicken	140	120	100	118	478	119.0	3.68
Asparagus	100	118	105	118	441	110.0	0.34
Potato	145	145	105	150	545	136.0	0.54
Lettuce	115	175	127	145	562	140.0	0.16
Tongue	50	55	50	55	210	52.5	1.57
Apple	115	120	110	115	460	105.0	0.00
Rice	20	20	20	20	80	20.0	0.23
Butter	47	28	35	47	157	39.25	0.16
Salt	4	4	4	4	16	4.0	
Sugar	35	40	38	35	138	34.5	
Junket, oz.	8	8	8	8	32	8	1.38
Olive oil, oz.	1	1	1	1		1	
Lemon juice, oz.	¼	¼	¼	¼			
Water, c.c.	2,500	2,500				2,500	
							11.44

EXAMINATIONS, NOV. 7, 1907.

Gastric Contents.—Character of meal, Ewald; removed in one hour; amount, 50 c.c.; appearance, fairly well digested; mucus, moderate amount; Congo test, present; total acidity, 60 (0.21 per cent.); free HCl, 40 (0.14 per cent.); lactic acid, none; rennin and pepsin, present; bile, absent.

Microscopically, negative.

Blood.—Hemoglobin, 87 per cent.; red blood corpuscles, 5,000,000; leucocytes, 9,280.

Urine.—Amount, 1,800 c.c.; color, light yellow; slightly cloudy; precipitation, none; reaction, acid; sp. gr., 1030; albumin, trace, none by Heller's test; acetic acid precipitate, none; serum globulin, albumose, sugar, acetone, phenol, bile, absent; indican, slight excess; Rosenbach's reaction, none; urobilin, trace; urea (Marshall), 16.49 gm.; ammonium nitrogen, not determined; uric acid, 0.44 gm.; total nitrogen, 8.41 gm.; volatile fatty acids, not increased.

Microscopically: No casts; few uric-acid crystals.

Remarks.—The chief points of interest in the clinical history of the patient are the long periods of rheumatism from which her mother suffered, the eczema which attacked one brother and one sister, and the patient's frequent attacks of tonsillitis, as well as eczema, which was apt to be worse when her eyes were better, and *vice versa.*

From the laboratory findings it is evident that there was secondary anemia; that, except a little mucus and on one occasion bile, the presence of which was not accounted for, the analysis of the gastric contents revealed nothing distinctly abnormal; that analysis of the bowel contents revealed thorough digestion of meats and starches, poor digestion of fats, a moderate amount of mucus, an alkaline reaction and an offensive odor. The over-digestion and odor are probably accounted for by the constipation. There was an entire absence of pus, blood and parasites.

In the urine, the apparently marked retention of nitrogen, the high ammonia output, the relatively low area, and the great variation in the uric acid eliminations, suggest deranged nitrogen metabolism.

Referring now to the question of intestinal putrefaction products, it is shown that their evidence in the urine is a decidedly higher proportion of ethereal (conjugate) sulphates to the preformed sulphates. Specimens of urine collected after the patient had been on a very simple diet for some days failed to show any excess of indican, no phenol and no excess of urobilin; but two specimens examined later, when this strict diet was not followed, contained an excess of indican and a slight excess of urobilin. On one occasion, it will be noted, that the volatile fatty acids were high, but not on other days.

Treatment and Progress of the Case.—In consultation with Dr. Fife, and based on his findings in the laboratory, the following treatment was suggested: Cutting down of proteids as much as possible, allowing milk and eggs (the white of eggs better than the yolks) to be the chief protein to be ingested; large quantities of milk, or better still, buttermilk or kumiss, were ordered, but practically no meat, and especially no meat of growing animals, such as veal, or of any glandular organs, such as sweetbreads, liver, etc. Vegetables, with the exception of peas and round beans, and those vegetables which habitually disagreed with the patient, were ordered to be taken freely. The patient was directed to drink enough water to make the elimination of urine about two and one-half or three quarts per day, and every other day the lower bowel was to be flushed out, these flushings, of course, not to be continued indefinitely. Proper laxatives were ordered, as needed by the condition of the bowels. The only medicine ordered was small doses of potassium iodid, indicated by the general condition.

The improvement of this patient was rapid and satisfactory. Except for one day, after the examinations had been completed and the treatment had been ordered, there was no return of the blurred vision of the right eye and of the muscæ, which had been particularly alarming just prior to her examination. The gain in weight was rapid and satisfactory, and within a few months she had added 20 pounds to her weight. Five months later the secondary anemia had practically disappeared, the hemoglobin being now 87 per cent., and the red cells 5,000,000 per c.mm. There were some slight dyspeptic symptoms (referable to hyperacidity, and the urine on two occasions contained an excess of indican, suggesting putrefactive products of intestinal origin. These were corrected by a renewal of appropriate diet, which had been for the time being set aside.

Remarks.—In this patient we have the interesting opportunity of comparing the results of what may be called the usual treatment of chorioiditis and its relapses with a treatment which was largely diatetic and intended to correct faulty nitrogen metabolism and probable moderate intestinal autointoxication. What the line of treatment was which she received during the earlier attacks of chorioiditis, and particularly in those attacks which occurred in the year prior to her coming under our care, we are unable to say, except that she was treated by most competent physicians, who doubtless adopted well recognized therapeutic measures, but who did not succeed, or at least the remedies employed did not succeed, in checking the recurrences, which ultimately so disordered the nutrition of the chorioid of the left eye that cataract formed, and it was only when this cataract began to appear, as well as the muscæ before the right or better eye became definitely manifest, that she was driven to seek additional advice.

Now almost a year has elapsed, during which the diatetic regimen already referred to has been strictly followed, with, perhaps, only one or two lapses, and there has been no recurrence of inflammation in the neighborhood of the old patch of chorioiditis, nor the development of new areas of inflammation in this membrane. True, she has taken during this year a certain amount of iodid—no other remedy, except at intervals, iron; but she also took in the preceding year all manner of alteratives, and yet in spite of them the recurrences occurred, with the result of the forming of cataract. It may be urged that the process in the left eye was more widespread, and, if you choose, more malignant than that in the right eye, and therefore, the remedies did not have as good an effect in this eye as they had in the other one. Nevertheless, it would seem that a certain amount of credit should be given to the therapeutic regimen which was evolved by a scientific examination from the laboratory standpoint. That it did good can not be denied for an instant, as is attested by the gain in weight, by improvement in general nutrition and by the loss of secondary anemia. All things considered, we feel that this case is a fair demonstration of the value of studies along these lines, and that the results thus far attained fully compensate for the trouble and time which such examinations required.

CASE 4.—*Relapsing Uveitis (Irido-Chorioiditis) of Ten Years' Standing; Irritative Nephritis; Autointoxication from Gastrointestinal Decomposition.*—Mrs. A. H., aged 26, the mother of one child, no miscarriages, applied for treatment Oct. 21, 1907.

Family History.—The patient's father and mother are living and well. Nothing is known of the maternal family. The paternal grandmother died of dropsy at the age of 79, the paternal grandfather at 60 of paralysis. There is no other history of heart, lung, nerve or constitutional disease in the family.

Past History.—The patient had measles, chickenpox, whooping-cough, all in mild degree, as a child. She never suffered from skin disease. At 6 years of age she had pneumonia, and on several occasions tonsillitis. The dates of these attacks are not obtainable. There is a history of muscular rheumatism, which occurred at frequent intervals, especially in the right shoulder. Lumbago is absent, and there is a vague history of pleurodynia. The patient has always "caught cold" easily. Menstruation was established at 14, and has always been regular and normal. From her seventeenth to her twenty-first year she was never very strong, working at this period very hard as a stenographer, with poor appetite and nervous disposition, and always very tired. At the age of 21 she married, and has had one child, now 2 years of age. Syphilis is definitely eliminated, and no evidence of tuberculosis has been uncovered. Calmette's test has not been used.

Past Eye History.—The patient's eye troubles began in 1898 or 1899, with an attack of uveitis of the right eye, which seems to have lasted for three months. This inflammation recurred in 1903, and in October of that year she paid one visit to the dispensary for diseases of the eye of the University Hospital, and the records show that there was a marked uveitis, with punctate keratitis and vitreous opacities confined to the right eye, the left one being normal. Vision at that time was 6/12. She was not seen again at this period, but reports that she had a number of relapses, until January, 1904, by which time the vision of the right eye was entirely destroyed.

The first intimation of inflammation of the left eye occurred in March, 1907, lasting only for about a week. In April of the same year, in association with blurred vision, muscæ appeared and synechiæ formed, which, according to her statement, were "broken up" by atropin. From June of that year until the late fall, she was under the constant care of a competent oculist, without, however, any definite relief, as the relapses were frequent and the results of therapeusis disappointing. She applied for treatment in the dispensary for diseases of the eye of the University Hospital for the second time on October 12, 1907, and two days later was admitted to the hospital, where she remained until November 16.

Examination.—The patient is a woman of small frame, but well proportioned. Her tissues were soft and flabby and the mucosæ pale. There was no lesion of the skin; the throat and nasopharynx were negative, as were also the lungs. Lymphatic enlargement was not demonstrable. There were no cardiac murmurs, but there was marked accentuation of the second aortic sound. The liver and spleen were negative and there were no areas of definite tenderness in the abdomen. The right kidney was palpable and slightly movable; the reflexes and station were normal. The teeth and gums were sound.

Examination of the Eyes.—V. of O. D., light perception in the periphery, with obliteration of the perception of light in the center of the field. The tension of the eye was slightly below normal, the iris discolored and adherent to a totally cataractous lens of chalky appearance. V. of O. S. 6/12, the pupil dilated under the influence of atropin, and remnants of synechia could be detected around the entire periphery. On the posterior surface of the cornea, in the usual triangular manner, as well as in a more scattered disposition, were free deposits of small mutton-fat drops, the keratitis punctata of ordinary parlance. The vitreous was full of thick floating opacities, and the fundus could be studied with difficulty, the chief change being the unusual enlargement of the retinal veins. No definite patches of chorioiditis were discovered.

LABORATORY EXAMINATIONS.

Blood Count.—Oct. 16, 1907. Erythrocytes, 4,650,000; leucocytes, 6,100; hemoglobin, 76 per cent.

Differential Count.—Polymorphonuclears, 61 per cent.; lymphocytes, 32 per cent.; large mononuclears, 4 per cent.; transitionals, 3 per cent.

Blood Pressure.—Systolic, 125; diastolic, 80.

Gastric Contents.—October 16. Quantity, 40 c.c.; appearance, upper 1/3 translucent liquid, lower 2/3 a white precipitate; digestion, moderate; free HCl, none; total acidity, 23.75; lactic acid, none.

Microscopic Examination.—Yeast and starch present; Oppler-Boas bacilli, sarcinæ and blood, absent.

October 29. Quantity 50 c.c.; appearance, upper 1/2 is a light brown translucent liquid, having some floating stringy mucus, the lower 1/2 is a fine gray sediment having specks of brown; free HCl, 10; total acidity, 34.

Microscopic examination: Starch well digested. Yeast moderate amount. Fat, small amount. No red cells. No Oppler-Boas bacilli or leucocytes.

Feces.—Four examinations revealed about the same conditions. Stools formed normally. Dark brown color; offensive; slight acid reaction; contained hydrobilirubin. None gave reaction for occult blood. Two contained a moderate amount of mucus, while two other specimens contained a very small amount of mucus. The macroscopic inspection revealed much sand; no excess of undigested meat; no starch; no fat; numerous vegetable fibers, chiefly skins and shells.

Microscopically, there were some striated and unstriated meat fibers, a moderate excess of vegetable cells, no undigested starch, no neutral fat, considerable soap, a few fatty acid needles, many triple phosphates, and numerous sand granules. No blood and no pus; a few leucocytes. The most striking abnormality was the large amount of intestinal sand in all specimens.

Average diet for six days: Eggs, 109 gm.; bread, 132 gm.; tomato, 152 gm.; baked potato, 312 gm.; steak, 138 gm.; beans, 111 gm.; apple sauce, 238 gm.; salt, 7 gm.; sugar, 26 gm.; milk, 744 c.c.

Urine.—Oct. 21, 1907. Constant diet for four days preceding collection of specimen equals about 15.4 gms. nitrogen per day. Amount in 24 hours, 900 c.c.; reaction, acid; sp. gr.,

·1024; color, light amber; precipitate, flocculent; odor, normal; albumin, trace by heat and acid test, acetic acid and potassium ferrocyanid, and a very faint trace by Heller's contact test; so-called nucleoalbumin (acetic acid precipitate) present in trace; albumose, serum-globulin, Bence-Jones albumin, negative; indican, moderate excess; sugar, negative; acetone, trace; diacetic acid, negative; bile, negative; urobilin, very slight excess; phenol, very faint trace; volatile fatty acids = 57.6 c.c., 1/10 normal solution (Blumenthal's method); total nitrogen, 13.0 gms. (Kjeldahl's method); urea (hypobromite method), 23.2 gms.; uric acid (Folin's modification of Hopkin's method), 0.70 gm.; ammonium nitrogen, 0.09 gm. (Steyer's method); chlorids (estimated as sodium chlorid), 5.13 gms.; total phosphates, 2.45 gms. (estimated as P_2O_5); earthy phosphates, 0.36 gm. (estimated as P_2O_5); alkaline phosphates, 2.09 gms. (estimated as P_2O_5); total sulphates (estimated as H_2SO_4), 2.641 gms.; preformed sulphates (estimated as H_2SO_4), 2.312 gms.; conjugate sulphates (estimated as H_2SO_4), 0.229 gm.

Microscopic: Few short broad hyaline casts; a few coarsely granulated broad casts; cylindroids, a few; numerous mucus shreds; leucocytes, present; epithelium, normal; calcium oxalate crystals.

Oct. 23, 1907. Constant diet for six days equals about 15.4 gms. nitrogen. Amount in 24 hours, 730 c.c.; reaction, acid; color, dark lemon yellow; sp. gr., 1026; precipitate, flocculent; odor, normal; albumin, trace by heat and acid test, acetic acid and potassium ferrocyanid tests; none by Heller's contact test; so-called nucleo-albumin (acetic acid precipitate) present in trace; albumose, negative; Bence-Jones albumin, negative; indican, moderate excess; sugar, negative; acetone, trace; diacetic acid, negative; bile pigments, negative; phenol, very faint trace; volatile fatty acids = 124.8 c.c., 1/10 normal solution (Blumenthal's method); total nitrogen, 12.5 gms. (Kjeldahl's method); urea (hypobromite method), 29 gms.; uric acid (Folin's modification of Hopkin's method), 0.60 gm.; ammonium nitrogen, 0.08 gm. (Steyer's method); chlorids (estimated as sodium chlorid), 4.6 gms.; total phosphates (estimated as P_2O_5), 2.10 gms.; earthy phosphates (estimated as P_2O_5), 0.24 gm.; alkaline phosphates (estimated as P_2O_5), 1.86 gms.; total sulphates (estimated as H_2SO_4), 2.22 gms.; preformed sulphates (estimated as H_2SO_4), 1.999 gms.; conjugate sulphates (estimated as H_2SO_4), 0.221 gm.

Microscopic: Few short hyaline casts, a very few fine and coarse granular casts; cylindroids, a few; numerous mucus shreds; leucocytes, moderate number; epithelium, normal; calcium oxalate crystals.

Summary.—Commenting on these findings, Dr. Fife writes as follows: The urine measured for eight twenty-four-hour periods was never more than 900 c.c., the spetific gravity fluctuating normally with the amount of urine. Each specimen contained a small amount of serum albumin, a distinct trace of nuclear albumin, hyaline casts and cylindroids, and in three specimens a few granular casts. These findings, taken into consideration with the somewhat high blood pressure and the accentuated second aortic sound, would indicate kidney irritation, associated with arterial change. Whether this kidney lesion and the arterial tension are dependent directly on toxins can not be stated with definiteness.

The excess of indican, the presence of phenol, the slight excess of urobilin, the trace of acetone and the moderately high volatile fatty acids, suggest autointoxication from gastrointestinal decomposition products. This, however, was not confirmed by the determination of the conjugate sulphates in three specimens, the proportion of conjugate sulphates to preformed sulphates being 1 to 10, 1 to 9.4 and 1 to 12.2.

Referring to nitrogen metabolism, it may be said that the amount of urea is normal, but the uric-acid output was greater than the intake of uric-acid-forming substances would lead us to expect. This suggests an excess of endogenous purins, but only suggests it, as many more factors would be necessary to definitely confirm it. The total nitrogen output is less than the intake, allowing for a loss of about 1½ gms. of nitrogen in the feces. The chlorid output is less than the intake. This is probably dependent on nephritis. Dr. Fife makes special reference to the intestinal sand which he found in the stools, and which in at least one case of marked gastrointestinal autointoxication was a conspicuous feature. He also calls attention to the anemia of the secondary type and the hypoacidity of the gastric contents.

Treatment and Course of the Case.—After consultation with Dr. Fife, based on the analyses which have been submitted, a diet list was made out which as much as possible should contain foods of low purin content, but which do not decompose readily and are at the same time as rich in hemoglobin-forming properties as possible. Free drinking of water was advised, provided it did not increase the arterial tension, and the colon was flushed with large quantities of normal salt solution. Considering the character of the blood pressure, the secondary anemia and the possible changes in the arterial coats themselves, the administration of small doses of iodid of potassium was directeu. Locally, the eye was treated with dionin, atropin and hot compresses.

By November 4 the patient was greatly improved, the vitreous opacity had in large measure absorbed, and the vision, after correcting half a diopter of astigmatism, was 6/7.5 and part of 6/6; and on November 16, or just a month after admission, she was permitted to go home and to discontinue the atropin.

All went well until the latter part of December, when there was a decided relapse and vision reduced to large letters by a free deposition of mutton-fat drops on the posterior surface of the cornea, and a rapid redevelopment of thick vitreous opacities. The patient was admitted again to tne University Hospital on Jan. 2, 1908, and remained there for five weeks, again placed on as strict a diet as possible (which, however, had also been continued while she was at home, as had also the iodid of potassium), and treated with pilocarpin diaphoresis, which after the fourth sweat had to be discontinued on account of the intense nausea which it produced, and later with subconjunctival injections of saline solution, which acted very favorably. At the present time (March, 1908) there has again been some improvement. The vitreous, although far from clear, has lost most of its thick opacities and the K P has disappeared. The unusually large retinal veins are still a marked ophthalmoscopic picture. Patches of chorioiditis are not visible. The vision is 6/12.

Remarks.—This case indicates that although it may be assumed that an autointoxication from gastrointestinal decomposition was present, and that its correction by suitable diet was followed by an exceedingly rapid improvement in a relapsing uveitis of distinctly malignant tendency, such treatment was not enough to prevent a recurrence. Evidently autointoxication is not the sole cause, although it may be a contributing one. What the toxin is which is responsible for the relapses has not been demonstrated, and we assert only that the intestinal intoxication as one factor is worthy of consideration, because the relapses appear to have been much more susceptible to correction that those relapses which had occurred prior to the establishment of this strict diet, and which were responsible for the destruction of the vision of the right eye.

It may be maintained that such searching examinations of the secretions as have been recorded in two of the preceding cases would be likely to reveal one or other of the conditions which are associated with intestinal autointoxication or faulty nitrogen metabolism in any patient who has for a long period of time been a sufferer from a chronic or relapsing ocular disorder. Therefore, the following case, which from the ocular standpoint belongs in the same class with those which have preceded it, but which, in so far as laboratory investigations are concerned, is excluded from it, is recorded.

Case 5.—*Relapsing Iritis (Uveitis); Entire Absence of Evidences of Autointoxication.*—L. W., male, aged 62, came for consultation Feb. 28, 1907.

Family History and Past History.—Data in these respects are not recorded, as they have no bearing on the present question. The influence of rheumatism, tuberculosis and syphilis may be excluded.

Past Eye History.—Patient always myopic, has been wearing glasses since the age of 15. At the age of 22 he had an attack of iritis of an approximate duration of ten days. A second attack occurred at the age of 25, and from then on until about six years ago he has had an attack every two or three years, but during the past six years the attacks have manifested themselves every twelve to eighteen months. In 1897 iridectomy was performed on the left eye.

Physical Examination.—The patient is a spare man, with a small amount of adipose tissue, the muscles being moderately well developed. There was no distinct emaciation, the bones were small, the mucous membranes a little pale and slightly cyanotic; the head and neck were negative, the chest long and narrow, but of good expansion. The lungs were negative. The heart area was very slightly enlarged. There were no murmurs, but the second aortic sound was moderately accentuated. The abdominal organs were normal in size and position, the glands negative and the reflexes and station normal.

Eye Examination.—V. of O. D. with — 2.50 c. axis 105, 4/15. The pupil under the influence of atropin was a vertical oval, 5 by 4, the anterior chamber deep and the lower and inner and outer margin of the pupil is fringed with gray exudate. There was a slight peri-nuclear haze and some pigment on the capsule of the lens, together with a fine deposit of dots on Descemet's membrane. Remnants of synechia were visible at the outer part of the pupil. In the vitreous moderately developed string-like opacities were visible. The disc was a horizontal oval, with a scleral ring broadening below into a superficial crescent. There was general epithelial chorioiditis, and in the macular region there were delicate grayish-white lines, with small pigment dots and smaller white dots. The tension was normal and the field of vision normal. V. of O. S., with — 6 D., fingers at 24 inches. There was a narrow upward coloboma, with well-placed edges, and the pupil transmitted a red reflex. To a mass of lymph just behind and above the pupil the margins of the coloboma were adherent. The iris was tremulous; there was no rise of tension and no view through the cataractous lens of the fundus.

LABORATORY EXAMINATIONS.

Blood.—Erythrocytes, 4,900,000; leucocytes, 6,560; hemaglobin, 70 per cent. Systolic blood pressure, 112; diastolic pressure, 85.

Examination of stomach contents showed contents well digested, small amount of mucus, free hydrochloric acid, 26; total acidity, 48.

Urine.—March 2, 1907. Quantity, 24 hours, 1,410 c.c.; color, dark straw; cloudy; sediment, flocculent; odor, slightly putrid; reaction, acid; sp. gr., 1010.

Quantitative determinations: Total solids, 30 gms.; serum-albumin, serum-globulin and glucose, none; total nitrogen (Kjeldahl), 11.23 gms.; urea (Doremus), 21.75 gms.; uric acid (Folin-Hopkins), 0.31 gm.; ammonia nitrogen (Steyer's apparatus), 0.15 gm.; volatile fatty acids (Blumenthal's method), 54.0 c.c., 1/10 normal solution; total chlorids, estimated as NaCl, 7.65 gms.; total phosphates, estimated as P_2O_5, 234 gms.; earthy phosphates, estimated as P_2O_5, 0.416 gms.; alkaline phosphates, estimated as P_2O_5, 1.924 gms.; total sulphates, estimated as H_2SO_4, 2.941 gms.; preformed sulphates, estimated as H_2SO_4, 2.636 gms.; conjugate sulphates, estimated as H_2SO_4, 0.305 gm.; purin nitrogen, 0.23 gm.

Microscopic examination: Small amount of mucus; few uric-acid crystals; no casts.

March 3, 1907. Quantity, 24 hours, 1,450 c.c.; color, deep straw; appearance, faintly cloudy; sediment, none; odor, normal; reaction, acid; sp. gr., 1010.

Quantitative determinations: Total solids, 32. gms.; serum-albumin, serum-globulin and glucose, none; total nitrogen (Kjeldhal), 12.70 gms.; urea (Doremus), 18.0 gms.; uric acid (Folin-Hopkins), 0.33 gm.; ammonia nitrogen (Steyer's apparatus), 0.42 gm.; volatile fatty acids (Blumenthal's method), 56 c.c., 1/10 normal solution; total chlorids, estimated as NaCl, 8.85 gms.; total phosphates, estimated as P_2O_5, 3.96 gms.; earthy phosphates, estimated as P_2O_5, 0.53 gm.; alkaline phosphates, estimated as P_2O_5, 3.34 gms.; total sulphates, estimated as H_2SO_4, 3.00 gms.; preformed sulphates, estimated as H_2SO_4, 2.784 gms.; conjugate sulphates, estimated as H_2SO_4, 0.216 gm.; purin nitrogen, 0.23 gm.

Microscopic examination: Small amount of mucus; no casts.

March 4, 1907. Diet, special; quantity, 24 hours, 1,636 c.c.; color, pale amber; appearance, faint cloud; sediment, flocculent; odor, normal; reaction, acid; sp. gr., 1012; serum-albumin, very faintest trace possible.

Quantitative determinations: Total solids, 38.0 gms.; serum-albumin, very faintest possible trace; serum-globulin, none; glucose, none; total nitrogen (Kjeldahl), 14.78 gms.; urea (Doremus), 22.10 gms.; uric acid (Folin-Hopkins), 0.35 gm.; ammonia nitrogen (Steyer's apparatus), 0.38 gm.; volatile fatty acids (Blumenthal's method), 38.0 c.c., 1/10 normal solution; total chlorids, estimated as NaCl, 10.0 gms.; total phosphates, estimated as P_2O_5, 3.09 gms.; earthy phosphates, estimated as P_2O_5, 0.81 gm.; alkaline phosphates, estimated as P_2O_5, 2.18 gms.; total sulphates, estimated as H_2SO_4, 3.43 gms.; preformed sulphates, estimated as H_2SO_4, 3.16 gms.; conjugate sulphates, estimated as H_2SO_4, 0.27 gm.; purin nitrogen, 0.29 gm.

Microscopic examination: Small amount of mucus; few uric acid crystals; no casts.

Remarks.—Commenting on these examinations, Dr. Fife points out that the urine examination was practically negative. On the first two days of observation equilibrium of nitrogen metabolism was not established, the intake being greater than the output and the patient normally gained one pound in weight, but on the third day the equilibrium was just about established with a weight variation of only two ounces. It will be noticed there is no increase in ammonia nitrogen coefficient, in the volatile fatty acids, or in the proportion of the sulphates; no phenol, acetone, excess of indican or urobilin. The uric acid and purins are perhaps a little high and the urea a little low, but nothing in the urine suggests autointoxication. The amount of albumin was so slight that it could scarcely be detected with the heat and acid test and not at all by the contact test. Examination of the feces was negative, the digestion of all food elements being good. Occult blood was present, probably due to rare meats.

The patient did not remain for treatment, and therefore the subsequent history of the case can not be given. It is quoted only, as before stated, as an example of entirely negative results in so far as the discovery of intestinal autointoxication is concerned, and, indeed, as the discovery of any toxin or infection may have been responsible for the relapsing iritis.

CASE 6.—*Central Exudative Chorioiditis of the Right Eye of the Plastic Type, with One Patch of Peripheral Retino-Chorioiditis; High Irregular Astigmatism; Furunculosis; Questionable Autointoxication.*—L. L., a boy, aged 15, came for consultation on March 31, 1906.

Family History.—The patient's father and mother are living and the father is in good health; the mother in recent years has been a chronic neurasthenic. Two brothers are living and healthy. The family history of more distant date is fairly good, and the grandparents lived to old age. One uncle died of Bright's disease. There is no reason to suspect specific taint in any of the blood relatives.

Past History.—The patient has always been a fairly healthy boy, having had scarlet fever, but of moderate degree. There is no history of tonsillitis and none of rheumatism. In August, 1907, but more than a year after the eye troubles began, furunculosis was evident, the active pustules being chiefly situated on the right side of the face and also on the arm, and these lasted, coming in various crops, until December of that year.

Past Eye History.—For the earlier data of the patient's eye conditions I am indebted to the courtesy of Dr. Posey, whom he first consulted April 18, 1902, for asthenopic symptoms, which were relieved by the correction at that time of a simple hypermetropia, which yielded normal vision, and there were no pathologic ophthalmoscopic changes. Three years later, with a renewal of the asthenopic symptoms, an astigmatism of half a diopter against the rule was discovered after atropin mydriasis, and later, following an attack of acute catarrhal conjunctivitis, there was a tendency to spasm of the right ciliary muscle and the astigmatism had increased to double the quantity. Four months later, in association with a renewal of the asthenopia and a marked increase of the astigmatism of the right eye, which was now + 1.75 D. axis 5, a granular condition of the right macula was first noted. Again, five months later the patient returned with metamorphopsia and decided macular chorioiditis was evident, although at that time the vision was still normal, but the astigmatism had risen to 2.25 D. axis 180. A month later vision had fallen to 5/6, and in spite of restriction in the use of his eyes the chorioiditis had apparently increased.

Examination.—The patient is a well-formed boy whose nutrition seems to be exceedingly good and whose weight is 115 pounds. A careful examination by his physician at that time, Dr. Louis Starr, failed to reveal any organic lesions, but only such conditions as in general terms suggested lithemia, to which diathesis he was entitled by direct inheritance. The teeth were sound and the rhino-pharynx healthy.

Eye Examination.—V. of O. D., counts fingers at 50 cm., this marked reduction of vision having taken place within a month prior to his examination. The ophthalmometer revealed an astigmatism of 6 D., there were no deposits on the posterior surface of the cornea, thick opacities floated through the vitreous, the disc could be seen only dimly, but appeared not to be swollen, the retinal veins were large and irregular, and the center of the eyeground directly in the macular region was occupied by a large, circular, greenish-white exudate pushing forward into the vitreous from 3 to 4 D. above the level of the eyeground and gradually sloping into its surrounding area. The field of vision was normal in its periphery, but in the center there was a scotoma corresponding to the chorioidal deposit just described. Far in the periphery of the same eyeground in the outer and lower outer region there was a very large area of pigmented retino-chorioiditis.

V. of O. S., after the correction of half a diopter of astigmatism against the rule, was normal, and the ophthalmoscope failed to reveal any pathologic lesions. The patient was admitted to the Orthopedic Hospital, where for two days there was a slight rise of temperature, never going beyond 100 F., and subsequently returning to normal, where it remained.

LABORATORY EXAMINATIONS.

Only the blood and urine were examined. The former was normal in all respects, and the latter gave an average specific gravity of 1014, was amber in color, alkaline in reaction, and showed a persistent increase of indican. Casts were not discovered. Unfortunately, none of the thorough examinations of the urine previously reported were made, nor was there any analysis of the gastric contents or of the feces.

Treatment and Progress of the Case.—The treatment consisted in the internal administration of iodid of sodium, daily diapnoresis in a cabinet bath, light massage and a strict diet, with the elimination of all sweets, pastries and easily decomposed foods. At the expiration of five weeks, during which period sixteen vapor baths were taken, the vitreous was entirely clear, the greenish exudate in the chorioid had contracted, although it was a little more elevated and had assumed a somewhat cone shape, the apex of which was + 5 D. It now became surrounded by a ring of erosion twice as wide as the retinal vein. No change was visible in the peripheral patch of retino-chorioiditis, which was certainly of ancient date. Vision was now with some difficulty 6/60 and eccentric. The boy was taken from school, sent to live in the country and given only from time to time small doses of biniodid of mercury.

Little or no change took place in the eyeground, except a gradual absorption of the greenish exudate, which now became pigmented on its margin, while the collar of erosion widened. Occasionally, fine hyalitis was visible. Little by little, with widening of the eroded collar, the central areas of exudate disappeared until at the present time the sclera is exposed in a white patch and the vision remains as before, approximately 6/60 eccentrically.

During the summer of 1907, as previously noted, furunculosis appeared. At this time the patient was under the care of Dr. E. G. Beardsley, who reports the urine to be normal in every respect, as well as the blood, namely, erythrocytes, 5,200,000, leucocytes, 7,200. There was a slight increase in the polymorphonuclear neutrophiles. Dr. Beardsley, referring particularly to the acne pustules on the face, writes as follows: "I have been interested in observing the relation of the opsonic index of the serum of the blood to the various strains of staphylococcus which I have from time to time isolated from the acne lesions. When the index was first estimated it was decidedly low, being .51, and varied from time to time, but never reached a point above .62, except following the injections of cultures of the germ in question. The treatment of the acne lesions by bacterial vaccines proved disappointing, although there was improvement at first, the index rising above 2.2, but with almost total disappearance of the local lesions, with the discontinuance of the vaccines, however, the resistance of the serums dropped back to below 1 and a few new pustules appeared."

During the period of the acne eruptions there was no marked change in the right eye nor in the left, but on their disappearance in December, 1907, the patient began to complain of blurred vision in the left eye, with asthenopia, some epiphora and some dread of light. These symptoms, ordinarily unimportant, were alarming on account of the history of the right eye. With absolute cessation of eye work, a two weeks' period of atropin mydriasis and the internal administration of Fowler's solution and renewal of a stricter diet, they disappeared and the vision became accurately normal in the left eye. At present there are no signs in any portion of the left eyeground of any chorioidal disturbance.

Remarks.—Except for a persistent increase of indican during the period of active chorioiditis, there were no signs of intestinal fermentation, but also no elaborate examinations of the urine or of any other of the secretions of the body were made. Moreover, the treatment was that ordinarily applied to cases of chorioiditis of this type plus the regulation of the diet, with special elimination of food-stuffs known to be unhealthy. In other words, the treatment did not differ from that which may be called routine in cases of this character. It is recorded here for the purpose of calling attention in a later paragraph to the relationship of the furunculosis to the chorioidal changes.

CONCLUSIONS.

I come now to consider what conclusions may be deduced from the studies just presented.

1. Is there any known disease of any of the histologic systems of the eye which of itself would justify the inference that an intestinal autointoxication is present? Certainly not, because, in the first place, we have no definitely certain knowledge of any specific intoxication depending upon the non-elimination of metabolic products, and, in the second place, the clinical pictures of ocular diseases, for example, of the uveal tract, may be identical, although their etiology may be widely different.

2. Have laboratory examinations isolated any definite toxin to the influence of which could be attributed any of the diseases of the eye at present under consideration? They have not. Hence, if such a criterion of the diagnosis of an autointoxication is necessary, as I have already stated, none of the cases recorded could be regarded as expressions of metabolic disorders.

3. Is it worth while, negative answers having been given to questions 1 and 2, to pursue the line of investigation in the cases under consideration? It would certainly seem so. At least we find or do not find the evidences of intestinal putrefaction and become acquainted with the patient's nitrogen metabolism. If the metabolism is abnormal it may be restored to the normal by a dietetic regimen, which could not be worked out in the absence of the data furnished by such examinations, with brilliant results, as, for example, in cases 1, 2 and 3, and striking, if not brilliant, in case 4.

What I particularly wish to emphasize is that while there must be, again to quote Taylor, no loose interpretation of the facts of metabolism and their relation to disease, certain uveal tract and corneal affections should be sharply separated from the perfunctory examinations which they have only too often received, and from the equally perfunctory and insufficient therapeutic measures which have been accorded to them, and that the investigations along lines already indicated, which have also been urged by Elschnig, Kraus, Groyer, Stephenson, Spicer, Cross and other writers, should be commended and pursued. As Dr. Goldthwaite recently stated in a most scholarly and illuminating address on the treatment of non-tuberculous joint affections, investigation of each case and not routine medication is what is required. If, as he has demonstrated, many cases of non-tubercular infectious arthritis, formerly vaguely attributed to rheumatism, are really due to foci of infection in the accessory sinuses, the teeth, the tonsils, and possibly to bacterial activity in the intestines, and that removal of such foci opens the way to cure, the same may be true of the ocular diseases now being considered. Indeed, we well know that some of them, notably cases of uveitis, are caused by infections which pass from the pharyngeal ring, the tonsils, the alveolar processes and the air sinuses.

To make our investigations complete we should add

to them such data as may be gleaned from chemical examinations of the body secretions, notably those of the kidney and the intestinal tract, but these examinations must be thorough, and in order to indicate the thoroughness and care with which they should be undertaken, the detailed laboratory results have been recorded.

Finally, I wish to call attention to another matter, which has not escaped the attention of other clinicians, and to which I have[3] made reference on another occasion, namely, a certain relationship which exists between the outbreaks of uveal tract disease, notably chorioiditis, and lesions of the skin. This was a noteworthy feature in case 3. In this patient when the skin affection was evident the eyes were better, and *vice versa.* Among those patients to whom reference is made in a previous paper, one for example, had in the right eye a localized plastic chorioiditis near the macula. Two years later an exactly similar lesion developed in the fellow eye, and again two years later a sharp attack of herpes zoster, and on this occasion the chorioid remained unaffected. In another patient plastic chorioiditis appeared to alternate with an attack of eczema of the face, while in the last case recorded in the present series, during the development of facial furunculosis, the eye was quiet, but on the subsidence of the furunculosis the earliest symptoms of chorioidal change began, which yielded, however, very promptly to active treatment, without the development of pronounced lesions in this membrane. This association of eczema, herpes zoster, acne and chorioidal disease appears to be more than a coincidence. If it be true that an intestinal intoxication may sometimes be interpreted in an effort of elimination by the development of a skin disease, for instance, one of the three named is it not probable it may have a similar interpretation by the development of a chorioiditis or uveitis, and that sometimes the toxin is responsible for the skin lesion and on another occasion in the same patient for the uveal tract affection?

---

3. Ann. Ophth., 1906, xv, 513.

MEMORANDA

THE EYE AS A CONTRIBUTING FACTOR IN TUBERCULOSIS.*

F. PARK LEWIS, M.D.
BUFFALO, N. Y.

The almost universal prevalence of tuberculosis, the enormous death rate, together with its possible prevention and cure, have focused the attention of the world on this disease in a way and to an extent unique in the history of medicine. The opportunities for infection are so frequent, and the number of recoveries in which the healed lesions are recognized only postmortem are so numerous, as to justify the German-folk saying, *"Jedermann hat am Ende ein bischen Tuberculose."* It is evident, then, that some other element than that of infection merely must influence the course of this disease, otherwise, as almost every one is exposed to infection, the world would become a mortuary from this cause alone. It is generally recognized, however, that any condition which lowers the vital resistance or increases what Jonathan Hutchinson calls the "vulnerability," predisposes to infection and retards recovery.

Among the earliest symptoms of beginning tuberculosis are increased pulse rate and a loss of weight. Even before a local lesion has become sufficiently pronounced to be detected the rapid pulse and malnutrition are signals of the on-coming storm.

The importance, then, of recognizing any other existing conditions that can increase the pulse rate or interfere with digestion and nutrition will be self-evident. It may have a bearing, too, that it is by no means a settled question that the respiratory tract is always the port of entry of the bacillus in pulmonary tuberculosis.

* This paper has been accepted by the Executive Committee of the Section on Ophthalmology of the American Medical Association, to be presented before the Section at the Chicago Session, June 2-5, 1908. Publication rights reserved by the American Medical Association.

J. Vernon White[1] says that "the investigations of a number of recent authorities seem to show that tuberculous infection through the alimentary canal is of very frequent occurrence," and that "tuberculosis due to the bacillus that enters the lungs with breathed air is an unknown affection." As both these opinions are based on the same facts, known to all pathologists, it is evident that there are unknown factors which prevent agreement in the interpretation of what is already known.

This paper is based on the following propositions:

1. Errors of refraction, or marked muscle imbalance, may so disarrange the nervous functions that gastric or intestinal disturbances may result, and metabolism be retarded in consequence, with lowered resistance and increased susceptibility to infection.

2. The continued existence of such conditions, especially in the neurotic, may so lower the vitality as to retard recovery from tuberculous infections of the lungs.

3. Relief of the abnormal visual conditions is a necessary prerequisite to recovery from pulmonary disease.

4. In view of these facts the complete examination of a suspected tuberculous patient has not been made until the condition of the eyes, including the refraction and dynamics of the ocular muscles, has been investigated and carefully recorded.

The conclusions on which these premises are based have a practical application.

The following two cases, which are typical of many, will illustrate, first, the causative relation of eyestrain to disturbed digestion and assimilation, and, second, the importance of both in tuberculosis:

Case 1.—Eyestrain due to anisometropia causing gastric and intestinal indigestion.

Patient.—F. L., aged 33, principal of high school.

History.—About ten years ago he began to have severe pains in stomach. These would be relieved after eating, but would recur, with increased severity, in a few hours. This gradually grew less for four or five years, when he began to have attacks of nausea after eating, with a disagreeable "sour feeling" in the stomach. His digestion was always better when he did not use his eyes. Absolute rest for one day from close work was always followed by relief of the stomach symptoms. While walking on the street at times he would have blind attacks, with pain in and about the eyes. After half an hour, the blur

---

1. New York Med. Jour., Nov. 2, 1907.

would disappear, and he would become nauseated, with intense headache. Dietetic and medicinal treatment seemed to afford him little relief.

Examination.—A cycloplegic test showed hyperopic astigmia with anisometropia. R. V., + 0.50 D. cyl. ax. 75 V. = 20/20. L. V., — 0.37 D. cyl. ax. 120 V = 20/20. Muscle balance was normal.

Subsequent History.—After wearing corrective glasses for a week all these disagreeable symptoms disappeared and did not return. After six months, a slight acidity of the stomach suggested a re-examination of his eyes, when a change in the axis of the cylinder of the right eye was found, it having turned from 75 to 90 degrees. Since wearing the glasses, his metabolism had so improved that he had gained fifteen pounds in weight. The indigestion could be brought on again at any time by leaving off his glasses, if only for a few hours.

The second case shows the influence with a like condition exercised when associated with tuberculosis:

CASE 2.—Compound hyperopic astigmia-anisometropia, causing impairment of digestion and metabolism, and preventing recovery in pulmonary tuberculosis.

Patient.—Mrs. J. S. P., female, aged 25.

History.—In 1905 she developed a tuberculous condition in the apex of one lung, and was immediately sent to the Adirondacks and put under competent care. The usual treatment, that of an absolutely outdoor life, with superalimentation, was followed. She suffered constantly from intestinal indigestion and malassimilation, continued to lose weight, and in October was much worse than in May. It was determined that she should spend the winter in California, and *en route* came from her father's home in Rochester to Buffalo for relief of an eyestrain of which she had recently become conscious.

Examination.—Under cycloplegics, the following condition of anisometropia was found: R. V., + 0.50 D. sph. ⊂ + 0.75 D. cyl. ax. 165 V. = 20/20; L. V., + 1.00 D. sph. ⊂ +1.75 D. cyl. ax. 165 V. = 20/20. Esophoria of 3 degrees was present. For nearly three months she had suffered persistently from nausea, with constant intestinal indigestion. She was so weak and nervous that she was obliged to lie down for several hours before she could have her refraction taken. Her pulse was exceedingly rapid and weak.

Subsequent History.—It was found that she could take a full correction, and two days later started for New Orleans. The nausea immediately disappeared. For the first time in her life she was able to take a railway journey without suffering from car sickness. With a disappearance of the nausea the indigestion ceased, assimiliation became normal, weight increased, and she returned in the spring, having gained fifteen pounds and fully recovered in every way. She can not go with-

out her glasses without having a return of her old symptoms of indigestion.

If the theory advanced in this paper is correct, that the effort to use abnormal eyes may disturb the nervous currents elsewhere, and if the proportion of tuberculous people who suffer from eyestrain is at all large, its bearing on the general problem of tuberculosis is one of enormous importance. It is a generally accepted truism that any agent or condition which undermines the integrity of the nervous system will increase the susceptibility to disease, and the neurotic appears to be peculiarly vulnerable to tubercular infections.

In support of this contention, Clifford Albutt, discussing a variety of phthisis, says: "I began to find in my own practice and in the writings of alienists how large a part phthisis plays in neurotic families. Even then, however, it did not occur to me to associate any particular form of phthisis with neurotic disorder until a few striking cases of unclassable variety occurred in neurotic families under circumstances which spoke too eloquently to be overlooked. If we go a step further and ask for a pathologic explanation of these facts we approach a land of darkness."

It is not the purpose of this paper to discuss tuberculosis as a neurosis, but to demonstrate how important nervous conditions are in this disease, and to indicate that the eyes may be an important element in producing these conditions. Concerning the truth of this proposition, the mass of confirmatory testimony is so great that it is now very generally accepted, both by ophthalmologists and practitioners of internal medicine. Baker[2] reports 100 cases of migraine relieved by the correction of errors of refraction, and Musser has said that "functional gastric disorder is very rarely a primary trouble." Stockton was the first to point out the relation of eyestrain to digestion. In 1894 he said that the causes of functional gastric disorders are usually some reflex irritation or some toxemia. Max Einhorn, in 1893, described, under the title "achylia gastrica," a most important condition of the stomach, later described by Dr. Allen A. Jones as "gastric anacidity." The majority of the cases reported by Dr. Jones, together with several

---

2. A statistical inquiry as to the Relief and Cure of Migraine by the Correction of Errors of Refraction, Academy of Ophthalmology and Oto-Laryngology, 1906.

others included in the above-mentioned series, were examined as to the existence of eyestrain. Without a single exception, there was found to exist a definite and relatively uniform ocular defect, viz., unsymmetrical astigmatism of high degree, varying from one to five diopters. Cohn[3] emphasizes this by saying: "The visual apparatus is in closest connection with the other higher nervous mechanism, and the slightest disturbance of the visual portion may produce irritation in the entire motor, sensory and psychic systems." It may be conservatively stated, then, as the conclusion of the best American investigators, that eyestrain is a frequent cause of impaired metabolism.

The importance of eyestrain in the tuberculous being recognized, the natural inquiry which would follow is as to its frequency. Here we have absolutely no statistics. In none of the institutions established by public or private beneficence for the investigation or treatment of tuberculosis, in none of the reports which have been issued by individuals or associations, and by none of the authorities, so far as it has been possible to learn, has an exact examination with record of the condition of the refraction and of the dynamics of the eye muscles been considered an essential part of the anamnesis.

It can not be assumed that the tuberculous are more free from visual defects than are the non-tuberculous, and Gould says that he has never yet seen a mechanically perfect eye. How general visual disturbances, of such an extent that they may not be considered negligible quantities, are, is evidenced by the fact that refractive tests constitute from 60 to 70 per cent. of our daily work as ophthalmologists, while the attempted adaptation of lenses to eyes requiring their help occupies practically the entire time of opticians.

It is absurd, then, to ignore the existence of focal defects in the tuberculous or to minimize their importance. Yet in the Henry Phipps Institute, Philadelphia, where the examinations are conducted with the most scrupulous care and the reports are most detailed, the requirements seem to be met by recording the color of the eyes (an item of questionable value), and noting whether or not the pupils are dilated or unequal. Concerning the latter, the observations are most interesting and it would seem to lead one to think of further

3. Physiological Therapeutics.

investigations: "The matter of dilated pupils and of unequal pupils as symptoms of tuberculosis," says the report of 1906, "receive our support from the table, but only in regard to frequency of occurrence. No light is thrown on the cause of the phenomenon nor on the relationship of the disease. It is not even clear that they actually are symptoms of tuberculosis. Occurring in some cases and not in others, it is possible, and even probable, that they may be due to mixed infection or some complication."

The third report, that for 1907, shows that among 885 new patients 208 had dilated pupils, 399 had not, and of 278 no record was made. In 55 patients the pupils were unequal. "Dilated pupils," says the report, "for this year have occurred in about one-third of the patients of whom a record has been made as to the pupils. Unequal pupils have been recorded infrequently. Much has been said as to the condition of the pupils in tuberculosis by some writers, and statistics are here presented with a view of getting some light on the subject. So far we can draw no conclusions. We do not even know to what the phenomenon is due. Usually it is ascribed to muscular weakness." One year, therefore, we find the accommodative weakness manifesting itself in enlargement of the pupils, ascribed to a toxemia which must have a remarkable predilection for particular nuclei of the third nerve, and the next year to a muscular weakness which is equally speculative.

Is it not amazing that with such a specific assurance that the visual mechanism is in trouble, investigation should cease and vague and variable surmise serve as a basis from which to guess the etiology?

A dilated pupil is often associated with myopia. Astigmatism is the turnstile, as Risley says, through which the eye passes in achieving myopia. Exophoria and dilated pupils are definitely correlated, and this combination works such disaster in the midbrain as often to be nerve wrecking. It is not essential that we should know the channels through which the irritation is carried in order that we may appreciate the fact that eyes organically unlike, in an endeavor to blend images in the cortex, will cause nausea, vertigo, hyperacidity or subacidity of the stomach, and intestinal indigestion.

These are matters of daily experience in the practice of every ophthalmologist. That long neural band, the fasciculus longitudinalis, originating anterior to the nuclei of the third nerve and extending back till it is lost in the medulla is probably the medium by which the root organs of the various cerebral nerves are connected. That some such connection exists has been clinically demonstrated. When the eyes are organically different an excess of energy, equal to the difference between the better and the most abnormal eye, must be sent to both. Under such conditions the endeavor to maintain the parity between accommodation and convergence results in ciliary spasm or ciliary relaxation. It is probable that the one is associated with esophoria, the other with exophoria. The unconscious effort or paresis, as the case may be, of one set of muscles or fibers is reflected to other and remote sets. If one makes a strong effort to clench one hand very tightly he will find that he is unconsciouly closing the other. The effect of tension within the eye, or of relaxation, seems to be reflected particularly to the non-striated muscular tissue, and as a result a contraction or a relaxation of circular fibers follows. This is true of the vasodilators or vasoconstrictors of the capillaries, of the circular fibers of the stomach or of the intestines, of the urethra and of the uterus. Hence follow local congestions or local anemias, cramp of the stomach or catarrh of the stomach, constipation or diarrhea, incontinence of the urine, and in several instances I have seen pregnancy, after many years of sterility, follow the relief of an eyestrain that could be explained only on the basis of a relaxation of a persistent contraction of the circular fibers of the cervix. With these far-reaching nervous involvements, inadequacy of metabolism as an element in tuberculosis assumes an added importance whether or not Ravenel[4] is correct in his contention that "the alimentary tract is a frequent port of entry for the tubercle bacillus," for the same conditions that disturb the nervous functions of the digestive tract will involve nerve supply of all of the essential organs, and given a neuropathic diathesis we have the conditions prepared for the reception and culture of the infective organism.

---

4. Am. Jour. Med. Sc., October, 1907.

CONCLUSIONS.

The essential propositions which these conclusions warrant are:

1. The inadequacies of focus or the motility of the eyes may give rise to and be responsible for disturbances of digestion and assimilation.

2. Lowered vitality, especially in the neurotic, predisposes to tuberculous infection, and as superalimentation is of first importance in effecting a cure, an exact and complete examination of the refraction and of the motility of the eyes should constitute an essential part of the examination of every patient suspected of having this disease.

3. If these are the views of the ophthalmologist on this subject they are of such vital importance to a vast number of sufferers that resolutions to that effect should be adopted, and the recommendation made to this Association that it is the sense of the members of this section that no examination for tuberculosis can be considered complete until it shall include the refraction and the motility of the eyes.

THE CALMETTE OCULAR REACTION TO TUBERCULIN.*

HARRY C. PARKER, M.D.

Associate Professor of Ophthalmology, Indiana University School of Medicine.

INDIANAPOLIS.

Wolff-Eisner[1] and Calmette,[2] working independently, were the first to suggest the conjunctival tuberculin reaction as a diagnostic test for tuberculosis. Since their earliest reports in the spring of 1907 the medical journals in this country and abroad have contained the reports of many observers working along the lines suggested by Calmette. Wolff-Eisner at first used a 10 per cent. aqueous solution of tuberculin which produced a marked conjunctivitis in tuberculous patients, while the non-tuberculous did not show any conjunctival reaction. Calmette used but a 1 per cent. aqueous solution prepared by the precipitation of crude tuberculin with 95 per cent. alcohol, the precipitate being collected and dried. He claimed that in this manner the glycerin and beef extract salts were removed, which in themselves might cause a conjunctival irritation.

Most observers have used the solution prepared in the manner described by Calmette, although several observers, notably MacLennan[3] and Webster and Kilpatrick.[22] have obtained equally good results with a 1 per cent. aqueous solution of "old" tuberculin. MacLennan tested 25 cases with a 1 per cent. aqueous solution of "old" tuberculin of Koch. Of 14 clinically tuberculous patients. 12 reacted positively; 10 of the positive cases had previously reacted to the Calmette solution.

---

* This paper has been accepted by the Executive Committee of the Section on Ophthalmology of the American Medical Association, to be presented before the Section at the Chicago Session, June 2-5, 1908. Publication rights reserved by the American Medical Association.

1. Berl. klin. Wochschr., 1907, xliv, p. 700.
2. Compt. rendus de l'Acad. des Sc., June 17, 1907.
3. Brit. Med. Jour., Dec. 7. 1907.

Calmette[4] described the reaction as follows: "From the third hour onward the eye in which a 1 per cent. aqueous solution of tuberculin had been applied became reddened, and in the course of several hours showed all the appearances of a more or less pronounced attack of mucopurulent inflammation of the conjunctiva. The maximum was seen within six or seven hours after the instillation of the tuberculin. All traces of inflammation had disappeared in two or three days. The plan is free from danger and causes the patient scarcely any discomfort."

Various observers recommend solutions of different strength. Schenck and Seiffert,[5] who make their dilutions with a 3 per cent. solution of boric acid, recommend three different strengths. If the 1 per cent. solution of tuberculin produces no reaction, a 2 per cent. solution is tried, and if this fails a 4 per cent. solution is used.

Comby[6] uses a 0.5 per cent. solution in children, which, he says, is sufficiently strong to produce the reaction and is not harmful. In 132 unselected hospital cases he obtained 62 positive reactions. Ten of the tested cases later came to autopsy, 4 of these had reacted and 6 had manifested no reaction. The postmortem findings confirmed the value of the tuberculin reaction.

Baldwin[7] recommends 0.33 and 0.5 per cent. as the strength of the solution to be used at first. If these fail a stronger solution is used in the other eye. In a personal letter Dr. Baldwin informed me that he avoids the stronger initial dose and also avoids using the same eye twice, because of a possible severe inflammation. These sequelæ will be considered below.

From the study of nearly 2,200 tested cases taken from the medical literature of the past year it is safe to assert that in the ocular tuberculin reaction we have a test which is equal, if not superior, to any other one test; its application is extremely simple; it almost never produces any constitutional disturbances, and, if the initial dose at least is under 1 per cent. strength, little or no danger can possibly come from its use. A positive reaction almost invariably means tuberculosis, even though the case clinically has not been so diagnosed.

---

4. Presse Méd., June 19. 1907.
5. Muench. med. Wochschr., 1907, liv, p. 2269.
6. Presse Méd., Aug. 10, 1907.
7. The Journal A. M. A., Dec. 14, 1907.

The clinician can not always exclude a latent or old tuberculous focus. More postmortem reports on tested cases, both positive and negative, will be awaited with interest.

Cohn[8] obtained 8 positive reactions in 12 cases of typhoid tested with tuberculin. He explains these findings by the fact that typhoid cases have a special hypersensibility to bacterial albumin in general as well as to typhoid bacillus extracts. He concludes, however, from a study of 310 cases other than typhoid, that a positive reaction to the ocular tuberculin test is presumptive evidence of tuberculosis. He obtained 38 positive reactions out of 41 cases in the first and second stages of tuberculosis, and only 22 positive reactions out of 45 cases in the third stage of tuberculosis. His observations in this respect agree with many others.

Many observers have obtained positive reactions in all clinically tuberculous cases, while others, like Cohn, have often failed to obtain the reaction in advanced cases. This is explained by the fact that the opsonic index of these patients is low and they offer no resistance to the tuberculin. In this connection it is interesting to note the observations of Smithies and Walker,[9] one of whom obtained a reaction in his own eye after he had been subjected to a subcutaneous injection of 1 mg. of tuberculin. The ocular test in this instance has been negative previous to the injection of tuberculin. These observers also agree with the majority, that cases of acute miliary tuberculosis and advanced and moribund cases in which there is no doubt of the condition often react negatively.

COMPARATIVE DIAGNOSTIC VALUE OF THE SUBCUTANEOUS INJECTION, VACCINATION AND OCULAR REACTIONS TO TUBERCULIN.

Baldwin[7] has stated that, while it is too early to compare the value of the ocular and subcutaneous tests, a close similarity in the results have been obtained. Cohn[8] compared the ocular reaction with Koch's method of subcutaneous injections in a series of doubtful cases which resulted in favor of the ocular test. Mainini[10] applied the cutaneous test of von Pirquet[11] in 208 cases

8. Berl. klin. Wochschr., Nov. 25, 1907.
9. The Journal A. M. A., Jan. 25, 1908.
10. Muench. med. Wochschr., Dec. 24, 1907.
11. Berl. klin. Wochschr., May 20, 1907.

and the Calmette reaction in 100 cases. He was impressed with the constancy of the reaction in patients with certain tuberculosis, except those in the advanced stage. He found the cutaneous reaction six times more frequently among patients merely suspected of having tuberculosis than the ocular reaction. von Pirquet,[11] in 360 tests with the cutaneous reaction in children, found a marked difference between the hyperemia produced in tuberculous and non-tuberculous children under 2 years of age. In older tuberculous individuals the reaction was slight.

Comby[12] found the age of the child materially influenced the ocular reaction. Under 1 year of age no reaction was obtained, either in tuberculous or non-tuberculous infants; in the second year the reaction was very uncertain; beyond 2 years of age the results were similar to those obtained in adults. It is interesting to note that von Pirquet found the cutaneous reaction uncertain over 2 years of age, and Comby found the ocular reaction uncertain under 2 years of age.

Warfield[13] reports 169 cases tested by vaccination, and his conclusions agree with those of Mainini in that the cutaneous test is harmless and is of value in the pretuberculous stage.

Lenhartz[14] tried both the cutaneous and ocular reactions in 111 cases, 37 of which were undoubtedly tuberculous. Of the 37 tuberculous patients, 15 had been previously treated with subcutaneous injection of tuberculin. Of these the cutaneous test was negative in 6, well marked in 4, distinct in 2, and doubtful in 3. The ocular test was positive in 11, doubtful in 2, and not tried in 2. The better results in these cases with the ocular test may have been due to the previous injection of tuberculin, as Smithies and Walker[9] obtained an ocular reaction in a non-tuberculous patient after tuberculin had been injected subcutaneously. In 11 of Lenhartz's cases, clinically non-tuberculous, the ocular and cutaneous reactions gave about the same results. Of 63 suspicious cases, 23 were positive to both, 40 negative to the cutaneous, and 36 negative to the ocular test (this test being omitted in 4).

---

12. Rev. Méd. de la Suisse Romande, 1907, xxvii, p. 888.
13. The Journal A. M. A., Feb. 29, 1908.
14. Muench. med. Wochschr., Nov. 26, 1907.

IS THE OCULAR TUBERCULIN TEST HARMLESS?

Calmette[15] has recently claimed that in more than 10,000 cases already tested its harmlessness has been proven. Delorme, in his discussion of Calmette's paper, cited 39 cases of excessive conjunctival reaction.

De Lapersonne,[16] in his investigation of alleged injury to the eye from the instillation of tuberculin, found six cases of ulcero-vascular keratitis, which were, with one exception, in patients having a pre-existing lesion of the cornea. All recovered with good vision. He found in two other cases intraocular sequelæ which took the form of iridocyclitis. De Lapersonne advises against the use of the ocular test until both eyes have been thoroughly examined. He also advises against using this test in differentiation of lesions of the eyeball, whether deep or superficial, although it might be used in the diagnosis of diseases of the lids, orbit and lachrymal organs. The complications noted by De Lapersonne did not become manifest until from ten to twenty days after the instillation.

Netter[17] has recently protested against too much enthusiasm for the ocular reaction, because of its liability to be followed by serious consequences. He said that he knew of several instances in which Parisian ophthalmologists had been treating severe eye trouble following the instillation of tuberculin.

Eisen[18] reports two serious conjunctival reactions in 45 tests. Both patients had suffered from conjunctivitis in youth. The reaction in these patients was so severe that they were turned over to an ophthalmologist for treatment.

Feer's[19] experience with both the ocular and cutaneous tests leads him to warn against the use of the ocular test in scrofulous children, for the reason that it is liable to incite a severe and lasting conjunctivitis.

Weins and Gunther[20] report several instances of serious trouble in their experience. In one case, a child of 3 had a severe chronic conjunctivitis following the instillation of the tuberculin which was still evident after many months. In another case the instillation was followed by swelling and suppuration of the conjunctiva,

---

15. Bull. de l'Acad. de méd., Jan. 14, 1908.
16. Presse méd., Dec. 7, 1907.
17. Soc. d'Ophth., Paris, 1907.
18. Pelt. z. Klin. d. Tuberk., vii, No. 4.
19. Muench. med. Wochschr., Jan. 7, 1908.
20. Ibid., Dec. 24, 1907.

and this, in turn, was followed by the formation of phlyctenular ulcerations which were present for over three months. In another case the reaction soon subsided, but it was followed by conjunctival hemorrhage and inflammation, the latter lasting over a week. In 38 cases tested with 0.5 per cent. solution the reaction was negative in all but one. In this case a pre-existing mild conjunctivitis became much aggravated, with membrane formation, hemorrhages. keratitis, and severe subjective disturbances. The end-result, however, in this case was complete recovery.

H. Truc[21] declares the ocular test to be entirely harmless even when applied to individuals with ocular lesions. The reaction occurred with equal intensity in the diseased as in the sound eye, and, so far as he could judge, had no bad effect on the diseased eye.

Baldwin[7] gives acute or chronic conjunctivitis, blepharitis, keratitis, trachoma, or any disease of the cornea and internal structures of the eye as contraindication to the use of the ocular tuberculin test. In a personal letter Dr. Baldwin cites the case of a colleague on whom the reaction was tried: "The instillation was followed by edema of both eyelids and great swelling of the bulbar and palpebral conjunctivæ. In over 200 individuals there have been at least five severe reactions, ranging from deep injection and tumefaction of the entire conjunctiva and edema of the lids to ecchymoses, which have occurred in two instances."

Dr. Frank Smithies, of Ann Arbor, in a personal letter, stated that a more intense reaction was obtained in patients having a pre-existing conjunctivitis. One patient under his observation, a syphilitic with an old arthritis, reacted so strongly to a second instillation that the inflammation was cleared up with difficulty.. This patient at the time was taking iodids.

Webster and Kilpatrick[22] mentioned one case of phlyctenular conjunctivitis following recovery for the ocular reaction. They reported 121 cases tested with the 1 to 100 "old" tuberculin solution.

THE OCULAR REACTION IN OPHTHALMOLOGY.

Stephenson[23] was one of the first ophthalmologists to apply this test for the differential diagnosis of ocular

21. Soc. d'Ophth., 1907.
22. Brit. Med. Jour. Dec. 7, 1907.
23. Brit. Med. Jour., Oct. 19, 1907.

lesions. He says in his report: "The preponderating part unquestionably played by syphilis in the production of many ocular affections has, perhaps, tended to render some of us a little blind to the influence of other causes, prominent among which, as I believe, stands tuberculosis. How often do we meet disseminated chorioiditis indistinguishable by ophthalmologists from the form due to syphilis in patients in whom there is no evidence whatsoever of a specific taint, acquired or inherited? I feel confident that no small number of such non-syphilitic cases are in reality due to tuberculosis."

Stephenson's cases are:

1. *Phlyctenular Keratitis and Conjunctivitis.*—Six cases of long standing in children. Only two of these cases manifested other tuberculous lesions. All gave positive reaction; one recent case of phlyctenular keratitis gave a negative reaction.

2. *Chorioiditis.*—Three cases in young women without syphilitic taint, and presenting no other tubercular lesions. All three tests positive.

3. *Interstitial Keratitis.*—Eight cases tested; five showed typical signs of inherited syphilis. These five cases gave no reaction; the other three cases gave positive reactions.

4. *Episcleritis.*—Three cases tested; one positive case, which showed enlarged glands, the other two cases negative.

5. *Tubercle of Iris.*—One case in a girl of 12, who had had severe inflammation of left eye for six months. Anterior chamber filled with dense exudate. No general clinical signs of tuberculosis or syphilis. Case gave positive reaction.

6. *Tubercle of Cornea.*—One case in girl of 12. Cornea showed patchy deposits, rest of cornea hazy. Posterior synechiæ. Ophthalmoscope revealed areas of yellowish-white exudate in cornea. Reaction positive.

7. *Chronic Iridocyclitis.*—Two cases, both positive; one case was in a child of 9, the other in a woman of 34.

Painblau[24] reported two cases of tuberculosis of the conjunctiva which reacted positively. Brunetiére[24] reported three negative reactions in cases thought possibly to be tuberculous, keratoiritis, interstitial keratitis, and exudative chorioiditis. Later Brunetiére affirmed the diagnostic value of the ocular tuberculin reaction as a means of differentiating ocular lesions.

Aubaret and Lafon[25] report the use of the ocular reaction in 18 ophthalmic cases with positive reactions. These cases included intraocular tuberculosis, phlycten-

---

24. Ophth. Provinciale, August, 1907.
25. Gazette Hebd. des sciences méd. de Bordeaux, Aug. 4, 1907.

ular keratitis, episcleritis, interstitial keratitis, lachrymal affections and optic neuritis.

H. Truc[21] tested 23 patients with various ocular lesions, 4 having certain or suspected tuberculosis gave a positive reaction, 4 other reactions were positive in patients showing no clinical signs of tuberculosis. The other 15 cases gave no reaction.

Dr. George Derby, of Boston, was kind enough to send me the results of his experience with the Calmette reaction up to Jan. 21, 1908. He had tested 24 cases, 8 of which were controls. Two of the controls gave a positive reaction, one having a tuberculous family history, and the other could not be followed up. Of the 16 remaining cases, 15 had ocular lesions which might have been tuberculous. Among the cases manifesting ocular lesions there were 5 cases of phlyctenular keratitis, one of which gave a positive reaction, later confirmed by subcutaneous injection, and one gave a doubtful reaction, the remaining 3 cases were negative. Two cases of recurrent sclerokeratitis were positive. Three cases of interstitial keratitis giving specific history were negative. Three cases of scleritis gave one positive reaction, later confirmed by subcutaneous injection. One case having corneal ulcer and another with chorioretinitis were negative.

Derby advises against the instillation of the tuberculin in a diseased eye. He mentioned one case in which the tuberculin had been instilled into an apparently normal eye to find on more careful examination an old corneal scar. The reaction in this case was followed by a mild episcleritis which lasted several weeks.

My own experience with the test has been so limited that a summary of my cases seems hardly worth while. Dr. John R. Thrasher obtained the cases of certain or suspected tuberculosis for his clinic in the Indiana University School of Medicine; he also made the sputum examinations and aided me in following up the cases. I made 31 tests, 7 of which were second tests in cases in which the first reaction was negative. The Calmette solution, 1 per cent., was made from tablets furnished me by the experimental department of Parke Davis & Co. In the 24 cases tested, 3 were positive and 1 doubtful. One positive reaction was obtained in a colored woman having a subacute bronchitis and enlarged cervical glands; sputum negative. The doubtful reaction was obtained in a case of long tuberculosis; sputum positive. Three cases of advanced tuberculosis showing numerous bacilli in the sputum gave a positive reaction in one case; the other 2 cases gave negative reactions. Of the 24 patients, 5 had ocular lesions, but were in other respects apparently normal. One case of optic atrophy was negative; one case of hyalitis with deposits on Descemet's membrane was negative; a case of phlyctenular keratitis in one eye gave a positive reaction when the solution was instilled into the sound eye; one case of interstitial keratitis, undoubtedly specific, was negative, and one case of central chorioretinitis was negative.

FREQUENCY OF TUBERCULOSIS OF THE EYE.

Helbron[26] claims that 0.5 per cent. of 15,000 ophthalmic affections in the Berlin eye clinic were due to tuberculosis. Stock's[27] report of 59 cases of chronic iridocyclitis, of which 61 per cent. reacted to the subcutaneous injection of Koch's "old" tuberculin, shows the great number of this class of cases caused by tuberculosis. Verhoeff[28] and Bull[29] have within the past year called our attention to the tuberculous nature of many cases of scleritis and episcleritis. These tuberculous cases have reacted to the subcutaneous injection of both the "old" tuberculin of Koch and the tuberculin T.R. Prof. Carl Hess,[29] in the discussion of Bull's paper, said that he used tuberculin for diagnosis in about 100 cases and over 50 per cent. of these cases had given a general reaction. Török[30] reports 16 cases of tuberculosis of the eye treated with tuberculin injections. These cases included tuberculosis of the conjunctiva, sclera, iris and chorioid.

Chance,[31] in a paper on iritis in general disease, makes the assertion that tuberculous iritis is much more common than it was formerly supposed to be.

Brücker[32] cites 38 eye cases in which tuberculin was injected for diagnostic purposes. Of 12 acute cases of iritis only 2 reacted, while in 14 cases of chronic iritis or iridocyclitis 11 reacted.

---

26. Muench. med. Wochschr., Jan. 7, 1908.
27. Tuberculose als aetiologie der chronischen Entzündungen des Auges und seiner adnexæ besonders der chronischen Uveitis, Leipzig, 1907.
28. Boston Med. and Surg. Jour., March 14, 1907.
29. The Journal A. M. A., Aug. 3, 1907.
30. Arch. Ophth., September, 1907.
31. Therap. Gaz., August, 1907.
32. Arch. Ophth., September, 1907, xxxvi, 647.

CONCLUSIONS.

1. The Calmette ocular tuberculin test is of as great diagnostic importance as any other single test.

2. A positive reaction is indicative of a tuberculous focus somewhere in the body.

3. The test is uncertain in patients under 2 years of age, in whom the cutaneous test of von Pirquet is most certain.

4. The test fails in advanced cases of tuberculosis, when there is little need of the test for diagnostic purposes.

5. The initial instillation should be preferably under 1 per cent. strength, in order that severe inflammatory conditions may not follow its use.

6. If necessary to make the second and stronger test the instillation should be made in the eye not previously used.

7. The consensus of opinion seems to be against using the test in an eye not wholly normal.

8. After-complications have occurred from the use of the test, but these have entirely cleared up in a varying length of time. These conditions are not so frequent when the initial test is made with a solution under 1 per cent. in strength.

9. Recent investigations have shown a greater number of ophthalmic affections due to tuberculosis than formerly supposed, and in the Calmette reaction we have a simple means of differential diagnosis which should be thoroughly tried.

10. The ocular reaction is especially valuable for ascertaining the tuberculous nature of cases of phlyctenular keratitis and conjunctivitis, episcleritis and scleritis, chronic iritis and iridocyclitis, interstitial keratitis, and chorioiditis.

11. A 1 per cent. solution of Koch's "old" tuberculin is nearly as good as the Calmette solution for diagnostic purposes.

12. The test in the hands of various observers has given such uniformly excellent results that its value is practically assured.

OCULAR COMPLICATIONS OF PREGNANCY.*

HIRAM WOODS, M.D.

BALTIMORE.

In dealing with the ocular complications of pregnancy, I shall try to present the bearing of recent pathologic investigations on the cause of serious eye disturbance. Medical literature shows that there is scarcely an eye disease which has not been more or less directly traced to the pregnant state. Some of these we now know are not distinctively so caused. Pregnancy, at most, increases liability by lessening resisting powers. Power[1] published three interesting papers, claiming that, among other complications, pregnancy produced a definite type of superficial central ulceration of the cornea. With our present knowledge of the rôle of infection in corneal ulceration, it seems more natural to attribute to pregnancy only such influence as is seen after any other severe tax on the system.

The same is true of the supposed tendency to phlyctenular ophthalmia. Asthenopia, with its defective accommodation, short of absolute paralysis, varying muscular anomalies, occasional blurring of vision, may be laid at the door of the general nerve tax under which the pregnant woman lives. One must take into account, too, from the same cause, an increase in a preexisting hysterical habit. Thus, Knies[2] reports cases of temporary blindness, without urinary abnormality or ocular lesion, occurring after unusually painful labor. A patient of Szili's became suddenly blind from the opening of a window in a darkened room, and recovered only after six weeks. Then there are the considerable

* This paper has been accepted by the Executive Committee of the Section on Ophthalmology of the American Medical Association, to be presented before the Section at the Chicago Session, June 2-5, 1908. Publication rights reserved by the American Medical Association.

1. Lancet, Lond., May 8, 15, 22, 1880.
2. The Eye in General Diseases.

classes of metastatic ocular infections, of amblyopia from excessive hemorrhage, of lighting up of a latent syphilitic lesion, which would probably have remained quiet but for the overtaxed metabolism. I have seen specific chorioditis relapse during pregnancy. But in all these cases there is, so far as I can see, nothing that is not observed after numerous other conditions.

Apart from temporary functional derangement, hysterical or neurotic, and diminished tissue resistance, there are certain ocular troubles of intensely serious significance to eyesight and even to life, which are observed with sufficient frequency during pregnancy to make the relation of cause and effect almost certain. For purposes of study, they may, I think, be divided into four classes, based on clinical manifestations: (1) The so-called uremic amaurosis, or sudden and complete blindness, without ophthalmoscopic lesion; (2) The hemorrhagic, exudative and degenerative changes in the retina, occurring in connection with albuminuria, and termed albuminuric retinitis of pregnancy; (3) Temporary or permanent loss of central vision or some portion of the visual field, without retinal lesion, the fundus either appearing normal or showing pallor of some portion of the optic disc; (4) A definite neuro-retinitis, with hemorrhages and exudates. but not resembling the albuminuric retinitis.

We may consider each of these separately.

1. *Uremic Amaurosis.*—In its association with pregnancy, the term has the same meaning as in nephritis: sudden occurrence of total blindness (usual form), or great impairment of vision. There may be associated other nervous symptoms, such as headache, vomiting, etc. Pupillary reaction is usually maintained, and Fuchs thinks this proves "that the location of the affection can not be in the eye or the optic nerve, but higher up, i. e., in the brain, which is poisoned by the excretory matters retained in the blood."

No lesion is found in the eye, and while this form of blindness has the gravest possible significance in chronic nephritis, and may be serious in pregnancy, it is usually transitory in the pregnant woman, provided she survives other complications. So far as my observation goes, it is confined, when occurring in pregnancy or parturition, to eclamptic cases, and follows the convulsion. The cause of this blindness is usually attributed to uremic poisoning, dependent on kidney disease.

The name, uremic amaurosis, is applied to cases incidental to pregnancy and parturition, because of the similarity of symptoms in the nephritic and parturient forms of blindness, the usual co-existing albuminuria, and the deeply grounded belief that it is through the medium of the kidneys that pernicious vomiting, puerperal convulsions and blindness occur. Difference in the prognostic significance of nephritic and parturient blindness is generally attributed to the fact that in the former the kidneys are in an advanced stage of disorganization, while in the latter the cause of blindness terminates with labor; but that parturient blindness is uremic and that derangement of kidney structure and function is essential to its production seems the fixed teaching of to-day, so far as our text-books go.

2. *Albuminuric Retinitis.*—The characteristic silvery-white, radiating spots, seen in the perifoveal region and at the disc margin are too well known to need description. In both chronic nephritis and pregnancy the appearances are practically identical. As is well known, in the former these spots are considered of grave significance, and a fatal termination usually comes within two years. In pregnancy, they may appear as early as the third or fourth month, but usually they are seen toward the close of pregnancy.

According to Fuchs these white patches are made up of "fatty degeneration of the retinal elements and of the cells of the exudate." De Schweinitz states that in the retinitis of pregnancy the type is most often inflammatory, and that with the termination of gestation these inflammatory deposits may subside. It is on this possibility of absorption of inflammatory exudates before destructive processes have occurred in the retina, that we base the better prognosis in this form of retinitis. Hence, there is a practical unanimity of opinion that the only logical treatment is induction of labor. While, however, this is true, and while the kidney lesion of pregnancy, to which the retinal inflammation is attributed, is, as Fuchs says, "benign," there is not in our ophthalmic literature much suggestion of any other pathway from the uterus to the eye than through the kidney. Is this a logical or correct position in view of teaching from modern pathologic investigation?

One finds in treatises on obstetrics uniform warning about the increased danger from pregnancy to a woman who has chronic nephritis. She is certainly more liable to show remote complications of kidney inflammation than she would be if the extra burden of pregnancy were not put on her. But if she develops uremic blindness or albuminuric retinitis during or at the close of pregnancy, the latter condition can no more be blamed for the complication than other influences which are known to exert a bad effect on chronic nephritis. At most, gestation is only an exciting cause and the complication is really dependent on the antecedent nephritis. The same is true of acute nephritis, from any of its usual causes, developing during gestation. Danger of remote complications or even of a fatal ending are greater. But this is not equivalent to saying that pregnancy can cause real nephritis, or that, in a woman, free from kidney involvement before pregnancy, the latter can so influence kidney structure and function as to produce through them grave ocular complications. Indeed, the weight of opinion seems the other way.

In the American Text-Book of Obstetrics the author of the chapter on the pathology of pregnancy says: "An acute inflammation of the kidney can not be caused by pregnancy, and is only observed in the rare cases where infective bacteria find entrance to the genito-urinary tract of the pregnant." J. Clifton Edgar states that "the kidney is affected in pregnancy by lesions which stop short of actual nephritis." This lesion is "purely a disease of the renal epithelium which undergoes more or less fatty metamorphosis—a deposit and not a degeneration."

It may be well to speak a moment of the so-called "kidney of pregnancy," a condition to which we are apt to attribute too much importance. J. Whitridge Williams mentions it only incidentally in the first edition of his book. and in the second edition says: "It is a slight degree of nephritis. . . . Such conditions are nearly always connected with the various disturbances of metabolism which will be taken up under toxemia of pregnancy." Edgar says: "There is an affection to which the term 'pregnancy kidney' is familiarly restricted, and which is certainly not due to pressure, nor has it anything in common with ordinary nephritis, whether pre-existent or developing during gestation as a result of exposure or infection. In one sense, the notion of pregnancy-kidney is a negative one, formed after the exclusion of other renal lesions, and including numerous conditions which present little in common." Hirst seems to attach more importance to it than most modern writers, and says: "There is often albuminuria in advanced degrees of the condition. Hyaline and granular casts, with epithelium filled with fat, may be found. The kidneys may prove physiologically insufficient, and there may appear all the symptoms of renal insufficiency observed in true nephritis." Hirst also differentiates between chronic nephritis and the kidney of pregnancy, and says that in the latter the kidney symptoms are usually confined to the last months, while in nephritis they are pronounced at an early stage; and, again, that so far as his experience goes, albuminuric retinitis does not appear in the kidney of pregnancy, unless symptoms point to chronic nephritis.

The question I am trying to present is—are ophthalmologists justified in limiting their conception of the etiology of pregnancy-blindness or retinitis to renal lesions? Pregnancy does produce temporary blindness, and sometimes permanent impairment of vision in women previously healthy. It does cause retinal spots of exudation and degeneration in the same class, and the retinal lesion is usually accompanied by albuminuria. But is albuminuria the pathway to the retinal disease, or is the blindness essentially uremic? The recognized authorities from whom I have quoted might be multiplied, but such a course would only confirm the opinions expressed: (1) That pregnancy itself does not produce nephritis; (2) That the so-called kidney of pregnancy is usually insignificant in its effects, and recovers; (3) That it does not produce what we term "albuminuric retinitis."

We may now study the matter from another point of view. The dimness of vision or blindness in cases which do not show retinal lesion usually comes toward the close of gestation, during or after parturition. Again, the visual defect is one of a symptom-group of which headache, somnolence, convulsive seizures, etc., are members. This array has received the name of eclampsia, and convulsions are its prominent manifestation. As is well known, puerperal eclampsia, or convulsions, was generally thought, until late years, to have a renal origin. This opinion was based on the close resemblance of the puerperal to the nephritic seizures, and the usual presence of albuminuria.

Beyond mention of a few facts it is needless to discuss the reasons for abandoning this theory. Briefly, the insignificant renal changes often found at autopsy, and absence during life of symptoms of renal involvement in cases of eclampsia, started investigations which have led away from the renal theory. Edgar agrees with Williams that the pregnancy kidney is most probably a mild product of toxemia. He adds :"The all-important subject of the connection between this renal lesion and eclampsia is best accounted for by attributing the latter to the toxic state and not to the kindey lesion, which is itself the result of the same or an allied toxemia. There is, moreover, every reason to believe that this unknown toxic state of the blood is not uremia."

In the last edition of his work on obstetrics Williams reviews at length his own work on the pernicious vomiting of pregnancy, first published as a monograph in 1906, and includes the work of Prutz, Schmorl and others. A brief summary of conclusions may be given. In pernicious vomiting there are found hepatic changes identical with those found in acute yellow atrophy of the liver. There is profound necrosis of the central portion of the lobule, while the periphery remains intact." The lesions differ from those observed in eclampsia in which the process is essentially one of thrombosis and begins in the peripheral spaces. Williams urges that the hepatic changes in both pernicious vomiting and eclampsia may account for at least part of the urinary changes through the non-conversion of nitrogenous material into urea and its excretion as ammonia. He continues, "It should not be believed that the essential process consists in the hepatic or renal lesions, but in an underlying toxemia, to which they are due."

To summarize those parts of the work which touch ocular problems it seems to be the prevailing opinion (1) That eclampsia of parturition is not uremic; (2) That both eclampsia and pernicious vomiting are results of a toxic substance circulating in the blood whose nature, or natures, are unknown; (3) That these toxic substances are capable of profoundly affecting the liver, and do so in a much more characteristic way than they do the kidneys; (4) That these substances can produce thrombosis in many of the smaller vessels with consequent degenerative and necrotic changes in various organs.

This conception of the serious complications of pregnancy, if confirmed, will put renal complications in the list of toxic effects. It will also influence our conception of these renal complications as the cause of ocular disturbances. The question will arise whether the toxemia which produces the renal, hepatic and other lesions may not also produce the ocular disturbances and lesions. If eclamptic convulsions are not uremic, except in cases of aggravated pre-existing nephritis, it seems more logical to attribute the temporary blindness of eclampsia to the toxemia of the latter, than to bring in an uremia whose existence is at the most hypothetical. A toxic substance capable of causing such profound nerve disturbances as convulsions and many of the sequelæ might affect the optic centers as well. And, as a matter of fact, we know that these centers are often affected, sometimes permanently, by toxic agents having no connection with uremia.

SECONDARY EFFECTS OF TOXEMIA.

The secondary effects of a toxemia are many; edema, exudation, thrombosis, apoplexy, etc., are among them. They affect the nervous system as well as other parts. Among 65 eclamptic autopsies Schmorl[3] noted thrombi in the smaller cerebral vessels in 58. Edema, hyperemia, etc., were practically constant.

Bearing these facts in mind, we may for a moment look at what we term the albuminuric retinitis of pregnancy. I think all of us have seen nearly identical appearances in patients without albuminuria. I have seen them in a chlorotic girl, with functional menstrual trouble, clearing up with improvement in general health. There was no albuminuria. I have seen them in an apparently healthy boy, without known cause, who later developed a choroiditis of exudative type in the other eye. In a case of neuro-retinitis from venous thrombosis during pregnancy the characteristic retinal spots were evident. Yet there was no albuminuria.

---

3. Williams' Text-Book.

Dr. James Bordley has been making careful study of ocular changes in cases of brain tumors at the Hopkins Hospital. He tells me that he has studied two hundred cases, but at this writing has tabulated only half. Yet in sixteen he found spots in the retina which he would have called albuminuric. The urine was normal. Diagnosis of intracranial neoplasm was confirmed by operation or autopsy. He and Dr. Cushing attribute the retinal changes to pressure, edema, exudation and consequent degeneration without inflammatory processes. All these are logical results of toxemia.

We have, then, the facts that other conditions than albuminuria can produce the characteristic clinical retinitis which has been called albuminuric; that among these are effects produced by toxemia, and that it is to

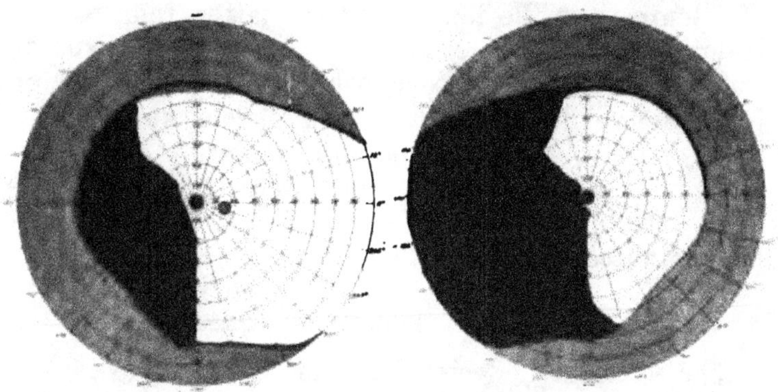

Figure 1. Figure 2.

Figs. 1 and 2.—Case 1. Fields showing loss of a portion of visual field without retinal lesion.

a toxemia that kidney changes in pregnancy are attributed; that in cases in which premature labor has been induced, cure of the retinal lesion has followed. I do not think it is going too far if one urges, with evidence at hand, that we cultivate at least an open-mindedness regarding the causation of what we have always termed the albuminuric retinitis of pregnancy. Such a state of mind has one very important bearing on therapeusis. So long as we interject an albuminuria into our thinking we will be in imminent risk of sacrificing eyes. There is but one remedy that will cure the disease—prompt emptying of the uterus. But if there is no albuminuria, and we believe this to be an essential pathologic factor, we will miss our only opportunity to save vision, and subject the patient to the risks of a profound toxemia, already evidencing its presence in a most dangerous form.

3. *Loss of central vision or some portion of visual field, without retinal lesion.* In 1902,[4] I reported a case, the fields of which are here reproduced (Figs. 1 and 2). Her history is given here as Case 1. At the time I was able to find only one such case reported in medical literature, but another has since been found,[5] and it is more than possible that there are others, under one name or another.

Case 1.—Patient was 33 years of age, in her first confinement. From the sixth month there had been traces of albumin, and careful watch had been kept. Her pregnancy was closed abruptly toward the end of the ninth month by instrumental delivery, after a single convulsion. Recovery was without incident, except that for four days she had transient visual disturbances, and then, with an atrocious headache, she suddenly lost the left field of vision. This was in September, 1901, and the loss has been permanent. Dr. Whitridge Williams recently furnished me with the following data concerning the urine. Its importance was not duly appreciated by me when the original report was made: "For the week prior to the eclampsia the daily amount of urine varied from 43 to 64 ounces, while the albumin and urea content varied from 0.5 to 1.5 grams and ·7 to 10.5 grams, respectively. For the week following the eclampsia the quantity of urine varied from 33 to 65 ounces, the albumin occurred only in traces, while the urea content varied from 15 to 21 grams per day." The significant element is diminished output of urea.

Case 2.—In this case the fields were taken in May, 1903, and again in March, 1908 (Figs. 3, 4, 5 and 6). Central vision then, as now, was 20/20. The papilla now is slightly pale (?). The following history was furnished by Dr. Williams: "The patient is a well-nourished woman, 37 years of age. Her fourth pregnancy began March 16, 1902. In July she complained of some headache and diminished urinary output. At this time the daily quantity of urine was 29 ounces, which contained no albumin and only 10 grams of urea. She was immediately put on a milk diet, and in the course of the next few days the urinary output had increased to 67 ounces, and the urea to 16 grams per day. Following this all symptoms disappeared. A 24-hour specimen, seen December 12, contained no albumin and 20 grams of urea. The patient went into labor on Jan. 1, 1903, and had an easy spontaneous delivery after eight hours of labor pains. The child was normal and weighed 7½ pounds.

---

4. Proc. Am. Ophthal. Soc.
5. Brit. Med. Jour., Sept. 30, 1893.

"The third day after labor the patient began to complain of flashes of light in her right eye, and the next day of intense neuralgic pains, particularly on the right side of the head. (The defect in the visual field occurred two or three days later.) January 13 there was a feeling of numbness on the left side. Closer examination showed a complete hemianesthesia. At the same time the muscular forces were considerably diminished as compared with those of the opposite side. On the seventh day of the puerperium the urine was negative, but on the thirteenth day it contained a trace of albumin, but no casts. A 24-hour specimen on the nineteenth day amounted to 50 ounces, and contained 42 grams of urea and a marked trace of albumin, with a few casts." Blood examination showed 4,240,000 red cells, 11,500 white cells, hemoglobin 50 per cent.

She was put on iron and made a complete recovery, except for the hemianopsia and nervous symptoms on the left side. There is still, five years later, marked impairment of sensation in the left hand and diminished muscular force, as compared with the right hand.

Dr. H. M. Thomas saw this lady in 1903, and I append a report he made in 1905: "She has, two years after the attack, marked sensory disturbance over the whole left side. Touch is perceived nearly normally, but painful stimuli with the point of a pin are not felt as sharp pricks, but at times are painful. There is marked disturbance in the perception of hot and cold stimuli. Heat is usually not perceived at all, and cold is only felt as pain and not as cold. Muscular sense is somewhat disturbed in the hand, and there is a complete loss of the stereognostic power. There is also some ataxia in the movements of the left hand. The symptoms, I believe, are the result of softening in the posterior part of the internal capsule and the region just posterior to it, probably due to a thrombosis of the posterior cerebral artery."

Case 3.—The patient had had five miscarriages, but was delivered of a full-term dead child Sept. 26, 1906. The history suggests syphilis. Her physician being dead, no particulars of gestation, etc., are obtainable. However, she had never noticed any visual defect until she was up after this confinement. Then she found herself running into chairs, etc., on the right side, and consulted Dr. J. J. Carroll, of Baltimore, who found normal central vision and the fields shown in Figures 7 and 8. She was in excellent health.

As stated, when I reported my first case in 1902, I found but one case on record, and this showed temporary right hemianopsia. F. Pick, who investigated the case, thought the visual disturbance resulted from a toxic paralysis of the central tracts of the optic nerve, with more marked involvement of one hemisphere.

R. Lawford Knaggs[5] reported the case of a woman, 40 years old, who for eight years had been blind in the left eye. The blindness was first noticed after confinement. Though not stated in the report, it is evident that she was pregnant when she applied for refraction cor-

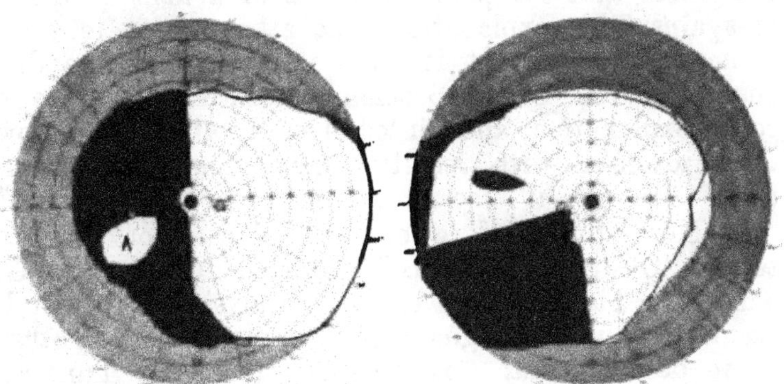

Figure 3. Figure 4.

Figs. 3 and 4.—Case 2. Showing visual fields as found in May, 1903. A, Dim area.

rection for the right eye. In the course of six weeks vision failed, while the field, taken before abortion, is shown in Figure 9. There was no albuminuria. Eleven months after abortion central vision was normal, and

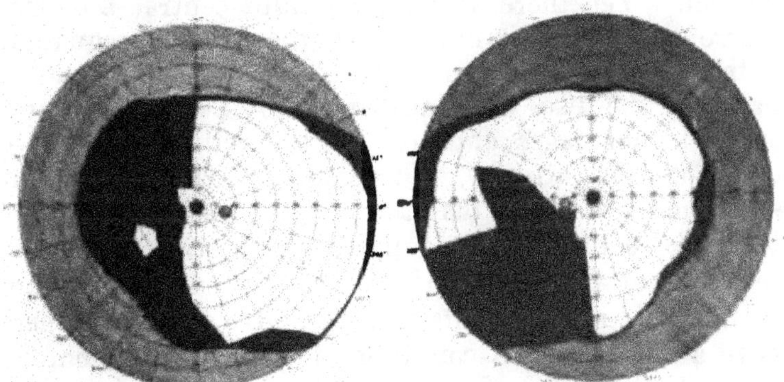

Figure 5. Figure 6.

Figs. 5 and 6.—Case 2. Showing visual fields as found in March, 1908. The light area within the solid black in Figure 5 indicates the dim area.

the field showed loss of vision in the right lower quadrant (Fig. 10). The reporter thought the case one of reflex amblyopia, and quotes this explanation from Mr. Priestly Smith, "A peripheral stimulus acting through the sympathetic nerve leads to a vasomotor effect within the eye, and the defects of sight are produced through the medium of the vessels of the capillary layer of the chorioid. . . . . The amblyopia is due to the impaired nutrition of the rods and cones." Mr. Knaggs recognizes that the permanent loss of a field quadrant is against this explanation, but attributes it to commencing atrophy. It is noteworthy that in the discussion E. F. Drake Brockman took exception to a reflex explanation, and hinted strongly at what we now term toxemia, with resulting hemorrhage or thrombosis. He calls it "the altered character of the blood."

J. Herbert Fisher[6] reviews several cases of what he terms "Obstetric Neuritis," reported by Dr. H. G. Turney.[7] Fisher adds a case of paralysis of one pupil, occurring during pregnancy, in connection with other nerve derangement. Incidentally, he quotes Turney's criticism of Knaggs' case, Turney attributing the blindness to a retrobulbar neuritis of toxic origin.

Mention may be made, finally, of a case reported by Dr. Charles J. Kipp, of Newark.[8] The patient lost vision in the right eye after four pregnancies, in each of which there had been ocular trouble. Dr. Kipp saw her first after her third confinement. Except for a slight loss of transparency in the region of the disc the fundus was normal. Yet there was an absolute central scotoma. There was no albuminuria. In the fourth pregnancy, with reduction of vision to light perception, there was pallor of the disc, with indistinctness of outline. Later small hemorrhages appeared in the retina. The case ended in total atrophy. Dr. Kipp says that to him "it seems most probable that the pregnancies caused a disturbance in the vascular supply, a congestion at or near the apex of the orbit, and that this produced pressure on the optic nerve and its sheaths." He says that others have attributed such conditions to autointoxication.

In all these cases, I think, nephritis can be excluded. The vascular supply and reflex explanations do not seem reasonable. From what we now know of the toxemias of pregnancy, of the results of toxemia in producing edema, thrombosis, exudation and necrosis, of the frequency of involvement of the nervous system in this

---

6. Ophth. Rev., xvii, p. 317.
7. St. Thomas' Hosp. Rep., xxv.
8. THE JOURNAL A. M. A., June 30, 1906, p. 1986.

toxic process, it seems to me that we abandon an adequate and ready explanation when we leave this field. For instance, Dr. Kipp's case, with its central scotoma in the third pregnancy, partial recovery between pregnancies, preservation of peripheral vision throughout, seems to be a typical picture of a recurrent toxemia.

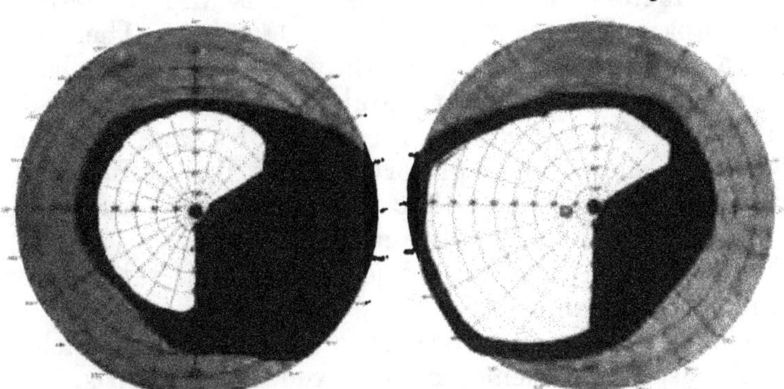

Figure 7. Figure 8.

Figs. 7 and 8.—Case 3. Showing visual fields as they appeared shortly after confinement.

These fields are worthy of more than passing notice. In some of them the entire half is obliterated. In others, where part of the affected retinal half is spared,

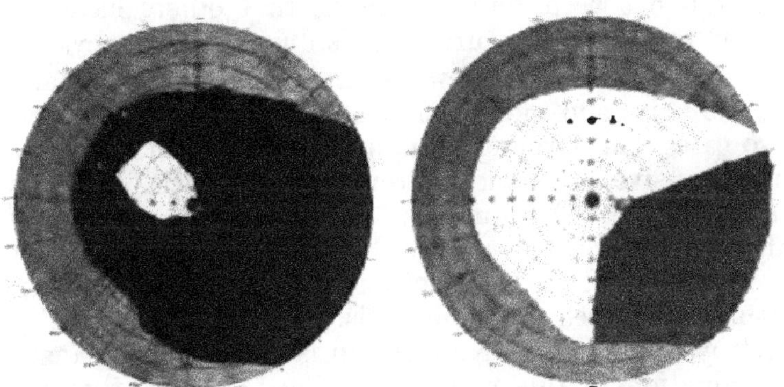

Figure 9. Figure 10.

Fig. 9.—Knaggs' case. Visual field taken just before abortion occurred.

Fig. 10.—Knaggs' case. Visual field taken eleven months after abortion.

the tendency is decidedly toward permanent involvement of the lower quadrant. I do not know why this should be. But it has, possibly, some bearing on etiology. Assuming, as I think we should, that toxemia is the basis of the lesions, the fields indicating total obliteration of a retinal half are probably the result of a necrotic process, while those showing preservation of a quadrant are more likely the result of toxic neuritis, certain fibers ultimately escaping, while others were destroyed. Thrombosis, necrosis and neuritis are essential factors of deep toxemia. It is also interesting to compare Figures 3 and 5, and 4 and 6. There are taken five years apart, from the same eyes. The large "dim area" in the lower nasal quadrant of Figure 3, taken in 1903, is found in the midst of a large scotoma. Figure 5 shows some preservation of this seeing spot. Figure 4 shows that in 1903 there was a scotoma in the upper temporal quadrant, and five years later (Fig. 6) this has broken through and joined the obliterated lower temporal quadrant.

The last ocular complication of pregnancy of which I shall speak is a hemorrhagic, exudative retinitis, and does not suggest the type known as albuminuric, I have seen only two such cases, and these within the past four weeks. I have not had time to make as complete a study of the literature as I should like, and hope at a later period to present the cases in a more thorough manner. However, the little research I have been able to make justifies classifying them as complications of pregnancy. Enough has been found to prove that others have observed this form of neuroretinitis during pregnancy.

There is a brief review[9] of an article by Paul Bar[10] on the poly- and mono-neurites of pregnancy. He cites two cases, one a young woman of 22, who lost both eyes in successive pregnancies from neuroretinitis. In this case there was albuminuria. In a second case, dimness of vision had been experienced toward the close of a first pregnancy, but little attention was paid to it. Later, Panas diagnosed optic neuritis. A second pregnancy destroyed both eyes. No mention is made of the urinary examination in this review, but Puyo,[11] states that the second case did not present symptoms of kidney involvment. Groenouw[12] says: "But retinal diseases, and hemorrhages in the retina in particular, also occur in the pregnant woman whose urine is free from sugar and albumin and who has no cardiac disease. Te-Mais

9. Ann. d'Oculistique, 1904.
10. Bull. de la Soc. d'Obstet., 1904, 4, 180.
11. Des Nevrites Gravidiques Par. Thes., 1905.
12. Graefe-Saemisch, p. 184.

reports on four such cases, of which three were completely cured after delivery. In the fourth case, hemorrhages of the conjunctiva appeared in the third month of pregnancy, and two months later in the retina."

Puyo studied the neurites of pregnancy thoroughly and goes over some of the cases mentioned in this paper. He concludes that the underlying cause is a toxemia of unknown nature, and excludes the kidney. The renal lesions, when present, he thinks secondary.

With this brief review of published cases, which seems sufficient to establish the existence of a pregnancy-neuroretinitis, I want to give clinical notes of the two cases recently observed, with special reference to the methods of diagnosing their toxic origin.

Case 4.—*History.*—Feb. 20, 1908, I was consulted by a lady, 35 years of age, from the South, for blindness of the left eye. She was the mother of five healthy children. In November, 1907, when she thought herself pregnant, she had, from some cause which could not be satisfactorily determined, a hemorrhage, which was diagnosed as a miscarriage. She made a prompt recovery. The December menstrual period was shorter than normal, and that in January was missed. Her own conclusion was that she had become pregnant shortly after her menstruation in the first week of December, and the usual appearance of morning sickness confirmed her opinion. In all her previous pregnancies she had been unusually well, but in this she had not felt well, with inclination to avoid exertion, etc. As nearly as she could place the date, her first eye symptoms had appeared on January 8, when she noticed that the lower field of vision was obliterated. She was sure that this was confined to the left eye. In a day or two this cleared up, but after an equal interval she became conscious that the left eye saw poorly, and soon sight was lost altogether. She consulted a local oculist, who correctly diagnosed neuroretinitis. Mercurial treatment had been without avail. The right eye was normal.

Examination.—I found extensive retinitis, with hemorrhages and large exudates over the entire fundus. There was also considerable swelling of the papilla. The veins were tortuous, thrombosed, broken in places, and there was no difficulty in determining that a venous thrombosis was at the bottom of the neuroretinitis. Syphilis was absolutely excluded. There was no reason to think that brain tumor or intracranial inflammation was the cause. Yet I felt that the salvation of the right eye, if possible at all, demanded discovery of the underlying cause of the thrombosis. In this connection I recalled Williams' work on toxemic vomiting of pregnancy.

Secondary results of the toxemia, which Williams claimed produced this condition, were found in the central nervous system, and I wondered if it were possible that, without the stage and symptoms of this sort of vomiting, serious nerve lesion might exist. I sent the patient to the University of Maryland Hospital for examination. Dr. Bull, of New York, to whom I submitted the history, agreed that this was the most promising line for investigation. While the urinary examinations were in progress, with the aid of Dr. Friedenwald, who saw the case with me, the literature was searched with the results already outlined.

The line of investigation may be best given by quoting from a paper on the Toxemic Vomiting of Pregnancy by Williams.[13] He first divides the subject into three varieties—neurotic, reflex and pernicious vomiting. The neurotic is often hysterical and when correctly diagnosticated can be controlled by suggestion and various simple means. Reflex vomiting is due to some malposition or other lesion connected with the pelvic viscera, and is subject to amelioration, when the toxic variety is excluded. But physical examination, to determine a reflex origin, chemical, to decide toxic origin, are needed before the neurotic variety can be accepted as the diagnosis. He says: "The urine, while diminished in amount as the result of scanty intake of fluids, does not contain albumin or casts until shortly before death, and may apparently present a normal amount of urea, as determined by the Doremus method, so that its casual examination gives no clue to the gravity of the condition. In reality, on the other hand, more detailed chemical examination at an early period reveals changes which are indicative of a profoundly altered metabolism. These consist of a decided decrease in the amount of nitrogen excreted as urea and a marked increase in the amount put out as ammonia. Accordingly, while the total nitrogen output may be practically normal, the percentage of nitrogen eliminated as ammonia is greatly increased, and this so-called ammonia coefficient, instead of being 4 or 5 per cent. as in normal pregnancy, may rise to 20, 30 or 40 per cent. . . . In my experience, if the latter (i. e., the ammonia coefficient) exceeds 10 per cent., the diagnosis of toxemic vomiting should be made, and the pregnancy immediately terminated, as there is no likelihood that the process can be checked by therapeutic measures, if it once leads to the production of the characteristic hepatic lesions."

The urine of my patient was subjected to such examination. The daily output was measured, tests for albumin, sugar and casts were made daily, and the urea and ammonia estimated quantitatively. At no time was there a trace of albumin, or sugar, and once the examiner, Dr. Adler, of the University staff, found, as he thought, a few hyaline casts. For the first three days the output was only 21, 19 and 23 ounces.

---

13. Am. Jour. Med. Sciences, September, 1906.

Forced intake of water made very little alteration. The total urea output during these days, from February 22 to 29, varied from 4.7 to 5.5 grams, while the ammonia coefficient was persistently 14 to 15 per cent. In a word, urinalysis gave exactly what Williams had described as the diagnostic basis of pernicious vomiting. Yet there was very little nausea and no vomiting. But there was a destructive neuroretinitis, dependent on venous thrombosis, and thrombosis is a recognized result of pregnancy toxemia.

I had little hope of improving the left eye, but, after consultation with Dr. Friedenwald and Dr. L. M. Allen, I advised premature delivery as the best method of safeguarding the right eye. This was accomplished by Dr. Allen on February 29. Recovery was uneventful. Dr. Allen thought the fetus indicated a pregnancy of at least three and a half months, which throws some doubt on the supposed miscarriage in November.

There was on March 5 a urinary output of 80 ounces, with 13.75 grams of urea. Since then the daily output has not fallen below 93 ounces per day, with excretion of urea varying from 7 to 13 drams. This is still below normal, but three examinations of the ammonia coefficient show 8.3 per cent., 5.6 per cent. and 6.1 per cent. The patient has improved generally, and it is worthy of note that from having in the left eye no light perception or pupillary reaction before delivery, both are now present in certain parts of the field. Incidentally, I may add that when I dilated the left pupil for ophthalmoscopic direct examination I found at the foveal region numerous spots which I would not have hesitated to attribute to albuminuria, but at no time was it present.

Case 5.—Tne patient was 22 years of age, in her second pregnancy. I saw her through the courtesy of Dr. Williams. She was admitted to Johns Hopkins Hospital February 5. The history shows persistent vomiting from February 5 to 17. Rectal nourishment was employed. Slight jaundice on February 16. On the 7th the ammonia coefficient was 36 per cent. On the 10th it was 20 per cent., at that time still more than double the amount on which a diagnosis of pernicious vomiting could be made. I do not know why Dr. Williams did not operate then, but he postponed doing so until the 17th. On the 16th the ammonia coefficient reached 40 per cent., and the next day the uterus was emptied. Ammonia output continued high, and the patient was intensely septic for several days. The ammonia output fell steadily, reaching 11 per cent. on March 9.

The day of first involvement of the eyes is not given, but on February 28 it is stated that the patient "could just barely count fingers when the eyes were worst." On March 2 Dr. R. L. Randolph found hemorrhagic neuroretinitis and large hemorrhages in both eyes, especially in the left eye. Exudates were scattered throughout the retinæ. On March 7 Dr. H. M.

Thomas found definite symptoms of multiple neuritis, into which I need not enter for present purposes. Life was almost despaired of, but the woman has survived, and when I saw her on March 10 she seemed to have good promise of preserving both life and vision. The exudates were nearly absorbed, and so were the retinal hemorrhages. The nerves and retinæ showed no special abnormality, and there was good pupillary reaction. She saw objects in the yard and counted fingers at ten feet.

SUMMARY.

Apart from the various nervous symptoms incidental to pregnancy, which often affect the eye functions, there are four serious ocular manifestations seen more or less frequently during pregnancy or after parturition. These are: (1) The so-called uremic blindness, which is usually seen in connection with eclampsia. (2) What has always been termed the albuminuric retinitis of pregnancy. These are the most common complications. Rarer forms are (3) loss of central or peripheral vision, due, so far as symptoms point, to a retrobulbar neuritis, and (4), a form of neuroretinitis, not essentially suggestive of the albuminuric type, but showing numerous retinal exudates and hemorrhages. The clinical symptoms of these conditions are reviewed, and the classes are studied from the standpoint of recent pathological investigations in the obstetrical field. There is, in view of these investigations, doubt as to whether the term uremic should be applied to the blindness occurring in connection with puerperal eclampsia. The same is true regarding the renal origin of what is termed the albuminuric retinitis of pregnancy. There is good reason to think that both the renal and ocular complications are manifestations of the same process—a toxemia. The basis for this is set forth in the paper.

The third and fourth varieties of ocular complications of pregnancy are also, doubtless, the results of pregnancy toxemia, a toxic neuritis or toxic thrombosis probably being the active factor in causation.

THE RELATION OF OCULAR AND CARDIOVASCULAR DISEASE.*

MELVILLE BLACK, M.D.

Professor of Ophthalmology, Denver and Gross School of Medicine.

DENVER.

This subject, I am sure, is not new to you, but since we are learning more about it every day, a few of my personal ideas and findings may prove of interest. The estimation of blood pressure has brought about a more comprehensive knowledge of cardiovascular disease. The remote disturbances which follow this important condition, and the etiologic factors which gradually lead up to it, are now receiving much attention. It is a well-recognized fact that a man may be on "his last legs," so to speak, from cardiovascular changes, and yet feel no serious bodily discomfort. He may have, therefore, no urgent reason for consulting his physician, but may have reason to consult his oculist, and we should constantly be on the lookout for ocular evidences of these vascular changes.

The recognition of these early changes in the retinal circulation may enable us to give many years of life to a considerable number of our patients. The "optometrist" will always be incompetent to recognize these danger signals in the eye, and it is one more urgent reason why he should not be licensed to practice his would-be profession. While the ophthalmologist keeps pace with the body of the medical profession in its new discoveries, the technical knowledge and the equipment required to make a thorough examination of the urine, the blood, and an all-round physical examination of the individual goes beyond his province. He has served a most useful purpose, however, in having recognized the

* This paper has been accepted by the Executive Committee of the Section on Ophthalmology of the American Medical Association, to be presented before the Section at the Chicago Session, June 2-5, 1908. Publication rights reserved by the American Medical Association.

ocular signs which warrant such a physical examination, and has done his duty by seeing that the patient had such an examination made.

It is no disparagement to the general practitioner to say that he also is incompetent to make this examination. It has been my policy to refer such a patient to some one capable of making this all-round examination, and then send him to his physician with the full report of our findings. I must confess that my efforts have been several times thwarted by the family physician making light of the entire matter. He thumps the patient a little, listens to his heart through a few intervening thicknesses of clothing and directs him to "go about his business." A dilated heart can only be mapped out by the most painstaking deep percussion. The presence of a low blood pressure, polycythemia, and dilated, tortuous retinal veins, uricacidemia and indicanuria all point to a clear diagnosis of general venous stasis, which tends not only to shorten life, but also opens the way to many physical mishaps before the end comes. The cases I am about to report show how these mishaps may affect the eyes.

I believe it is generally accepted that high arterial pressure is a common cause of renal and arterial degeneration. It has been my observation that in chronic interstitial nephritis, with high blood pressure, where the retina is involved, the reduction of the blood pressure is all important, and that thereby several years can be added to the life of the individual (Cases 11, 12 and 13). Case 11 shows not only how life was prolonged when the patient was on the verge of uremic convulsions, but how useful vision was preserved until her death.

I have been especially impressed with the frequency with which general venous stasis was found present in many cases of degenerative ocular changes (Cases 1, 2, 3, 4, 5, 6, 7 and 9). Several of these patients I never saw again; consequently I am unable to report on the results of treatment, but they serve to show the relationship, as mentioned. If the vascular changes were not instrumental in causation, then the etiology was certainly indeterminable. At our altitude of one mile above sea level we undoubtedly see more cases of heart dilatation and venous stasis than do those living at lower levels. How much greater the relative proportion is I do not know.

It is now a recognized fact that four-fifths of the heart lesions are muscular and that one-fifth are valvular. The influence which impaired circulation, caused from a weakened heart, has on the economy is now being studied extensively. The ophthalmologist is in a position to see some of the very direct results of muscular heart lesions; he should, therefore, be thoroughly alive to the importance of this subject.

Case 1.—*Retinal Hemorrhage, Due to Dilated Heart, General Venous Stasis and Polycythemia.*—Mrs. J. G. M., age 37, Aug. 8, 1907. Has been feeling well physically, with the exception of some shortness of breath on exertion. Two months ago she noticed a blurring of vision in the left eye, which has undergone no improvement.

Status Præsens.—The retina of O. S. is highly engorged. The veins are tortuous and greatly distended. Flame-like hemorrhages are present everywhere along the veins. The nerve head is red, outlines indistinct and somewhat swollen above.

The appearance of the fundus of O. D. is practically normal. The veins are somewhat larger than they should be. O. D. V.= 20/20; O. S. V. = 2/200. She was referred to Dr. E. C. Hill for physical examination, who reports as follows: Pulse, 92, sitting; 110, standing. Heart, one-half inch to left of nipple and one-half inch to right of sternum. Blood pressure, 105; 107 after exertion. Hemoglobin, 95 per cent. Red blood cells, 7,800,000. Urine, 1,027 c.c. in twenty-four hours. With the exception of a slight excess of indican and uric acid it was normal.

Treatment.—Fifteen drops tincture of strophanthus before meals, and 1/30 gr. strychnia after meals. Diet: Not more than two and one-half pints of fluid daily. Meat once daily. No coarse vegetables, such as cabbage, corn, etc. Potatoes and bread restricted. Fruit and green vegetables freely. Generally speaking, her diet is to be very simple and she must eat sparingly. Results two months later: O. S. V. = 20/30. Retinal hemorrhages all absorbed. Veins more normal in size and appearance; nerve head a little muddy. Dr. Hill finds her heart normal in size. Blood pressure, 108. This lady lived in Ohio and was seen by me while on a visit to Denver, consequently our altitude had nothing to do with the production of her venous stasis.

Case 2.—*Optic Neuritis, Associated with Exophthalmic Goiter. Dilated Heart, General Venous Stasis and Autoinfection.*—Mrs. C. H., age 31, November, 1906. History of enlargement of the thyroid gland with some exophthalmic symptoms. The enlargement has about disappeared under electropuncture. Eyes have been paining her for two years. Has had a number of transient blind spells. Vision became permanently affected eight months ago. It has gradually been growing worse. Has not been able to read for three months.

Status Præsens.—O. D. V. = fingers at four feet. O. S. V. = fingers at six inches. Left pupil larger than right, reactions for light and accommodation slow. Fields: Not enough vision to take left field; the right is contracted equally in all directions to the 5 degree line. With the ophthalmoscope, the nerve head of O. D. is swollen 5 D. No retinitis. The left nerve is almost completely atrophic. She was sent to Dr. Hill for physical examination, who reports as follows: Heart dilated to one and one-eighth inches beyond sternum and two inches beyond nipple. Blood pressure, 129. Pulse, 108. Urine, great excess of uric acid and indican. Red blood cells, 4,480,000. Patient disappeared.

Case 3.—*Retinal Hemorrhage, Associated with Polycythemia and Autointoxication.*—Mr. B. D. S., age 44, Aug. 13, 1903. Very full-blooded, florid-looking man, who is apparently somewhat over weight. Claims to have always enjoyed good health. Is a heavy eater, but has no other dissipations. About six weeks ago noticed that vision of O. D. was poor; no improvement since.

Status Præsens.—O. D. V. = 3/40. O. S. V. = 5/6. The entire macular region of the right eye presents the appearance of numerous hemorrhages, with chorioiditis. The veins are very large and tortuous, and the nerve head is red. Sent him to Dr. E. C. Hill for physical examination, who reports that his heart is about normal, but that his red blood cell count is 8,200,000; that he is passing only about one-half the normal amount of urine in twenty-four hours, which contains a considerable excess of indican, and three times the normal amount of earthy phosphates. He advises that he drink twice as much water as he is now drinking, and that his diet be of the simplest form; that it be largely vegetable and that he be allowed only one full meal a day. He was given 10 gr. iodid of potassium, t. i. d., 1/32 gr. biniodid of mercury, t. i. d. In three months time his vision had improved to 5/15. The fundus shows a few scars. No new hemorrhages. I saw him last in February, 1906. He had O. D. V., 20/30. Almost no retinal signs of his former trouble. I had Dr. James Rae Arneill examine him physically for me. He found his blood pressure to be 135; hemoglobin, 105 per cent.; urine normal. A letter received from him a few days ago says the eye still remains well.

Case 4.—*Retinal Hemorrhage, Associated with a Weak Heart and General Venous Stasis.*—Dr. J. M., age 53, Aug. 21, 1907. Has noticed a dimness of vision in lower field of right eye for ten days. He has been actively engaged in country practice for many years. Has no dissipations, unless it be in his eating. He is a hearty, rugged looking man.

Status Præsens.—The upper temporal quadrant of retina of O. D. is covered with flame-shaped hemorrhages. The veins are very full and tortuous. Nerve head congested. He was referred to Dr. E. C. Hill for physical examination, who reports as follows: Blood pressure, 99 sitting, and 107 after exertion; hemoglobin 90 per cent., red blood cell count, 5,350,000; heart is not dilated but degenerated and weak; urine 26 ounces in twenty-four hours; uric acid, one-third above normal daily maximum; no excess of indican.

Diagnosis.—Passive congestion.

Treatment.—Strychnia and hydrastinin hydrochlorid, and correction of his diet. Dec. 24, 1907, he reported that the vision in the lower nasal field is much improved. Is feeling well. Thinks blood pressure is higher than it was.

Case 5.—*Recurring Retinal Hemorrhage, Associated with Dilated Heart, General Venous Stasis and Autointoxication.*—F. S. T., age 26, Sept. 26, 1905. Occupation, farm hand. Has always enjoyed good health. For the last three weeks he has seen a curtain hanging in front of left eye.

Status Præsens.—O. D. V. = 5/5. O. S. V. = 5/27. With the ophthalmoscope a membrane is seen lying in the anterior portion of the vitreous, which is fixed; also large floating pieces of membrane. The appearances are of a previous vitreous hemorrhage which is being absorbed. The fundus can not be seen. Sent him to Dr. E. C. Hill for physical examination, who reports: Blood tension, 165; heart normal; pulse, 88 sitting, 100 standing; hemoglobin, 90 per cent. Urine shows considerable excess of indican, uric acid and earthy phosphates.

It was decided to reduce tension somewhat by the use of a very simple diet, also to correct intestinal fermentation by giving him 10 grains of sulphocarbolate of sodium, t. i. d., and 3 grains of calomel once a week. A month later the vitreous was found almost clear and V. = 5/9. No fundus lesion could be found. He was told to continue treatment for another month and report. He was not seen again for nine months, when he came because of another vitreous hemorrhage, which had occurred six weeks previously. I found his vitreous full of floating membrane, and a retinal spot could dimly be seen below the macula. Dr. Hill went over him again and found his blood tension 115; heart, much dilated; no indicanuria. He was given 10 drops each of tincture of strophanthus and nux vomica, t. i. d.

Two months later Dr. Hill found his heart still somewhat dilated and had him continue the heart tonics. I found a little floating membrane in the vitreous, and that the spot below the macula was becoming atrophic. I did not see him again until two months later, when he came in with a corneal ulcer caused by the diplobacillus, which quickly healed under zinc.

The vitreous is now perfectly clear and O. S. V. is 20/20. There are three spots of atrophic retina to be seen, a small spot just to temporal side of disc, a large one below the macula and a third some distance below the disc.

Four months later he came in saying that the right eye had been blurring for ten days. O. D. V. = 20/70; O. S. V. = 20/20. The vitreous of right eye contained floating membrane and no fundus details could be made out. Dr. Hill found the heart so dilated that the heart border was one and one-quarter inches to the right of the sternum and one-half inch to the left of the nipple in the sixth interspace. Pulse, 92 sitting, 105 standing. Blood pressure, 132; hemoglobin, 100 per cent. Marked indicanuria. In four days the vitreous had so cleared that a retinal spot could be seen on the nasal side of the disc. He was seen again three months later, when vision in each eye was found to be normal. The blood vessels of the retina have not the appearance of sclerosis. Dr. Hill found the blood pressure 145 mm., and heart almost normal in size.

Three months later he had another attack in the left eye. The vitreous was muddy, but there were no large pieces of floating membrane. Dr. Hill found his heart again badly dilated with a blood pressure of 115. This case illustrates the relation in a young man between vitreous hemorrhage and venous stasis, and how between attacks of the latter his vascular condition was comparatively normal.

CASE 6.—*Asthenopia, Associated with Retinal Venous Congestion, Heart Dilatation and General Venous Stasis.*—Mrs. M. A. H., age 35, Jan. 9, 1906. Complained of eyes watering and tiring for near work. Thinks vision is poor.

Status Præsens.—The vision of each eye is 5/7.5, with —.50 cyl., ax. 180°. Both nerve heads are congested, and the medium-sized veins are tortuous. I sent her to Dr. Hill for physical examination, who reports as follows: Amount of urine passed in twenty-four hours is 8 ounces, which contains a trace of albumin. No excess of indican nor uric acid. No casts. Blood pressure, 121. Heart very much dilated and is leaking all around. The right border is one inch to right of sternum. Hemoglobin, 95 per cent. Diagnosis, general venous stasis.

She was referred to her family physician for treatment. Results, unknown.

CASE 7.—*Conjunctival Edema, Associated with Heart Dilatation, General Venous Stasis and Autointoxication.*—Mrs. F. H. B., age 52, February, 1906. Eyes have been inflamed and in about the present condition for three months. Has worn glasses for three years. Has always enjoyed good health.

Status Præsens.—The eyes look very red and watery. The ocular conjunctiva is edematous and rolls up in front of the lid margins when winking. The palpebral conjunctiva does not appear to be affected. Sent her to Dr. Hill for physical examination and for bacteriologic examination of the ocular secretions, who reports as follows: A smear of the ocular secretions shows fatty degeneration of the epithelial cells, some ordinary staphylococci and proteus bacilli, but no diplobacilli. Pulse, 87 sitting, 90 standing. Heart, one and three-eighths inches beyond left nipple and one-half inch to the right of the sternum; the apical sounds were somewhat weak. Blood pressure, 121. Red cells numbered 6,200,000; hemoglobin about 95 per cent.; no excess of leucocytes. The urine shows an excess of uric acid and indican. He believes her eye trouble is partly due to uricacidemia, but mainly to stagnant circulation at this altitude. The treatment prescribed was strophanthus and nux vomica, and a. s. and 6 pills. Jan. 4, 1908, a letter from her stated that her eyes are better.

Case 8.—*Asthenopia, Associated with Heart Dilatation, General Venous Stasis.*—Mr. G. M., age 42, April, 1907. Has been having so much pain in eyes and back of head that he has been compelled to stop work. His refraction was estimated to be + 1.50 W — 50 cyl., in each eye, with 20/20 vision. These glasses were ordered. In the macular region of each eye there were seen shimmering lines and irregular splotches of a yellowish color. The veins were greatly dilated and the arteries small. He obtained no relief from wearing the glasses. He was referred to Dr. E. C. Hill for physical examination, who found: Blood pressure, 111; right side of heart greatly dilated. Hemoglobin over 100 per cent. He was placed on appropriate heart tonics, and in the course of two weeks time his headache was relieved and he was able to return to work.

Case 9.—*Episcleritis, Associated with Dilated Heart, General Venous Stasis and Autointoxication.*—Mrs. R. C. D., age 38, March, 1907. Her left eye has been subject to attacks of inflammation on the temporal side of the cornea. The eye becomes intensely injected over this portion of the globe, and is very tender and painful. The attack subsides in a few days and the eye becomes almost white; another attack follows in about a week or ten days. She was referred to Dr. Hill for physical examination who reports that she has a dilated heart, which is extended three-eighths of an inch to left of nipple and one-half of an inch to the right of the sternum. Pulse, 95 sitting, 106 standing. Blood pressure, 102. The urine shows a large excess of indican and uric acid. She was placed on strophanthus and sulphocarbolate of sodium and simple diet.

Case 10.—*Retinal Hemorrhage, Associated with High Blood Pressure.*—Mrs. Henry W., age 72, Aug. 19, 1907. General habit, plethoric. Has no complaint to make physically. For three months she had had two spots before left eye and has been aware of a gradual failure of vision.

Status Præsens.—O. D. V. = 20/20 W + 2.00. O. S. V. = 20/70 W + 1.75. With ophthalmoscope numerous hemorrhages are seen scattered throughout the retina of left eye. There are no hemorrhages in the right eye, but the blood vessels show strong evidences of sclerosis. She was referred to Dr. F. W. Kenney for physical examination, who reports as follows: Blood pressure, 240; heart normal; no kidney disease. This patient is still under observation. Her blood tension is still high.

CASE 11.—*Neuro-Retinitis, Associated with Chronic Interstitial Nephritis and High Arterial Tension.*—Mrs. M. B., age 45, Jan. 19, 1907. Has been suffering of late with severe diffused pain in head. Eyes so sore she can scarcely move them. Has been aware of a central blind spot in right eye for several days.

Status Præsens.—O. D. V. = 20/40; not improved. O. S. V. = 20/20; not improved. With the ophthalmoscope a typical picture of albuminuric neuroretinitis, with hemorrhage, is seen in each eye. The condition was more advanced in her right eye. She was referred to Dr. E. C. Hill for physical examination, who found she was on the verge of uremic convulsions from chronic interstitial nephritis. Her blood pressure was 240. Active measures were taken to reduce the high blood pressure. When it came down to 200, her headache stopped. It was gradually brought down to 185 and 190. The neuroretinitis gradually improved. In two months time the retinal hemorrhages were all absorbed, but the striæ and spots of retinal degeneration, and the opaque sclerosed blood vessels were more marked than ever. Four months later there was scarcely a trace remaining of the retinal degeneration. Vision was 20/20 in each eye, with full fields. She died just a year after my first examination, and enjoyed a fair degree of comfort with good vision until the end.

CASE 12.—*Neuro-Retinitis, Associated with Chronic Interstitial Nephritis and High Arterial Tension.*—Mrs. J. I. G., age 50, March 27, 1905. Referred to me by an optician to have her eyes examined for glasses. Has little complaint to make about eyes or her physical condition.

Status Præsens.—O. D. V. = 5/9 : 5/6 W + 75. O. S. = 1/200; not improved. With the ophthalmoscope a typical picture of albuminuric neuroretinitis was seen in each eye, which was more advanced in the left eye. Numerous retinal hemorrhages in both. She was referred to Dr. James Rae Arneill for physical examination, who reports that she has a dilated leaking heart, blood tension 260. Urine shows albumin and hyaline casts. I never saw this patient again. She felt well and could not believe that she had chronic Bright's disease. Much could have been done to prolong her life had she been willing to follow directions. As it was, I learned that she died after a few months, and that she became almost blind before her death.

CASE 13.—*Retinal Hemorrhage, Hemorrhagic Glaucoma and Optic Nerve Atrophy, Associated with Chronic Interstitial Nephritis and High Arterial Tension.*—Mr. H. L., age 60, Nov. 16, 1903. Vision has been blurred for ten days. Has always enjoyed good health. Has been a dissipated man as regards alcohol and tobacco. Has not drunk any during recent years.

Status Præsens.—O. D. V. = 5/15. O. S. V. = 5/15. Tn. The field of O. D. is contracted temporally to the 5 degree line, the left is normal. The ophthalmoscope shows marked evidences of sclerosis of the retinal vessels in each eye. The disc of O. D. is cupped. In O. S. the nerve head is congested, the adjacent retina edematous, the veins engorged and tortuous, and numerous retinal hemorrhages occupy the inferior nasal quadrant. He was referred to Dr. Hill for physical examination, who reported as follows: Albumin, 1 2/5 per cent. by volume; hyaline, coarsely granular and disintegrated blood casts. Blood tension, 240. He was placed on a strict diet, and was given 3 grains sodium nitrite, t. i. d., and a pill composed of euonymus, aloes and belladonna.

Jan. 18, 1904.—Great loss of vision. O. D. = Fingers at two feet. O. S. = Hand movements. O. S. was inflamed. T + 1. Vitreous so hazy that fundus could not be seen. Iris sluggish and off color. Dr. Hill found the albumin in urine reduced to 1⅛ per cent. by volume, and his blood tension was 215. The left eye went from bad to worse.

Diagnosis.—Hemorrhagic glaucoma. Enucleation. The vision of his right eye was now so poor that he could not see to get about alone. This was due to a scotoma which encroached on central vision and extended below temporally and nasally, about 20 degrees in each direction. He has been using eserin in oil in this eye, but I can not see that it has been of any service. It is doubtful if there has been, at any time, any increase of tension. For some months this eye remained about the same, and then the central scotoma increased until it occupied the entire temporal field. He has had numerous hemorrhages, but they have not caused hemorrhagic glaucoma as they did with his left eye. I saw him last in July, 1907. He had perception of light only, and numerous retinal hemorrhages were present. Dr. Hill estimated his blood tension several times, and found it to range from 135 to 145. He had a small amount of albumin in his urine. This patient is alive to-day because of the reduction of his blood pressure. His ocular mishaps were most unfortunate, and had he been seen a year or so sooner they might have been prevented.

The above cases serve to show how important are the ocular changes in pointing to the existence of cardiovascular disease. A greater number would needlessly prolong this paper.

MEMORANDA

VOLUNTARY UNILATERAL NYSTAGMUS. WITH REPORT OF A CASE.*

WALTER L. PYLE, A.M., M.D.
PHILADELPHIA.

The case herewith recorded is one of extreme interest, in that it exhibits a combination of the rare anomalies of unilateral and voluntary nystagmus. Either condition alone is sufficiently infrequent to be worthy of extended report.

Patient.—A young woman, aged 22, in excellent physical condition, and of average size and proportions, consulted me for relief from frontal and sick headaches, which had not responded to extensive general medical and neurologic treatment.

Examination.—There was well-marked, chronic catarrhal conjunctivitis in the upper and lower eyelids of both eyes, with a troublesome edema of the left eyelids. There was also complaint of pain in the left eye, particularly in close work. The patient had never worn glasses, and until the last ten or twelve months had experienced no inconvenience in her visual labors. In fact, she had been remarkably free from ocular disturbances. There had never been any association of ocular affection with her headaches. It was only when other means had been exhausted that as a last resort she was advised to apply for ocular examination. Under homatropin cycloplegia, I found a small amount of compound hyperopic astigmatism at horizontal axes, equal in amount in both eyes. Both with and without optical correction, the visual acuity was normal. There was no heterophoria or other disturbance of the ocular musculature. In the course of examination, I noted a sudden unilateral convergence of the left eye, with subsequent rapid oscillation for about 30 seconds. In a few minutes this recurred, which circumstance determined me to make guarded inquiry into the phenomenon. I soon found that the oscillations could be inaugurated voluntarily and as promptly checked. Although the patient disclaimed any knowledge of her ability to effect

* This paper has been accepted by the Executive Committee of the Section on Ophthalmology of the American Medical Association, to be presented before the Section at the Chicago Session, June 2-5, 1908.

these maneuvers, she stated that she had never, for purposes of exhibition or self-experiment, produced the nystagmus. However, she exhibited no surprise at my demonstration of her extraordinary ability in this direction, which would lead to the natural inference that she was fully conscious of her power. Repeated experiments failed to show any such control of the right eye. The family history was good, and there could be obtained no records of any noteworthy ocular affection in two generations, with particular reference to any disturbance of the extraocular muscles. She could not remember any case of strabismus in the family.

Treatment.—The constant use of proper glasses was followed by prompt and complete relief from all the asthenopic reflex symptoms, and when the patient left me, a month later, she was quite satisfied with her ophthalmic experience.

Remarks.—A year later I directed a letter to the address that she had given me, but received no reply, and hence am not able to record the after-history. I am in hopes of discovering her whereabouts, however, and in such case will publish a supplementary note to these observations. During her last visit, at intervals of about 5 minutes, she three times gave a demonstration of her extraordinary faculty and seemed to effect the oscillations with as much ease as before. The only requisite seemed to be the act of convergence, which, however, did not necessarily have to be extreme. The oscillations could be easily produced while the eyes were fixed on type at the ordinary reading distance.

UNILATERAL NYSTAGMUS.

Although unilateral nystagmus is of rare occurrence, a number of cases are recorded in modern ophthalmic literature. Alexander Duane,[1] in a discussion before the New York Academy of Medicine, March 20, 1905, classifies the anomalous types of nystagmus under the following headings:

1. *Disjunctive Nystagmus.*—The two eyes move, not in parallel directions, but alternately and away from each other. The movements are symmetrical and equal in the two eyes.

2. *Dissociated Nystagmus.*—The movements of the two eyes are unsymmetrical and unrelated, one either moving much faster and further than the other, or moving in a totally different way.

3. *Unilateral Nystagmus.*—He regards this as a variety of the second form. He also refers to circumduction nystagmus as an extremely rare form of the affection.

---

1. New York State Jour. of Med., 1905, v. 245.

In common with Neustätter, Schapringer, Spicer and others, Duane believes that most cases of unilateral nystagmus are really of the bilateral type, the movement of the supposedly quiet eye being very minute, and thus escaping detection. In this connection it should be noted that in many instances the lesser forms of nystagmus are not made frankly manifest until an ophthalmoscopic examination is attempted, or the eyes are tested in extreme rotations.

Alfred Graefe[2] mentions a curious case of vertical nystagmus in one eye and horizontal nystagmus in the other, which at first sight might have been considered unilateral or alternating nystagmus. He ingeniously demonstrated the type of movements by the shape of the corneal images of a candle flame—in the horizontal form the image was broadened; in the rotary form, it was enlarged in all directions.

Duane states, however, that he has seen but two undoubted cases of unilateral nystagmus. He also records one case of unilateral rotary nystagmus, in which, however, there later developed bilateral movements. Simon records one case in which at first the nystagmus was unilateral and mixed (vertical and rotary), but subsequently became bilateral and horizontal. It is of interest to note that a nystagmus originally bilateral may become unilateral. According to Schapringer, in spasmus nutans the nystagmus may disappear in one eye only. Again, according to Simon, bilateral nystagmus due to bilateral corneal opacities may disappear from the eye which clears first. He reports two cases in which infantile unilateral nystagmus was caused by unilateral corneal opacities. In the case under discussion, the nystagmus was originally bilateral and disappeared, first in one eye, and then in the other as the respective cornea cleared. It is worthy of mention, however, that nystagmus seldom occurs in cases of unilateral amblyopia, strabismus being the usual consequent disturbance of the musculature. Heimann mentions the occurrence of unilateral nystagmus in an amblyopic strabismic eye; but, according to Duane, such occurrence should be recorded as an acquired optical nystagmus rather than one infantile in origin. According to A. Graefe, in some of the cases of nystagmus, infantile in origin, without demonstrable causative ocular lesion, the oscil-

2. Graefe und Saemisch Handbuch, vi, 1.

lation may be attributed to a congenital retinal hemorrhage, which subsequently cleared.

Cases of unilateral nystagmus have been reported by Neustätter, Schapringer, Krause, Heiman, Spicer, Duane, von Reuss, Eversbusch, Bouchaud, Norrie, R. Sachs, Nagle, Oppenheimer, Weber, Schwarz, Simon, Nettleship, Soelberg Wells, Fuchs, Noyes, and A. Graefe. Of 52 cases collected by Duane, 34 were vertical, 11 horizontal, 5 rotary, and 2 mixed. In none of the cases reported, however, was the condition of voluntary nystagmus mentioned.

Duane points out three varieties of tremor of ocular movements: 1. Searching movements. 2. Pseudonystagmus, or jerking movements, which he says are not infrequently unilateral, particularly if the affected eye has the relatively weaker muscles. 3. True nystagmus, in which the eyes make a series of very regular, short, quick oscillations about a central point.

Unilateral nystagmus, he says, may be associated in early life with spasmus nutans, or unilateral opacity of the media. In later life, it may arise from unilateral amblyopia and unilateral opacity of the media, unilateral astigmatism, and nervous diseases (especially multiple sclerosis). From his observations he deduces that unilateral nystagmus differs in no essential way from bilateral nystagmus, but represents simply a form of the latter.

Nettleship[3] mentions three brothers (children), all of whom exhibited unilateral nystagmus; two were subject to "fits" and were strabismic. He reports another case of unilateral nystagmus in an infant, with rhythmic movements of the head and corresponding arm. He observes that this type of nystagmus, and associated with rhythmic movements of the head and arm, is not exceedingly rare; and also that this association of epileptic convulsions and other important nervous affections is not uncommon.

Zehender[4] also describes the case of a child with unilateral nystagmus.

Related to corneal opacities as a cause of nystagmus may be mentioned astigmatism. Stevens[5] reports five cases of functional nystagmus, or, as he prefers to call

---

3. Royal Ophth. Hosp. Reports, xi, 75.
4. Klin. Monatsblat., 1870, 112.
5. Stevens (G. T.) : The Motor Apparatus of the Eyes, 1906, 439

it, talantropia (an oscillating), in one family; a brother, two sisters and two young cousins (a boy and girl), in all of whom there was a high degree of astigmatism. Although no such case is recorded, it is quite possible for unilateral nystagmus to be associated with high unilateral astigmatism, and I have seen, personally, a nystagmic patient in whom the oscillations in the highly astigmatic eye were much more marked than in its less ametropic fellow.

Bernheimer[6] reports a case of a hypermetropic patient in which nystagmus was produced after prolonged close work, and disappeared after the use of proper correcting lenses. I have seen similar relief follow the full correction of astigmatism in at least a half-dozen such cases. It is my custom in all cases of purely functional nystagmus, and even in cases in which there are pronounced intraocular changes, to prescribe for constant use full correcting lenses, after most careful subjective and objective examination of refractive conditions, when necessary, under complete cycloplegia. Often there follows almost immediate subsidence in the rapidity and extent of the oscillations. Even in cases of nystagmus associated with grave cerebrospinal disease, I believe such procedure advisable, but, of course, with much less hope for noticeable improvement.

VOLUNTARY NYSTAGMUS.

Inasmuch as the term nystagmus signifies an involuntary oscillation of the eyeball, it is perhaps awkward or at least illogical phraseology to speak of voluntary nystagmus. J. W. Smith[7] has suggested as a better name for this condition ophthalmodonesis, which he defines as a voluntary tremulous or oscillating movement of the eyeballs.

Mention of voluntary nystagmus is exceedingly rare in ophthalmic or neurologic literature, and in most of the related text-books little or no mention of this condition is made. Graefe believed that voluntary nystagmus could only occur in persons who were formerly the subjects of an involuntary nystagmus which had disappeared. However, I have been able to find sufficiently accurate and complete reports of cases of pure volun-

6. Bericht über die 29 "Versammlung der Ophthalmologischen Gesellschaft," 1901.

7. Jour. Ophth. Laryngol. and Otolog., N. Y., 1902, xiv, 308.

tary nystagmus by Benson, Lawson, J. W. Smith, W. E. Gamble, Noyes, Williams, Dodd, A. E. Davis, J. E. Colburn, Grimsdale, Ernest Clarke, and Fuchs.

A. H. Benson[8] records a case in a young woman of 24, who could cause oscillation of her eyeballs at will. The motion was very rapid, but the excursions were short. It is noted that the nystagmus was always bilateral and at no time were there involuntary oscillations. The patient was slightly hyperopic. George Lawson[9] mentions having examined a man who all his life had been able to control his eyeballs at will. In this as in the preceding case the motion was so rapid that the margins of the cornea could not be continuously defined. As in the previous case the voluntary nystagmus was always bilateral. Lawson refers to another case observed by him in the person of a former house surgeon of the Royal London Ophthalmologic Hospital. In this instance, the lateral movements were not so rapid and it was necessary for the patient to converge his eyes before the oscillation could be started. The movements were invariably bilateral and under complete volition. In 1882, J. A. Campbell[10] recorded the case of a presbyopic woman who could vibrate both eyes horizontally at will. This seems to be the first American case reported.

Ernest Clarke[11] records an unusual case of nystagmus, which, while not voluntary, is of sufficient interest for mention here. The patient was a youth of 19 who had been apprenticed to a jeweler three years before. While working at his trade, while the eyes were fixed for any object at any distance, the view was cut off from either eye by the interposition of an opaque object, horizontal nystagmus occurred in both, the oscillation being slow and jerky when the right eye was occluded and rapid and more regular when the left eye was blocked. It is also noted that extreme movement in all directions would produce nystagmus. H. B. Grimsdale[12] reported four cases in which occlusion of either eye produced nystagmus, which immediately subsided on the restoration of the binocular vision.

---

8. Royal Lond. Ophth. Hosp. Reports, 1880-1882, x.
9. Royal Lond. Ophth. Hosp. Reports, 1880-1882, x, 203.
10. Trans. Am. Homeo. Ophth. and Otol. Soc., 1882, vi, 70.
11. Trans. Ophth. Soc., U. K., 1895, xvi, 327.
12. Trans. Ophth. Soc., U. K., 1895, xvi, 328.

These cases are analogous to those reported in a paper on "Acquired Nystagmus in Occupations Other Than Coal Mining," by Simeón Snell.[13] This author has written extensively on miners' nystagmus, which he attributes to prolonged natural upward rotation rather than to insufficient illumination. In the paper under discussion he mentions the classical and interesting biographic note of Michael Angelo set forth by Condivi, which was corroborated by Vasari, the contemporaneous biographer of the celebrated decorative painter. It is authoritatively stated that during his lifetime Michael Angelo was so affected by his strained attitude in gazing up at the vaults in the Sistine Chapel, in which for many months he was engaged in the work of decorating with frescoes, that he lost for some time the power to read except when he elevated the paper above his head and raised his eyes. Further, it is stated that Michael Angelo wrote a sonnet describing the constrained attitude in which he was compelled to work and its consequent disagreeable sequels—translation of which has been made by John Addington Symonds. Symonds remarks that the autograph of this manuscript included a humorous little caricature on the margin, showing a man, with protruded stomach and head bent back, using his brush on the surface high above him. He also mentions that as far back as 1874 Nieden recorded a case of acquired nystagmus "in a plank cutter," a workman who, in standing under the tree, observes very exactly a line marked for cutting, while keeping the eyes in a strained condition and upward direction—work very similar to that done by a bottom-sawyer in England. In a letter to Snell, Nieden remarks that, although he has made investigation in many cases of painters and ceiling decorators, he has not been able to find a case of regular nystagmus, although the symptoms of muscular asthenopia were often complained of. In his paper Snell has personally collected 21 cases of acquired nystagmus occurring in different occupations, comprising 6 compositors, 2 metal rollers, a plate layer, a plank cutter, a saw maker, a sanitary tube maker, a fitter and iron founder, a worker in a "cage," 2 employés in a glass factory, a youth engaged in a confectionery warehouse, a man employed at the screens at the surface of a coal mine, a tool sharpener, and a

13. Trans. Ophth. Soc., U. K., xvi.

custodian of a harness room. In all these cases the occupations necessitated unusual strain on the elevator muscles of the eyeballs, causing at first a weariness and later oscillating movements. The nystagmus in these cases, however, was less intense than in the generality of cases met in miners. Snell also refers to the headaches of the visitors of the large art galleries and sightseers in churches and large public buildings, and, although he does not report distinct nystagmus, muscular asthenopia and instability were frequently noted.

In 1896 Gamble[14] reported to the Chicago Ophthalmologic Society a case of voluntary lateral nystagmus in a German-American medical student of 24. While attending high school at about the age of 15, he first discovered that he could produce at will lateral nystagmus, which, however, was never involuntary. No difficulty was ever experienced in starting the oscillations, but they could only be continued for less than a minute. The patient was not able to produce unilateral oscillations. The nystagmus was most pronounced when the eyes were fixed on an object six or eight feet distant, directly in front, but even in making the lateral excursion it could be continued with much less rapidity. Gamble notes that the rapidity of the oscillations were as great as he had ever seen in any case of involuntary nystagmus. It was more pronounced in daylight than under artificial light. The patient had never been ill and did not suffer from headaches or eyestrain, notwithstanding the fact that he had always been a student and teacher. His refraction was:

R. + Sph. 2.00 + Cyl. 0.50, ax. 180° = 20/20.
L. + Sph. 0.25 = 20/20 +.

The media were clear, the fundus healthy, the field of vision full, and the color sense normal. The patient had never worked in the mines nor lived in a mountainous country. He had never had writers' palsy, or other profound nervous manifestation. Gamble states that the one other case similar to his that he had seen reported was that by Noyes,[15] in a patient who had acquired the oscillations after having been confined to his room for several weeks suffering with ocular disease. Noyes remarks that in his experience this case was unique. In his text-book Fuchs mentions rare instances

14. The Jour. A. M. A., 1899, xxxii, 483.
15. Diseases of the Eye, 1890.

of persons who could produce nystagmus voluntarily. Gamble refers to Noyes' case, which he had seen through the courtesy of the elder Williams, of Boston.

H. W. Dodd[16] reports a case of bilateral voluntary nystagmus in a man, an organist, of 23. The patient could produce at will conjugate lateral movements of the eyeballs. When he desired to demonstrate this faculty he would fix his head, look forward, open widely the eyelids, and, as he expressed it, "simply wish" to cause the oscillation. No great effort was entailed and only occasionally was there resultant vertigo or headache. The oscillations could be produced while looking up, down or laterally, either at a distant object or at close range, and also while under the influence of a cycloplegic. The objects looked at moved from right to left, or *vice versa,* and it may be mentioned here that only in voluntary oscillation are subjective disturbances of vision, nausea, vertigo, etc., seen. In all cases of voluntary nystagmus the oscillations can only be continued over a short period, usually in one minute. Dodd's patient possessed the remarkable faculty of being able to converge vigorously, while continuing the oscillations. The power of voluntary nystagmus was first observed at the age of 9. The family history was negative in regard to nervous or mental diseases, and the patient was particularly exempt from any nervous affection. Vision and refraction were practically normal, although there was a patch of chorioretinal degeneration in the right eye, which was of at least eight years' standing.

Possibly the most complete published record of a case of voluntary nystagmus is that by J. W. Smith.[7] The patient was a male student of 21 of French, Huguenot and English parentage. The family history was good, and the only remarkable ocular affection was noted in a sister of 17, who exhibited apparent convergent strabismus of the left eye in near vision, but whose eyes were in normal balance when directed at distant objects. Beyond a slight inflammation of the eyes at the age of 7 or 8, which speedily subsided under the instillation of a common eye lotion, there was no history of ocular disturbance in the patient. There was absolutely volitional rapid oscillations of both eyes simultaneously in

16. Trans. Ophth. Soc., U. K., 1901, xxi, 244.

the lateral direction or in the horizontal plane. The oscillations could be started and stopped at the patient's will. A careful subjective examination of the eyeball showed no marked disturbances of refraction, muscle balance, accommodation, fields of vision, color sense, or visual acuity. Ophthalmoscopic examination was negative. There was no malformation of the globe or orbit. The innervation of both the intrinsic and extrinsic ocular muscles appeared perfect, and the patient experienced no asthenopic symptoms, even after long-continued, close vision. The eyes oscillated only in the horizontal plane, but the motions could be produced not only in the primary position, but in the secondary positions, such as extreme convergence, extreme divergence of either eye, and looking upward and downward. The oscillations could be continued during the entire excursion of the globes (circumduction). Oscillations could be produced when the lids were closed and also when the patient looked through a 20° prism placed before either eye, with its base in any position.

It may be remarked that it is generally accepted that visual sensation influences all the various movements of the eyeball; that is, the efferent motor volitional impulses are originated or are preceded by afferent visual influences. In comment on this statement, J. W. Smith with good reason remarks it is certainly apparent in his case that the patient did not depend on visual sensation for the movements of his eyeballs, for he could produce the movements without looking out or for an object, either real or imaginary, and, indeed, could produce the movements with his eyelids closed, or in the dark, or without fixing the object. Likewise he could produce the movements of his eyeballs whether he fixed on an object at near range or in the distance. This would seem to show the independence or volitional character of the movements, and thus by elimination, "visual sensations may be excluded as a factor or elements in the causation of the ocular movements in this particular case. Again, if this be true, efferent motor volitional impulses are not wholly dependent on those afferent." Smith believes that the oscillations in his case were dependent on efferent impulses affecting the nervous centers in control of the ocular musculature, or, perhaps, the co-ordinating centers in the corpora quadrigemina, in which case he believes that "if they are not due to visual impulses they must be connected with the kinesthetic or psychomotor cerebral cortex."

The longest period during which Smith observed the movements was thirty-five seconds. The patient stated that in producing the nystagmus there was a sensation of slight pressure on each eyeball, pushing or pressing it forward. Ordinarily, during the production of the oscillation, the palpebral fissure was abnormally wide and the upper lids a trifle unsteady, causing noticeable exophthalmos. There was never observed any change in the pupil during the oscillations. Objects viewed while the eyes were vibrating had a simultaneous movement. At distance, objects appeared to be constantly changing their position, and at close range they doubled and blurred. When the patient vibrated his eyeballs and fixed the object, it seemed double and the images appeared to approach and recede. The oscillations could be produced in daylight or in darkness and in the presence of artificial light, with equal energy and rapidity. The amplitude of the vibration was about one millimeter and the rate of motion approximately 5 or 6 vibrations a second.

A noteworthy feature of the case was the ability of the patient to arch the right eyebrow independently of the left, or to arch the right upper brow and draw the left down at the same time. He could also close the left upper lid over the eyeball without wrinkling the forehead or the skin of the eyelids, the upper lid apparently falling gently and smoothly over the globe, while the right eye remained open. The patient could also vibrate the alæ of his nose very rapidly and move either ear. All these movements were executed while under the control of the will. I may here mention that one of the most successful and entertaining tricks of a well-known American comic opera comedian is this power to produce bizarre disassociated movements of the eyebrows. None of his stage play is more convulsively humorous than the contortions of his forehead and eyebrows (exaggerated by his "make up" to accentuate the incongruous upper facial grimaces).

Another popular comedian owes much of his successful fun-making to his ability to move one eye independently of the other. Foster remarks that "very few persons are able by direct effort of the will to move one eye independent of the other, though some, and among them one distinguished both as a physician and oculist, have acquired this power." I have seen this faculty exhibited in the person of a negro lad of about 19, a frequenter of the Dispensary of the Emergency Hospital, Washington, D. C., during my service, 15 years ago, as resident surgeon of that institution.

Dr. George M. Gould, of Philadelphia, and Dr. William L. Phillips, of Buffalo, have described an extraordinary case of voluntary unilateral divergence in a man of 32 (see illustrations). The patient not only had binocular fixation, but also binocular vision, which, however, was markedly decreased in comparison to monocular vision, likely due to persistent non-use of the binocular position. A remarkable feature of this case was the ability to keep both eyes simultaneously in focus while in the strangely dissimilar positions—one eve straight in front, and the other in extreme divergence. While reading a test-card with the fixing left eye the patient promptly recognized facial grimaces made by the examiner standing in such a position that his face could only be seen by the divergent right eye. Immediately the patient said, "I see you! You can't come that on me." Dr. Phillips also describes another similar case in a man of 60. This patient had taught himself to set tvne and read proof at the same time without movement of the head. He had never had noticeable diplopia.

In both of these patients the lateral field of vision, when the eyes were diverged, was 220 degrees. The other points in common in these two cases were: The anomaly had existed since birth. They were able to move their eyes in any direction, having absolute control of their external ocular muscles. They were both myopic and had about the same visual acuity under cycloplegia as with the accommodation active, and whether one or both eyes were used in the visual act. When angry they used binocular vision. They were able to converge and diverge when looking either up or down, to the right or left, showing absolutely no deficient innervation of the musculature. Their retinas showed a similarity to the ungulates, in not having a highly developed area, which would suggest a true macula. Although light perception was more acute centrally, it was, however, quite serviceable in all parts of the retina. If it were possible to secure a careful

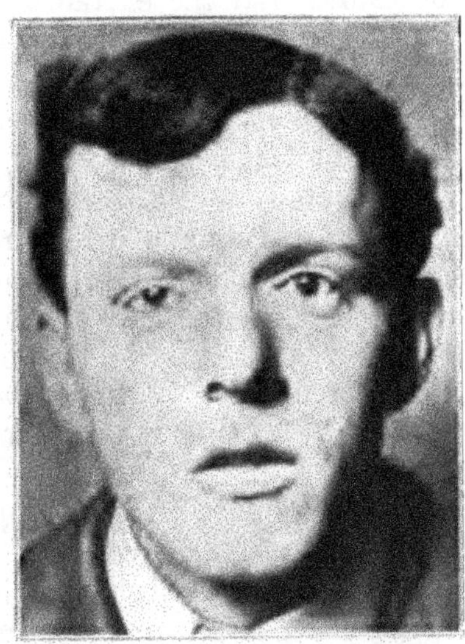

Fig. 1. Eyes in normal position.

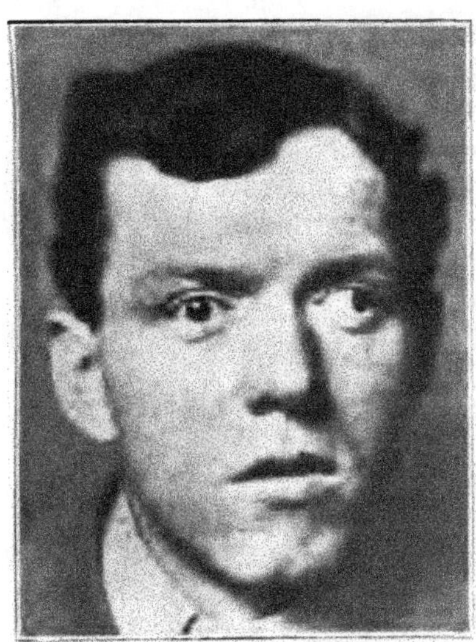

Fig. 2. Divergence of left eye.

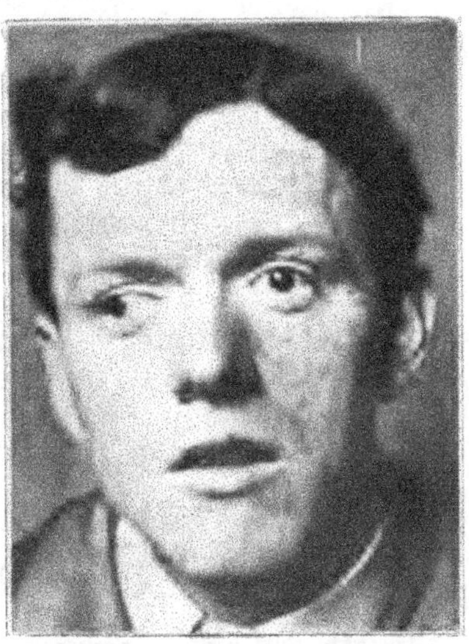

Fig. 3. Divergence of right eye.

GOULD AND PHILLIPS' PATIENT.

pathologic examination of these eyes, Phillips believes that it would be found that the extraordinary ability of ocular rotations was due to absence of a well-defined macula, which fact would afford evidence in support of the opinion that the macula is absolutely necessary only for binocular vision at the near point.

J. E. Colburn, quoted by Smith, reports a case of involuntary movement in one eye in an engraver of 28. He was accustomed to use his loup before the left eye with his tools distributed to his right side. He used his graver with his left hand and could changing the relation of his eye to his work. He had also acquired the habit of fixing with his left eye and rotating his right in any direction required, though not so rapidly and so steadily as when the loup was in position before the left eye. As a result of these curious ocular gymnastics there was produced an attack of cyclitis in the right eye, eight years before, which had recurred three years later, and again in two years. Each attack was more protracted than the preceding. Colburn also mentions the case of a girl, aged 18, who, following an injury to her head in a runaway accident, exhibited rotary nystagmus over which she had perfect control. However, when her attention was not fixed, the oscillations were continuous and considerable.

Such power as the foregoing would indicate inhibition of one eye with volitional innervation of the other, indicating, as Smith sets forth, that the coordinating centers of the two eyes must be influenced along different paths or by different stimuli, or by cortical impulses coming from different areas. He describes a so-called "Z-tract," the fibers of which extend from the neighborhood of the precentral sulcus—the motor area for the eyes—downward between the caudate nucleus and the lenticular nucleus (probably some fibers pass through the corpora striata), thence through the thalamus to the corpora quadrigemina and to the nuclei of the third, fourth and sixth nerves. He notes that nystagmic movements have been produced by passing a probe into the region of the corpora striata and optic thalami. It is remarked that incoordinated movements of the eyeballs are never intimately connected with lesions of the upper and more peripheral parts of the brain. Cerebral hemorrhage involving the basial ganglia often produces conjugate deviation of the head and eyeballs toward the unparalyzed side. Smith also calls attention to the fact that conjugate deviation of the eyeballs occurring as a symptom of cerebral lesion in the region of the basial ganglia is usually indirect and transitory, showing a temporary disturbance only in the tract of fibers connecting the cortex with a center of the brain. The natural conclusion is that in the projection system anatomic examination seems to indicate the connection between the cortical centers of the frontal lobe and with ganglionic centers of the thalamus, and of these with the nuclei of the nerves of the ocular muscles, and later with the coordinating centers.

MEMORANDA

ZONULAR OPACITY OF THE CORNEA.*

F. C. HEATH, M.D.

Professor Clinical Ophthalmology, Indiana Medical College; Secretary Indiana State Medical Association.

INDIANAPOLIS.

Zonular opacity of the cornea is described very briefly in the majority of text-books. Some do not mention it at all, a number dismiss it with a short paragraph, while a very few give it a page.

Nettleship contributed an article of about 25 pages on this subject to the *Archives of Ophthalmology,* in 1879, giving in detail 22 cases seen by various observers. Bock, Graefe, Usher, Best, Leber, and a few others have also investigated the subject quite extensively. The first description was given by Dixon in 1848, followed by Bowman, who went more deeply into the matter. Dixon called it calcareous film of the cornea, finding calcium carbonate and phosphate in the parts removed. Graefe named it band opacity, while Fuchs employs the term given at the heading of this paper. It has been more frequently designated as ribbon-like opacity, or keratitis, and calcareous keratitis.

Zonular opacity occurs in two forms, primary and secondary; the former in eyes otherwise normal, the latter in those blind from glaucoma, iridocyclitis or other intraocular affections. While neither form is common, the primary is much rarer than the secondary form.

It has been described as having the appearance of minute dots crowded together, "punctiform opacities," a gray stripe stretching across the cornea, most marked a little below the center, on the part exposed when the

* This paper has been accepted by the Executive Committee of the Section on Ophthalmology of the American Medical Association, to be presented before the Section at the Chicago Session, June 2-5, 1908. Publication rights reserved by the American Medical Association.

eye is open. The opacity usually begins about the same time at two points near the inner and outer corneal margins, meeting later in the middle line. Some cases have begun centrally. There is always a narrow, transparent zone about the margin.

The progress of the disease is extremely slow, usually continuing for years, although Wells saw one case develop in a few months. Sooner or later both eyes are almost certainly involved, but one may be affected quite a number of years before the other. In some cases there are spells of severe pain, while in others (probably the majority) there is no pain at all. There is no indication of ulceration, the corneal epithelium being smooth and unbroken, in the primary form.

This disease occurs principally in men and after middle age. In 14 cases tabulated by Nettleship, all but 4 patients were over 45 and only one patient was under 30.

The pathology of this affection consists in the deposit of hyaline masses and lime in the upper layers of the cornea, or, as it has been otherwise expressed, "hyaline degeneration of corneal cells that later become calcareous." Bowman's membrane may be the part first affected, and there may be also proliferation of connective tissue.

The etiology is obscure. The location of the trouble in the exposed portions of the cornea has led to belief in a local cause. But if this were true, why is it found in so few persons? Must there not be some predisposing tendency? In gouty subjects, or those with uric-acid diathesis, the nutrient fluid of the cornea, according to Leber, is supposed to be richer in lime salts and these may become deposited by evaporation. Swanzy says that in primary cases the cause of the degeneration is simply loss of vital energy in the cornea from vascular changes, attributed by Nettleship to gout, renal disorders and cardiac affections. Fuchs saw a case in a physician who had blown calomel into his eyes for years, and Toplanski met the disease in hatmakers whose eyes were irritated by flying pieces of hair. Graefe believed that, as the secondary form of this disease followed glaucoma, so the primary form was akin to the glaucomatous process or would eventually go over into glaucoma. As would be expected, these cases are made worse by atropin.

Sight has been restored or improved in some cases by scraping the cornea, the lime deposits coming away in flakes. In other cases iridectomy has proved of great advantage. May advises the use of carbonate of soda after scraping. Sellerbeck advocated the hourly use of 5 per cent. hydrochloric acid, while Nettleship tried nitric acid in one case without effect. Noyes stated that these cases rarely are benefited by any method, and Fox, in his text-book, in 1904, says treatment is of no avail. Guillery, of Cologne, has recently tried ammonium chlorid, beginning with a 2 per cent. solution and gradually increasing to 20 per cent. While his article[1] is headed "Calcareous Opacity of the Cornea," it is evident that he means opacity from lime burns, a very different thing from the subject of this paper.

The following case from my records, the only case of primary zonular or calcareous opacity of the cornea seen in 17 years of eye-work, will serve to illustrate the points of this disease. It is also worth recording on account of its rarity and the gratifying result of operative treatment. Indeed, all cases of such a rare disease, about which there is so little definite knowledge, should be reported fully.

Mr. W. W., born in England; first seen by me Feb. 23, 1897, when he was 34 years old. There was, then, a slight haziness of left cornea to the outer side, and he suffered considerable pain. He was a bricklayer and engaged at this time in the construction of sewers. On the theory that the keratitis might be malarial, he was given quinin, followed by arsenic. (De Schweinitz[2] described a peripheral annular parenchymatous infiltration of the cornea, of malarial origin, separated from the margin by a zone of clear tissue.) Our diagnosis seemed to be confirmed by the fact that the pain soon yielded to the antimalarial treatment. He was seen only a few times in 1897 and 1898, and then passed from observation for a number of years. The opacity evidently increased very slowly in extent and density.

September 1, 1904, he returned, complaining of pain in the right eye, the vision of which was normal, but there was a faint, almost imperceptible, haze near the outer margin and rather low down. The opacity of the left eye was now very dense and covered most of the cornea, being surrounded by a zone or rim of clear tissue, very narrow, and nearly the same width in all parts of the circumference, except the upper

1. Arch. Ophth., Sept., 1907.
2. Philadelphia Polyclinic, 1895.

margin, where it was a little wider. Vision in this eye was reduced to light perception only.

The opacity in the right eye progressed very slowly. Attacks of severe pain occurred at irregular intervals without a particle of redness of the ball. Tension was at all times normal. The pupil was round and responsive to light. He was given quinin and arsenic again, without any apparent effect. Analysis of urine showed no albumin or sugar. He had the appearance of being plethoric, was rather fleshy, with red cheeks. He was not a user of alcohol in any form, but was a great meat eater.

His internal treatment for a long time consisted in the alternate use of salicylate of sodium and iodid of potassium. Pilocarpin and holocain locally, with the addition of dionin a little later, seemed to modify the pain, and after a few months the attacks occurred at longer intervals and then ceased altogether. The dionin had no effect on the opacity. The cessation of pain and the long preservation of good vision led us to believe in the efficacy of the treatment. But it is more than likely that it was simply the naturally slow progress usually seen in such cases. A very weak solution of atropin was tried at the suggestion of one of my colleagues, who, however, advised its discontinuance at the next visit, noting some loss of vision. This accords with Graefe's view that atropin is contraindicated in zonular opacity. (In Nettleship's article mention is made of the use of atropin in several cases with no statement as to its effect further than that the pupils dilated readily.)

My patient was sent to Dr. James M. Ball of St. Louis, with a note asking if this were not a case of zonular or ribbon-shaped opacity, pictured and described on page 335 of his text-book. He replied that it was a typical case, and suggested an iridectomy downward and inward on the left eye. I could not see the advantage of this, as the rim of clear tissue in that direction was so very narrow. It looked to me that an upward iridectomy would be more promising, if any were done, as the rim was wider here than at any other part. But the patient was averse to any operation just then, the vision being still good in the other eye.

The faint opacity seen first in the right eye gradually extended upward and toward the center of the cornea, another band starting a few months later from near the inner margin and extending also toward the center. For a number of months the space directly in front of the pupil was not encroached on. Finally, a very faint haze appeared there, reducing distant vision from 20/20 to 20/40, where it remained for some time, falling to 20/70 for a while and then returning to 20/40. For nearly two years vision was good enough for his regular work as foreman in one of the departments of the Malleable Castings Company. But finally the opacity over the pupillary region deepened and extended a little higher, so that work had to be given up. He could not see enough to go about by himself.

Early in October, 1906, assisted by my colleague, Dr. F. A. Morrison, I proceeded to scrape off a space directly in front of the right pupil, and two weeks later made another scraping. this time assisted by Dr. W. N. Sharp, who examined some of the scrapings under the microscope, finding degenerated cells, probably hyaline, but no lime crystals. This did not flake out, as some have described it. Probably the other eye, in which the disease was more advanced, would have shown this. I regret that we did not try the effect of acids.

The scraping was followed by the use of weak carbonate of soda solution, as suggested by May, but, although we had scraped as much as we dared, there was no improvement of vision. In fact, it wás temporarily made worse.

After the inflammatory reaction had subsided, he was sent to the Indianapolis City Hospital, where I did an upward iridectomy, resulting in 15/40 vision with + 6. sph. = + 2. cyl., axis 180. This enabled him to return to work and earn as much as ever. This vision has been maintained now for more than a year.

About eight months ago he was helping a fellow workman, a sufférer from trachoma, drop medicine into his eye, and accidentally infected his own left eye, fortunately not the one I had operated on. Prompt treatment with strong solutions of silver nitrate at the office, and 1 to 4,000 bichlorid solution at home, controlled this well, and the good eye has never become infected.

It is interesting to note that there has been some improvement in the unoperated eye. At one time light perception alone existed, and in November, 1906, when the other eye was operated on, there was only faint shadowy perception of large objects, not enough to enable him to get about without being led, but the sight of this eye now is 10/200. Is this due to the internal use of salicylates and iodids? Has the local treatment for the trachoma or the irritation of that disease had any tendency to clear it up? Does the operation on one eye have any effect on the other? These questions are easy to ask, but very difficult to answer. I can give no satisfactory explanation. The opacity certainly looks less dense than formerly, especially directly in front of the pupil. In one of the cases given by Nettleship, Mr. Fairlie Clarke, under whose care the patient was, thought the central clear space in front of the pupil due to spontaneous chipping away of the film.

In view of the good result in this case, and in some of the cases reported by Bowman, Walton, Graefe, Nettleship and others, the statements of Noyes and Fox about the uselessness of treatment sound strange. Possibly they had in mind only the secondary form, occurring in eyes already blind, aside from the opacity, and therefore not amenable to treatment.

In conclusion, I would emphasize the interesting features of this case, the comparatively early age at which the affection began, the rather unusual pain in the first stages and the remedies therefor, the improvement in the vision of the unoperated eye, and the gratifying result of the iridectomy in the other. These circumstances, together with the rarity of this form of the disease and the paucity of the literature, seem to justify the detailed report of this interesting case.

427 Newton Claypool Building.

DIFFUSE INTERSTITIAL KERATITIS IN ACQUIRED SYPHILIS.*

A. E. DAVIS, A.M., M.D.

Professor of Diseases of the Eye, New York Postgraduate Medical School and Hospital.

NEW YORK.

Interstitial keratitis, the result of acquired syphilis, is a rare disease, if we are to judge from the number of cases reported in literature, only about one hundred cases having been reported up to date. and judging from the number of cases reported in American literature it is an extremely rare disease, only about a dozen cases having been published.

Members will be surprised to learn that not a single case of this disease due to acquired syphilis has been presented to this section since the foundation of the Association; certainly not since the establishment of THE JOURNAL, in 1883, as I have carefully looked over all the volumes since then for such cases, and have been unable to find any. Furthermore, to emphasize the extreme rarity of the reports of such cases, I may state that, so far as I have been able to ascertain, the volumes of the transactions of the American Ophthalmological Society, published first in 1864 and continuously since then, do not contain the report of a single case presented to the society, and the same is true of Knapp's Archives of Ophthalmology, begun in 1869; the American Journal of Ophthalmology, begun in 1884; Annals of Ophthalmology and Otology (now the Annals of Ophthalmology), begun in 1892, and Ophthalmology, begun in 1906. The Ophthalmic Record, begun in 1891, has the original reports of two well authenticated cases, and

* This paper has been accepted by the Executive Committee of the Section on Ophthalmology of the American Medical Association, to be presented before the Section at the Chicago Session, June 2-5, 1908.

of one doubtful case. Ellett,[1] Marlow,[2] and Hildrup,[3] report these cases.

I have not taken into consideration the annular or disciform varieties of keratitis or other unusual forms of interstitial keratitis, confining myself strictly to the diffuse interstitial keratitis, as is so commonly seen in cases of inherited syphilis. The small number of published cases is remarkable when we remember that these are the leading ophthalmic journals in America, and also the great length of time covered by them. Not only is there a lack of original cases reported in these journals, but, as would be expected under the circumstances, very rarely indeed is there an abstract of such cases from foreign literature. Why wonder, then, that some leading oculists doubt the existence of the disease at all from acquired syphilis.

When I presented my first case to the New York Ophthalmological Society, December, 1907, one of the oldest members of the Society, the late Dr. D. B. St. John Roosa, said he had never seen a single clear case of interstitial keratitis from acquired syphilis in his long practice of forty-eight years, either private or hospital; and in a personal letter to me subsequently, in support of his contention, he cited Hutchinson's classical Memoir,[4] as follows: "Although I will not make so sweeping an assertion that interstitial keratitis never occurs excepting in the subjects of inherited taint, yet I can not conceal from myself, and have no wish to do so from my reader, that such is my present belief. It seems, moreover, improbable that a peculiar disease, remarkably well separated from all its congeners, both by its symptoms and its progress, should acknowledge a specific cause in nineteen instances, and in the twentieth present precisely the same phenomena in total independence of such origin. It is only fair, in passing, to ask of those who are inclined to test the accuracy of this opinion that care be taken in the diagnosis."

In looking over the literature on the subject, however, I find that Hutchinson had occasion to change his mind later. In his retiring address[5] from the presidency of the Ophthalmological Society of the United

1. Ophth. Rec., ix, 283.
2. Id., xiii, 113.
3. Id., xiv, 214.
4. Ophth. Hosp. Rep., 1858, i, 231.
5. Tr. Ophth. Soc. U. Kingdom, 1886, vi, 517.

Kingdom, in commenting on a case of interstitial keratitis in acquired syphilis published by Mr. Morton,[6] he says: "So far as I know that case remains practically unique. I have seen a few doubtful and ill-marked parallels, but never one that could be properly placed by its side. Why keratitis should be so common in inherited syphilis, and so rare in the acquired disease is one of the pathological enigmas for which as yet we have no answer. Mr. Morton's case was not sent specially for his delectation; there are others like it if we could but find them, and to find them we want the help of the army of trained specialists now associated in this Society. Our volumes contain, so far as I know, no reference whatever to the occurrence of keratitis in acquired syphilis."

How near these words (spoken twenty-two years ago) come to describing accurately the condition now existing in American ophthalmic literature, is apparent from my opening remarks. Yet, we all know that interstitial keratitis from acquired syphilis is not extremely rare. If we would but look for such cases and report them, I am sure that many could be placed on record, and that is one of the obects of this paper, to direct attention to the importance of publishing such cases.

Callan, of New York, has reported several such cases verbally, although not publishing a single one. Several members of the New York Ophthalmological Society, in discussing the case shown by me, said they had seen anywhere from one to seven such cases in their own experience, yet not a single case have they thought worth while to report. Most of the present-day ophthalmic text-books (there are a few exceptions) speak of acquired syphilis as a cause of interstitial keratitis, but report no cases that I have been able to find. If I have overlooked cases, as undoubtedly I have, in my limited time to look up the literature on the subject, I trust that my confreres will be good enough to cite any they may know of. It is high time for some one to call attention to these hitherto neglected cases, and to urge the publication of the same, at least in sufficient numbers to remove doubt of the existence of such cases. I beg, therefore, to report two cases—the only two well-authenticated ones seen in my practice of sixteen years. Both

6. Moorfield's Hosp. Jour., 1874.

of these cases were seen this winter, one, in fact, while engaged in writing this paper.

CASE 1.—*History.*—Mr. C. M. M., aged 27 years. This patient came to me Oct. 5, 1907, because of pain and failure of hearing in the right ear. He gave a history of having the drum punctured six months previously because of an acute abscess.

Examination.—I found the drum membrane somewhat congested, shrunken, and a scar in the lower and posterior quadrant. Hearing had been reduced to 7/40. Bone conduction was normal; hearing in the left ear normal, 40/40; bone conduction and air conduction normal. There was a chronic laryngitis. By inflating the ear and treating the throat, the pain in the ear was completely relieved in a few days. On November 30, about two months after consulting me concerning his ear, he consulted me because of an acute inflammation in each eye, more pronounced in the left. At this time he admitted the history of syphilis of one year's duration, and a report from his family doctor who treated him from the beginning confirms this. The patient had a primary chancre followed by secondary eruptions and sore throat; in fact, was under treatment by his family physician when he first came to me, but of which he made no mention.

Present Condition.—There are absolutely no indications of inherited syphilis at all. The teeth are perfect and there are no scars about the mouth or other marks of congenital syphilis of any kind. The man is robust in appearance.

Local Condition of Eyes.—For the last two weeks the patient has complained that the eyeballs have gotten red at night, burned, and that the light hurt him very much; tears also ran from the eyes. At the present time both eyes are inflamed, there is a marked circumcorneal injection in the left eye, and almost the entire cornea is covered with a grayish haze of a typical ground-glass appearance, and deep in the corneal surface can be seen a number of punctate spots, together with a few fine blood vessels. The right eye is affected very much in the same way as the left, but to a lesser extent. Vision in the right eye has been reduced to 20/30 and in the left eye to 20/50, although his vision, he tells me, has been absolutely perfect before the present attack.

Treatment.—The patient was placed on atropin and hot water, locally, and the mixed treatment was pushed to the full limit. With the pupils well dilated under atropin, there were distinct changes in the chorioid to be observed far forward in each eye, and especially well marked in the left eye. After a few weeks' treatment the inflammation subsided rather rapidly, until the ground-glass appearance has almost disappeared.

March 7, 1908: The right eye is completely well, except for a slight circumcorneal injection; no infiltration of the cornea and no punctate spots remain. In the left eye all the gray haze has disappeared, together with most of the blood vessels, and but one very small punctate spot can be seen under the magnifying glass, and here and there a very fine blood vessel. The vision in the right eye was brought up to 20/20, and in the left eye to 20/40. There remains some congestion in the fundus of the left eye, and a few fine granular shreds floating in the vitreous.

CASE 2.—*History.*—Mr. G. B., aged 35 years. The patient consulted me first March 11, 1908 (consequently I have had him under observation about one week), with a history of his left eye being sore for the last two months, sensitive to light, running tears, and with rapid failure of vision in that eye. His family history is absolutely negative, in so far as can be obtained by me and by his family physician, the family physician assuring me there is no trace of syphilitic taint to be found in his family on either side. He is a married man and has a family. The first child died at the age of 8 months, the second child at the age of 6 months, the next two were miscarriages, and since then his wife has given birth to four healthy children, all now living.

He gives a history of a hard sore occurring on the penis three years ago. It was about two months in healing, but he denies any chance of infection except from his wife. Although there is this distinct history of the hard sore, there have been but few secondary symptoms. At the present time there is a slight enlargement of the glands in the neck and in the inguinal region. The man is robust in build, being about 5 feet 10 inches in height, and weighs about 190 pounds. He has absolutely none of the marks of congenital syphilis anywhere, and apparently is in perfect health.

Local Condition of the Eye.—The upper one-sixth of the left cornea is covered with the most pronounced salmon-patch I have ever seen; so deep, in fact, that it is almost liver-colored in appearance, while the rest of the cornea is completely covered with an intense grayish infiltrate. There is a slight circumcorneal injection, a very deep anterior chamber, and vision is reduced to counting fingers at six inches. It is as typical a case of diffuse interstitial keratitis as I have ever seen. The right eye is not affected; the vision is 20/40 without correction; the fundus appears to be normal. The fundus of the left eye could not be seen, because of the intense infiltration of the cornea. The patient gives a history of no other disease that would be likely to cause the present condition. There is no history of rheumatism, influenza, malaria, gout, etc. There is no previous history of an eye affection of any kind.

Wandel,[7] who gives Fournier the credit of reporting the first case of this nature, reports a case himself and reviews the literature of forty-five cases.

It is rare, indeed, in these cases to have the "salmon-patch." In fact, Trousseau says,[8] that the salmon-patch never appears in these cases, and Mr. G. Anderson Critchett[9] said he had never been able to persuade himself that there was a true salmon-patch in the cases observed by him. In the case reported by Marlow,[2] the appearance of the cornea was very much like that presented in my second case, and I venture to give, very briefly, the case as reported by him.

A woman, aged about 30, was brought to him with a chancre of the conjunctiva in the lower retrotarsal fold of the right eye, with the preauricular and submaxillary glands enlarged on that side. He prescribed antispecific treatment, and did not see the patient again for ten years, when she presented herself with a typical interstitial keratitis in the right eye, the whole cornea being occupied by a diffuse patch of haze, while the upper part, perhaps 1/5, was covered by the characteristic salmon-patch of Hutchinson. The left eye was unaffected. The scar of the chancre was plainly visible at this time. She was not seen again.

Lange[10] also has reported a case of interstitial keratitis following a primary sore of the ocular conjunctiva.

Another very well authenticated case of interstitial keratitis, with the distinct salmon-patch, due to acquired syphilis, is reported by J. B. Lawford,[11] with four others, two of which were of doubtful authenticity. The particular one to which I refer is as follows:

Woman, aged 39 years. Her right eye was affected by diffuse interstitial keratitis. In the upper part the cornea was vascular and gray, and at the extreme upper edge was a very distinct salmon-patch. The pupil was active and dilated circularly under atropin. In the left eye nothing abnormal was found. There was no history of a previous eye affection. History as to syphilis was uncommonly definite. Thirteen years before she had prolonged affection of the throat, a skin eruption and loss of hair, and one year previous to coming under observation she had perforation of the hard palate. She brought to the hospital her young daugter, Violet H., aged 8, suffering from typical interstitial keratitis in both eyes. Her

---

7. Wchnschr. f. Therap. u. Hyg. des Auges, December, 1903.
8. Ann. d'Ocul., 1895.
9. Tr. Ophth. Soc. U. Kingdom, 1900, xx, 67.
10. Tr. Ophth. Soc. U. Kingdom, 1892, xii, 74.
11. Tr. Ophth. Soc. U. Kingdom, 1900, xx, 67.

first child was living, aged 18. Five subsequent pregnancies resulted in stillbirths; then the daughter, Violet, and there are three younger children.

The patient was under observation four months, treatment being iodids and atropin. She was greatly improved. Mr. J. H. Herbert Fischer furnished the notes of this case for Mr. Lawford.

Mr. George Anderson Critchett, in discussing the case presented by Mr. Lawford, said he was glad to hear that a distinct salmon-patch had been met with in one case; that he had never been able to persuade himself that there was a true salmon-patch in any of his cases, though there was generally vascularity, but the opacity in the cases he had seen had not, as a rule, been so deep, so interstitial as in inherited cases. Mr. Griffith, in discussing the paper, mentioned the fact that Mr. Hutchinson had reported a case as a secondary manifestation in syphilis. He himself had seen four cases; in one of these the sight was lost—only the perception of light remaining, although he had given a favorable prognosis.

This point in regard to the loss of sight should be borne in mind by oculists in giving a favorable prognosis in these cases, although in most cases due to acquired syphilis the disease runs a much lighter and quicker course than in those of inherited syphilis.

Another interesting question has been brought up in connection with these cases, and that is whether it is possible for a man inheriting syphilis to acquire syphilis primarily himself, and the disease (interstitial keratitis) in this way be due to the inherited rather than the acquired taint. In this connection Fritz Mendel[12] reports the case of a young man whose mother was syphilitic, and who had suffered from this hereditary taint in the first year of his life, but acquired syphilis at the age of twenty-one, and had both eyes affected at this later date with a typical diffuse keratitis, which cleared up under free inunctions of mercury.

Mr. J. Herbert Fischer,[13] in a recent paper on some cases of interstitial keratitis from acquired syphilis, reports a number of cases. He expresses the opinion that interstitial keratitis from acquired syphilis is generally a tertiary manifestation; that it seems usually to attack

---

12. Centrlbl. f. Prakt. Augenh., January, 1901; Med. Press and Circ., December, 1907.

13. Ophth. Soc. U. Kingdom, November, 1907; also Ophth. Rec. (London), Jan., 1908.

only one eye, and that the infiltration frequently limits itself to a portion of the cornea only; that the keratitis, as far as it goes, is identical in clinical appearances to that due to the inherited disease, and that the statement made by Nuel, that it was usually secondary to irido-chorioiditis, was by no means accepted universally. He also expressed surprise that more cases had not been reported. Mr. Sidney Stephenson, in discussing the paper, stated that about one hundred cases had been reported in literature, and that the average time of the development of interstitial keratitis after the primary affection was 10.8 years. He also thought that the unilateral location of the affection was due to treatment and that the bilateral cases occurred in the untreated cases. In a very recent communication, Mr. Stephenson,[14] states that nearly every case of interstitial keratitis is secondary to disease in the anterior part of the uveal tract. This opinion coincides with Nuel's.

It is interesting to note that this disease has been produced experimentally in the lower animals—rabbits, monkeys, etc.—by scrapings from lesions, chancres of the human being, and that the spirochetes had been found in such lesions. Mr. Sidney Stephenson also mentioned the fact that he and other observers, Stock, Peters Römer and Babb, had found the spirochetes in congenital syphilis of the eye.

PATHOLOGY.

As to the pathology of the disease I shall say but little, except to quote briefly Mr. J. Herbert Parsons.[15] He says: "The cases of true interstitial keratitis, in the restricted clinical sense, which have been examined microscopically, are very few and are mostly complicated by other conditions which make it difficult to determine the anatomy of the disease. Even amongst the cases examined, a large proportion of those described as parenchymatous keratitis were undoubtedly tubercular. This raises the question of the true etiology of the disease. In England we are accustomed to lay the typical condition to syphilitic origin, and no satisfactory proof has been brought forward that this view is incorrect. . . . There is a difference of opinion as to the cases of true interstitial keratitis; V. Michel

14. Tr. Ophth. Soc. U. Kingdom, May 25, 1907.
15. The Pathology of the Eye, 1, 1, 191.

and others distinguishing between a primary and a secondary keratitis. In the former, a triangular opacity appears at the margin of the cornea and gradually spreads over the whole area; it is often followed by iritis, keratitis, punctata, etc., and is ascribed by V. Michel to syphilitic affection of the marginal loops of the blood vessels. The secondary form is distinguished by marked inflammation of the uveal tract, and often of the sclerotic, more particularly in the anterior part of the eye."

According to Stephenson, the cause of the keratitis is the deposit and multiplication in the cornea of the *Treponema pallidum,* which comes from the uveal tract.

DIFFERENTIAL DIAGNOSIS.

At times it is extremely difficult to say what is the true cause of diffuse interstitial keratitis. The tuberculous and the syphilitic forms are so nearly alike clinically that it is often impossible to distinguish between the two, and even difficult to arrive at a conclusive differentiation by microscopic examination. Bull[16] has classified the syphilitic affections of the cornea, due to acquired syphilis, into the following four classes:

(1) Diffuse parenchymatous, or interstitial keratitis.

(2) True keratitis punctata, of Mauthner; which is exactly the same as Hock's specific punctate keratitis.

(3) Keratitis punctata, with general clouding of the cornea.

(4) Gummatous keratitis.

It is well to bear in mind this classification, as it will be of service in arriving at a diagnosis and in classifying the cases.

Von Hippel, Jr.,[17] says: "The question as to whether there are certain subjective symptoms of the eye diseases that would prove the syphilitic or tuberculous character, has to be answered in the negative. The limited vessels in the deeper strata of the cornea and the chorioid, chorioiditic changes considered by Hirschberg as characteristic of lues, are also found in the tuberculous form."

It is evident, therefore, that we must depend chiefly

---

16. A System of Genito-Urinary Diseases, Syphilology and Dermatology, Prince Morrow, vol. ii, p. 550.
17. Twenty-fourth Rep. Ophth. Cong., Heidelberg, Aug. 18, 1895.

on the clinical history of the case and the symptoms found when the patient presents himself and the effect of treatment on such symptoms, to arrive at a diagnosis, as it is seldom, indeed, that an opportunity is presented for a microscopic examination on such cases. I would suggest that Calmette's test might be of service in clearing up the diagnosis in these cases.

CONCLUSIONS.

1. Diffuse interstitial keratitis may occur as a result of acquired syphilis.

2. It usually occurs as a late secondary sign of the disease or during relapses in the tertiary stage of the general disease. Stephenson gives the average time of development of interstitial keratitis as 10.8 years after the primary sore. Loewinson[18] has reported one case as early as three weeks after the appearance of a primary sore, while Ellett reports a case appearing as late as twenty-three years after the infection.

3. It almost invariably affects but one eye, although there are a few exceptions reported where both eyes were affected.

4. It runs a quicker and lighter course, as a rule, than the cases due to inherited syphilis, and is rarely harmful to the sight. It should be remembered, however, that Griffith has reported one case in which the sight was entirely lost.

5. True "salmon-patches" occur but seldom in these cases.

6. It is difficult to make a clinical diagnosis between the syphilitic and the tuberculous forms of the disease, and even a differential pathologic diagnosis is not always conclusive.

7. The prognosis is favorable, though it should be somewhat guarded from the fact that sight has been lost entirely in one case.

---

18. Loewinson.

OPACIFICATION OF THE CORNEA FOLLOWING CATARACT EXTRACTION.*

VARD H. HULEN, A.M., M.D.

SAN FRANCISCO.

The following case is the only one I have seen among 209 cataract operations, and seems worth placing on record:

History.—D. D., male, aged 81 years, retired furrier, native of England, entered the University of California Hospital Aug. 23, 1907, to be operated on for hemorrhoids. He was recovering from a carbuncle and lumbago. The medical report of his physical examination gives the heart action as being intermittent and irregular, with systolic and diastolic murmurs; the result of the blood examination was not significant. Senile breathing; lungs negative; urine gave trace of albumin; yet all his life he had been considered a very well man. The recovery from the general anesthetic and operation was prompt and uneventful.

Examination.—The patient being practically blind, I examined his eyes September 6. An interesting ocular condition was found with an uncertain history. He stated that for three months after birth his eyes did not open, also that he had a congenital cataract in the left eye. (If the former were due to ophthalmia neonatorum the latter was probably an anterior polar cataract.) The vision of the right eye was good for all purposes until he was 45 years old, when, after a fall on his head, glasses for reading became necessary. Attention was not attracted to his eyes again until 1893, when he had an attack of pain in the right eye, accompanied by failing vision. But even before this he thinks his sight was not perfect. Two years later the vision had gradually failed until reading was no longer possible. About this time a competent oculist told him that there was a chalky degeneration of the left lens which irritated the right eye somewhat and advised extraction of the lens. Vision of the left eye had never changed.

* This paper has been accepted by the Executive Committee of the Section on Ophthalmology of the American Medical Association, to be presented before the Section at the Chicago Session, June 2-5, 1908. Publication rights reserved by the American Medical Association.

Ten years ago an ophthalmic surgeon of national reputation operated on his left eye. A preliminary iridectomy was done, later the cataract was extracted without accident. Neither pain nor inflammation attended, but there was a turning in of the lashes. No vision was given by the operation.

Inspection revealed a spastic entropion of the right lower lid which was successfully controlled by repeated applications of collodion. For some conjunctival irritation due to the entropion a boric acid wash and the occasional use of argyrol were advised. Patient's general condition steadily improved. On September 20 he was transferred to my service in the hospital, and the following notes were made:

Status Præsens.—Left eye: Cornea rather thinly but entirely opaque, with patches of greater density, while the site of the corneal section, two millimeters from the limbus, is solidly white. The opacity appears to be in the stroma, but the epithelial covering is very irregular and steamy. The key-hole pupil is faintly visible. Tension normal; vision equals movement of hand in all directions. Right eye: Cornea clear and slightly anesthetic. Lens appears a dark amber color. The ophthalmoscope shows red reflex around the periphery of cataract when pupil is dilated. Tension normal. Vision equals perception of light; projection good.

Treatment.—I advised extraction of the cataract and performed the preliminary iridectomy on this date. Atropin instilled, bandage applied, rest in bed. No reaction whatever followed the operation, blood remaining in the anterior chamber after the cut of the iris promptly disappeared. Healing was normal and rapid. Pupil widely dilated; cornea perfectly clear; patient discharged.

October 17 he re-entered the hospital and was given the usual preparation. General condition and spirits decidedly improved. The right eye differed apparently in no wise from a normal cataractous one after an iridectomy, but owing to the history of the fellow eye unusual precautions were taken. October 18 operation was done with the patient in bed. A 4 per cent. solution of cocain was instilled three times, at intervals of five minutes. Section of two-fifths of limbus, raising small conjunctival flap above, from which was slight hemorrhage. Peripheric capsulotomy done with sharp cystotome; when the capsule was opened a small amount of clear fluid escaped. Speculum removed and the cataract, about two-thirds the size of an average lens, was expressed easily with the fingers. As a few flakes of soft lens matter remained in the pupil, the anterior chamber was gently irrigated with a special glass nozzle pipette, using a small quantity of a warm sterile physiologic salt solution. No further manipulation was required; there was no loss of vitreous or other mishap and even less than the usual traumatism. The patient behaved well and experienced no sensation during the operation. Atropin was instilled and a gauze bandage lightly applied over both eyes. Before closing the eye operated on, attention was called to the fact that the lips of the entire corneal wound were whitish.

After the lapse of twenty-four hours the eye was inspected though the patient had no discomfort. The wound was closed; anterior chamber fully restored; thickened capsule in pupil which is widely dilated, edges of coloboma free, but the entire upper half of the cornea was affected by the appearance of a well-marked typical "striped keratitis;" otherwise no evidences of reaction. At the end of the second day the striated appearance had extended the full width vertically across the cornea. Anterior chamber very deep; tension, —1. There were no subjective symptoms; no ciliary and but slight conjunctival injection; the wound was firmly closed. The bandage was left off and a light dressing was held in place by strips of silk plaster.

October 21, in addition to the striated opacities, the cornea was thinly and diffusely opaque, apparently due to changes deep in the substantia propria or endothelium. Pupil not distinctly seen, but was widely and evenly dilated.

October 27, the eye had remained entirely free from inflammatory reaction and the patient complained only of his lumbago. The general diffuse opacity had gradually increased, but was conspicuous only by focal illumination. The striated opacities seemed less marked and were broken so that a dark branching line about one millimeter wide appeared in the shape of a "Y," with the arms above extending to the extremities of the site of the corneal section and the thinner body reaching below within three millimeters of the limbus. Close inspection with oblique illumination revealed that the dark line did not mean entire transparency. The epithelium was undisturbed; the corneal surface was smooth and glistening. Tension normal; no subjective symptoms. Dionin and hot fomentations were commenced. General condition satisfactory.

November 2, as the eye seemed entirely well but for the corneal opacity, the patient was allowed to leave the hospital, with instructions to continue the dionin and hot applications, and to use atropin to keep the pupil dilated. He has been seen at intervals since, and at the last visit, March 8, the eye remained much the same. The striated opacities were still distinct and crossed irregularly by fine opaque lines, the "Y" appearance being but faintly defined. The deeper and diffuse opacification was less dense to the temporal side. The cornea was very slightly steamy. Vision 2/200. No change in tension, and had it not been for the corneal opacities the healing process could have been recorded as uneventful. Patient's health continued fair, appetite and nutrition good, but stayed in bed a great deal because of "misery in his back."

It is generally known that the use of a solution of bichlorid of mercury for irrigating the anterior chamber, as well as various accidents and complications, may be followed by corneal changes, nor would opacification be unexpected in a patient whose general condition and nutrition were undoubtedly bad. But in my case none of these elements entered into the causation, so far as can be determined. As it was impossible to obtain details from the first operator, I had thought it not unlikely that the opacification had been due to bichlorid, as that antiseptic was being used extensively about this period. Also there might have been some connection between the presence of the opacification and the section having been made far into the corneal tissue. And at this time, ten years before my operation, the patient's health was most excellent.

Had the cornea shown the slightest haziness following the preliminary iridectomy I should not have proceeded to extraction.

In the literature at my command only one or two text-books of ophthalmology mention general opacification following uncomplicated cataract extraction, and attribute it to the use of corrosive sublimate solution. So it seemed worth while to call attention to the subject. Hoping to make my paper of some value, the following questions were addressed to every member of the Section on Ophthalmology of the American Medical Association:

1. Have you had cases of general opacification of the cornea following cataract extraction; if so, how many (or if none) in what number of cataract operations?

2. To what cause or causes do you attribute its occurrence?

3. What appearance or forms did the opacity assume?

4. What part of the cornea seemed to be the seat of the lesion, and what the pathologic change?

5. To what extent did the opacity disappear, and how long before corneal changes ceased?

6. Kindly give separately the ultimate corrected vision in each case.

7. What preventive measures and curative treatment have you found of value?

8. What percentage of your cataract extractions has been followed by "striped keratitis"?

9. Have you ever seen striped keratitis fail to clear up so that the ultimate vision was affected by it; if so, what percentage did not clear completely?

10. Does your experience touch on any notable point outside your answers to the above questions?

To search case records for absolutely accurate replies was a task too laborious to be expected from any one, but I had hoped for a large number of approximate estimates of cataract extractions. This, with the data on corneal opacifications, should throw some light on an apparently obscure subject. However, I can not sufficiently express my appreciation for the generous and courteous responses made and regret that the limited space prevents my using more extensively the very valuable material gathered.

Out of the 227 heard from at this writing, 87 gave either the precise or estimated number of extractions, amounting to 19,821. From the figures given a conservative estimate of extractions by my correspondents would not be less than 50,000, and among these are only 39 cases of general opacification.

Concerning striated keratitis, there were great variations in statements. Sixteen correspondents reporting the exact number of cataract operations (the largest 397) aggregating 1,248 cases, had never seen this condition, while others gave large estimates, ranging from 50 to 100 per cent., depending, one says, on how closely we observe the condition of the cornea. The average of all answers is about 11 per cent. In my limited experience it has been about 3 per cent. and has always disappeared. Eleven reported cases of striped keratitis that affected the ultimate vision. One colleague wrote "Ribbon keratitis (Elschnig) or zonular keratitis (Salzmann) always heralds general bulbar degenerations," but I had reference to that well-known clinical appearance, commonly noted in case histories in a routine way by "striped keratitis present."

About 45 cases were reported as general opacification, but closer review determined that the process did not involve the entire area of the cornea. Distinct causes enumerated in all of these histories were identical with many of the known causes for the cases of complete opacifications. The pathologic conditions were probably similar, differing only in degree. One operator leaves the bandage on his myopic subjects twice the usual time. Another had frequently seen striped keratitis until he adopted the "open method" of treatment, but none since. Another of large experience states that since he had abandoned attempts at artificial ripening he had not seen a case of striped keratitis. And another advised, in cases of marked arteriosclerosis, to make the section in the limbus with a large conjunctival flap. Two interesting cases of partial opacification have been reported by Dr. Harold Bruns and one by Dr. H. Gradle.[1]

Following is a synopsis of the 39 cases reported of general (complete) opacification of the cornea.

Case 1.—Doubtful cause, syphilis. Specific treatment did no good.

Case 2.—Operations, 75. Causes given, senility and poor nutrition, blood count low. Ultimate vision, 5/200.

Case 3.—Operations, 150. Bichlorid getting into anterior chamber. Cleared up under atropin and alteratives. Vision, 15/50.

Case 4.—Alcoholism and debility. Cleared up about one-half.

Case 5.—Accidentally irrigated anterior chamber with bichlorid for saline solution. Ultimate vision, moving objects.

Case 6.—Operations, 100. "Infection," no treatment; cleared; vision, 20/50.

Case 7.—Cause doubtful unless incision too far in cornea. Vision, fingers 4 feet.

Case 8.—Operations, 21. Dislocated lens; general debility. Vision, fingers 2 feet.

Case 9.—Operations, 50. Section with poor knife. Corneal changes very similar to my case. Vision, fingers at one meter.

Case 10.—Caused by infection more than a week after operation. Leucocytic infiltration of substantia propria. Opacities permanent.

Case 11.—No cause. Partly cleared, dionin. Vision, 20/120 after five months.

Case 12.—In another's practice, due to bichlorid solution.

Case 13.—Operations, 200. Much lens matter left in anterior chamber produced irritation. Slight opacity only after three months. No treatment.

Case 14.—Operations, 100. Traumatism and possibly syphilis. Vision P. L.

Case 15.—Continued hemorrhage from "abnormal retinal vessel."

Cases 16 and 17.—Operations, 80 to 100. Caused by irrigation of anterior chamber (with what not stated), both cleared completely in two weeks, hot applications, atropin and dionin.

Case 18.—Operator of large experience. Patient in good health, aged 58 years. Perfectly smooth operation, simple extraction, no rational cause discovered. Rapid opacification of

1. Ophth. Rec., 1905.

entire cornea, apparently in parenchyma. Under long continued subconjunctival injections it cleared up in a measure, but no useful vision was obtained.

Cases 19, 20, 21 and 22.—Operations, 1,000. La grippe, followed on second day after operation. Very feeble patient. No cause known. Debility.

Case 23.—Operations, 20. Senile debility, age 83 years.

Case 24.—Operations, 400. Caused by using strong solution (4 per cent.) holocain in place of a 1 per cent. solution. Disappeared in four months. Used hot applications, atropin and dionin ointment, 5 to 10 per cent.

Case 25.—Striped keratitis, involving entire cornea, that never cleared. Patient in good health, age 79 years. No cause known.

Cases 26, 27 and 28.—Operations, 200. All said to be due to "lessened nutrition of cornea;" all cleared practically, he believes, after several months.

Cases 29, 30, 31, 32, 33 and 34.—"Many hundred operations." All due, he thinks, to lack of "constitutional vigor."

Case 35.—Operations, 50. Caused by extensive (three-fifths of circumference of cornea) section and to action of bichlorid on endothelium. Vision, 20/200.

Case 36.—Hypermature cataract. Great loss of vitreous. Vision, fingers three feet.

Case 37.—Operations, 100. Caused by accidental introduction of alcohol into anterior chamber. Vision perception of light ultimately.

Case 38.—Operations, 100. Cause, severe iridocyclitis. Vision, perception of light. As this is the only case in which the pathology given is based on the microscopic findings, it is a great satisfaction to copy the report in full: "The whole cornea looked like ground glass. There was a deep white change with no disturbance of the superficial epithelium, not the so-called ground glass dots, but a general white opacity. Sections of the eye showed that the endothelial lining was replaced by a mass of dense new connective tissue, possibly one-third as thick as the original cornea. This new tissue, I believe, was the result of the iridocyclitis—masses of organized exudate. The proper substance of the cornea was unchanged, and the epithelium was normal. My colleagues and myself looked on this case as one of general opacification of the cornea. The whole appearance justified the expectation that the microscope would reveal interstitial changes."

Case 39.—My own.

One operator only out of the twenty-nine reporting cases could include the history of the other eye, also operated on for cataract with useful vision obtained, but lost two years later through infection, and emphasizes the rarity of my case in which the second eye, ten years later, almost paralleled the course of its fellow through its peculiar and unexplainable history of opacification.

CONCLUSIONS.

The deductions that I would make from my study of this subject are that treatment is of but little or no avail, and that there is no indication at present known which enables us to determine beforehand when general opacification of the cornea may follow cataract extraction. But with the warning from such a result in one eye, the cause undetermined, I should favor some method other than extraction for the remaining cataract, and would suggest this as one of the very few conditions where couching may be a justifiable operation.

THE SURGICAL TREATMENT OF ORBITAL COMPLICATIONS IN DISEASE OF THE NASAL ACCESSORY SINUSES.*

ARNOLD KNAPP, M.D.

NEW YORK.

The orbital complication referred to in this paper is the subperiosteal abscess. When disease of the nasal accessory sinuses extends to the orbit, the infection passes through the os planum of the ethmoid or through the floor of the frontal sinus. Two clinical pictures will be present, depending on whether the perforation occurs suddenly or gradually—acute or chronic. In the former, the local symptoms are those of an acute abscess with cellulitis. The orbital manifestation may disappear with intranasal treatment or the pus works its way to the surface and discharges spontaneously. The acute symptoms may then abate, the fistula closes or remains open and a purulent sinus persists which leads into the frontal or ethmoidal cavities. In the second variety there is a greater or less defect in the orbital bony wall of the frontal and ethmoidal sinuses, and with the orbital periosteum a large abscess cavity is formed, causing marked exophthalmos which usually brings the patient to the eye clinic.

In children, the acute perforation takes place through the ethmoidal plate. A curved incision is made along the inner and upper orbital margin, the orbital periosteum and contents are retracted and the opening in the os planum can then be seen. This should be enlarged. and the adjoining cells curetted according to the amount of disease found present.

---

* This paper has been accepted by the Executive Committee of the Section on Ophthalmology of the American Medical Association, to be presented before the Section at the Chicago Session, June 2-5, 1908. Publication rights reserved by the American Medical Association.

In the chronic cases with exophthalmos and in the other cases with acute perforation which do not improve on the restoration of intranasal drainage, the method of operating is as follows: It is a distinct advantage to remove the anterior half of the middle turbinate a day or two before the external operation, though this procedure is condemned by some; thus Killian claims that the virulence of the infection is thereby increased. I have never seen any ill effects from this preliminary operation.

Under morphin-ether narcosis, the external excision is made (Fig. 1) along the upper orbital border midway between the eyebrow and the bony orbital margin,

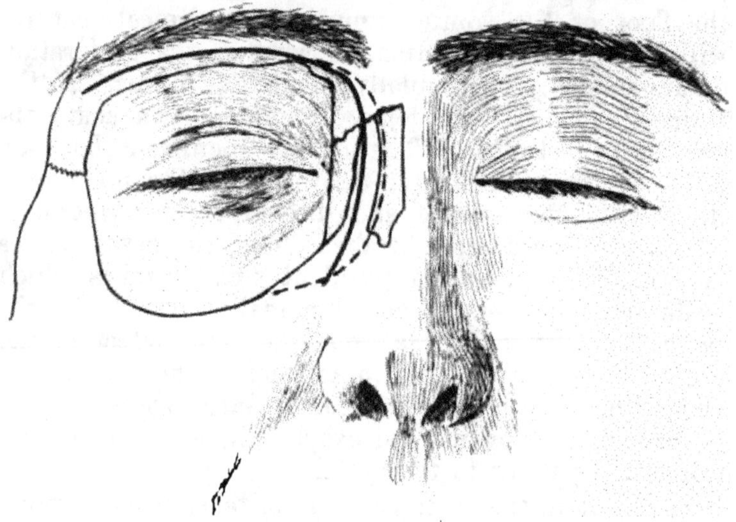

Fig. 1.—Showing line of cutaneous incision and (interrupted line) the resection of bone.

then down along the inner wall and the side of the nose to the floor of the orbit. This incision in my opinion is preferable to the incision through the eyebrow (Killian) as it permits external drainage of the frontal sinus if this be found necessary without making another incision. I have not found that packing the nose with gauze or insertion of a postnasal plug is necessary. The periosteum is divided just at the orbital margin above and in line with the cutaneous incision along the nose. The periosteum is retracted with a rather sharp elevator. After the firm adhesion of the periosteum to the orbital margin is separated, the soft parts with the orbital contents and the lachrymal sac are gently detached and free access is given to the roof and to the inner wall of the orbit (Fig. 2).

The pulley of the superior oblique is carefully detached from the trochlear fossa. It is important not to disturb the relation between the tendinous ring through which the tendon passes and the periosteum to which it is adherent; the periosteum later becomes attached in its normal position by the healing process and interference with the superior oblique muscle is avoided. This important relation can best be preserved by dislodging the pulley from the trochlear fossa by a blunt periosteotome working from behind forward. An examination of one hundred skulls has shown me that in four out of five

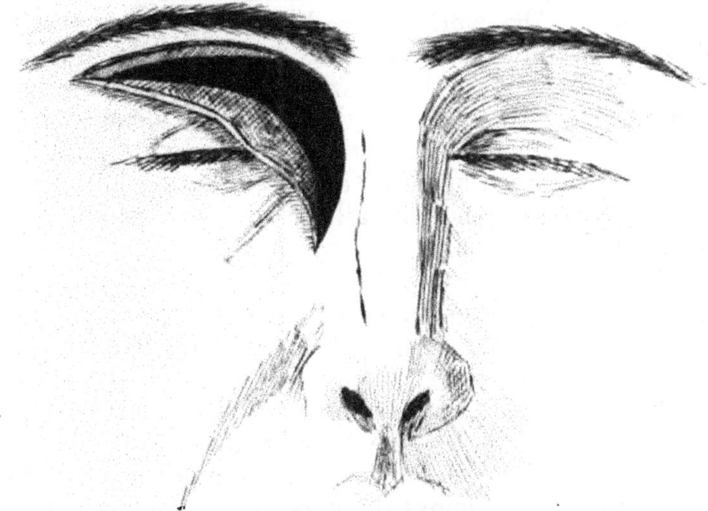

Fig. 2.—Complete detachment of the orbital contents and removal of floor of frontal sinus and of internal orbital wall.

the pulley is attached to merely a slight depression in the bone; in the remainder a well-developed spine directed straight down and occasionally slightly forward, was present just posterior to this fossa. It is evident that in the cases in which a spine is present the periosteum with the pulley can only be sparingly detached by following the above-described procedure.

The entire floor of the frontal sinus is then easily removed with the chisel and hammer, the diseased mucous membrane is curetted and the bony septa in the frontal sinus are carefully eradicated. A portion of the orbital margin can be removed without causing any deformity if the normal curve be preserved. The nasal process of the superior maxillary, the lachrymal bone and the ethmoidal os planum are then resected, giving broad access to the middle meatus of the nose and to the ethmoidal labyrinth. Work in this region is facilitated by suitable retractors for the orbital soft parts. The two which I use are a curved, shovel-shaped retractor and one shaped like a tongue depressor. The ethmoidal labyrinth is completely removed with the curette, Jansen's forceps or Hartmann's conchotome, remembering that the anterior ethmoidal foramen, which is a constant landmark, indicates the base of the skull and that as one proceeds back the ethmoid becomes broader laterally. The remaining part of the middle turbinate may now be removed and the sphenoidal cavity entered if necessary. The work is facilitated by introducing a finger well into the nose which serves as a guide and prevents some of the blood from running into the nose. The final curetting of the ethmoid is best done with the head low down and when the patient is partly revived. As broad an opening into the nose as possible is made, in addition to removing all disease, to insure proper drainage.

If the frontal sinus extends unusually high up, as it is apt to near the median line, and the upper limit can not be curetted from below, the cutaneous flap with the eyebrow is forcibly retracted upward, a window is cut in the anterior bony wall similar to the Kuhnt and Killian methods (Fig. 3), leaving a broad bony supraorbital margin covered with periosteum; the purpose of this window is not to remove the greatest part of the anterior bony wall but should be only large enough to treat properly the upper parts of the cavity under direct inspection. Marked subsequent sinking in of the forehead can thus be prevented. The cutaneous wound is not sutured, the soft parts approximate of themselves, a single wick of gauze is passed from without at the nasal angle into the frontal sinus. There is drainage not only into the nose but externally. Slight packing is introduced through the nose to the ethmoid region, if bleeding demands it; this is removed after twenty-four hours.

The patient occupies a partly upright position in bed. The external wound usually closes primarily; the small opening for the drain is left at the inner orbital angle for from seven to ten days. The nasal cavities are left undisturbed. In some cases diplopia was noted for a few days. This always disappeared and all patients were carefully examined for diplopia with a colored glass and a candle, especially in the lower part of the field.

I have performed twenty-two operations according to this method which can be described as a modified combination of the Jansen and Kuhnt methods. In recent years, Killian's method has become deservedly popular. It has seemed to me, however, that the Killian operation has certain objections, at least for this class of cases.

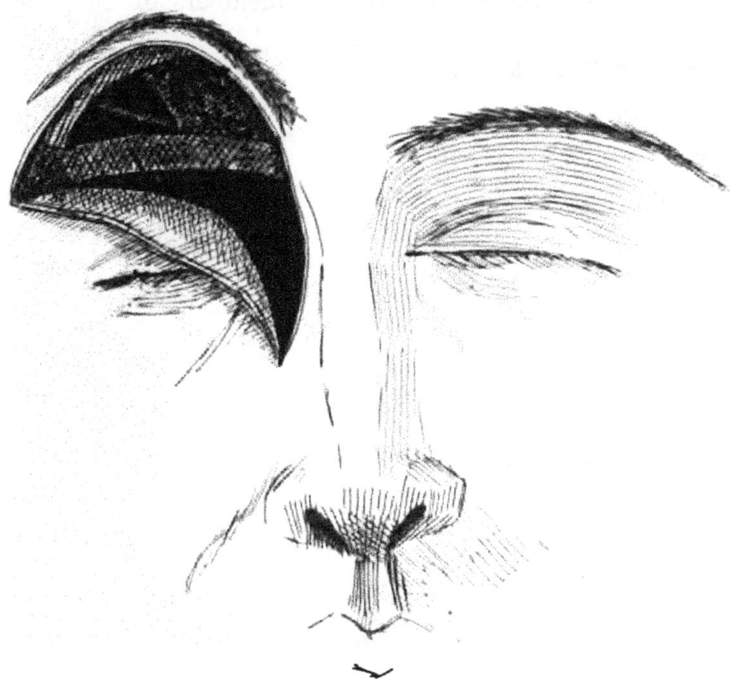

Fig. 3.—Partial resection of anterior wall in the cases in which the sinus extends high up.

Thus it can be simplified if the trochlea be systematically dislodged. The entire floor of the frontal sinus can then be easily removed from below. In the healing process it is also of advantage if the entire bony floor is removed for then the cavity, especially at its outer part, has a better chance to obliterate. In many patients with a broad access from below a window resection of the anterior bony wall of the frontal sinus is not necessary unless the sinus is an unusually high one. This window does not need to include most of the anterior bony wall, but should be sufficiently large to permit thorough curetting of the uppermost limit of the frontal sinus. This is an improvement cosmetically. Complete removal of the ethmoidal structures is also facilitated when the orbital contents can be well retracted.

The elements of success in operations of this kind depend upon the use of a proper light (either with mirror or electric forehead reflector), the control of hemorrhage and a knowledge of anatomy. These should surely not deter the ophthalmic surgeon from continuing in the development of this important field where the first advances were made by members of our specialty.

26 West Fortieth Street.

SOME CLINICAL ASPECTS OF LENTICULAR ASTIGMATISM.*

EDGAR S. THOMSON, M.D.
NEW YORK.

The subject of astigmatism has for its keynote the astigmatism of the lens. This is not only of interest from a scientific standpoint, but it is also of vital importance in the management of cases. It is not sufficient that we know the total astigmatism of an eye, unless we wish to prescribe glasses largely from the anatomic standpoint. In order to obtain a correct idea of the conditions present in each given case, we must separate the comparatively fixed quantity, the corneal astigmatism, from the fluctuating and uncertain one, the astigmatism of the lens. Leaving aside the differences in the corneal surfaces and the eccentricity of the visual axis, both of which quantities are so small as to be negligible from the clinical standpoint, the two broad facts to be determined are the amount of corneal astigmatism and the amount of lens astigmatism.

The corneal astigmatism, which is congenital in the vast majority of cases, may be determined accurately by the ophthalmometer of Javal and Schiotz. It may be stated in the beginning, however, that we have at present no accurate means of measuring the lens astigmatism, either as regards its quantity or its axis, but must depend on the subtraction of the corneal from the total astigmatism, as obtained by one of several methods.

VARIETIES OF LENS ASTIGMATISM.

Lens astigmatism may be either static or dynamic, and is probably far oftener the latter than the former. It would otherwise be difficult to explain the occur-

* This paper has been accepted by the Executive Committee of the Section on Ophthalmology of the American Medical Association, to be presented before the Section at the Chicago Session, June 2-5, 1908. Publication rights reserved by the American Medical Association.

rence of so many cases of corneal astigmatism of low degree (0.5 diopter) accurately compensated by the lens, especially in hyperopic cases with a well-developed ciliary muscle, and it hardly seems logical to attribute the cause of this to static astigmatism when we consider how small the measured change must be. In support of this, we have the clinical fact that low degrees of corneal astigmatism in myopic cases are much less frequently compensated by the lens; that is, they frequently accept cylindric glasses entirely at variance with the ophthalmometric reading, and this we should expect, because the ciliary muscle is relatively weaker, and because accommodation has no effect in increasing the visual acuity in use of the eyes for distance vision.

We are more apt to find this variation in the lens astigmatism the higher the total myopia and the weaker the ciliary muscle. That there exists a primary static astigmatism of the lens can scarcely be doubted, but that it exists unchanged in many instances may be very much doubted. Donders[1] found in his own eye astigmatism produced by the tilting of the lens, and that this can occur must be acknowledged by those who have seen astigmatism produced by a partial luxation of the crystalline lens. Children frequently learn to overcome low degrees of astigmatism by tilting the head, and presumably tilting the lens in relaxation of the zonula during accommodation. It is also a matter of common experience to see a patient with spherical glasses overcome an astigmatism by looking obliquely through the lens. Aside from these exceptional cases, however, which usually have rather pronounced clinical features, dynamic lens astigmatism is, in all probability, most frequently caused by partial contraction of the ciliary muscle in the meridian of least refraction, allowing that meridian of the lens to become, within certain degrees, more convex.

If the tilting of the lens were a frequent cause of dynamic astigmatism, we should expect it to appear fully as frequently in presbyopes as in the young. Exactly the reverse is true. Astigmatism in presbyopia becomes manifest just as certain other errors do, unless, of course, we have a static astigmatism of the lens, and it is doubtful if dynamic astigmatism occurs at all after the age of 50.

---

1. Accommodation and Refraction, p. 532.

Lens tilting argues an even higher individual development of control over the ciliary muscles, inasmuch as the mechanism by which it is produced must be the drawing forward of a certain set of ciliary fibers confined to a very small area. It is doubtful if this highly specialized action of the muscle exists frequently. Indeed, all the cases of lens tilting that have come under my observation have been, I believe, due primarily to the action of gravity in the twisted positions of the head which such patients assume.

Aside from the cases of lens tilting due to partial luxation of the lens, I have never seen a case where lens tilting seemed to occur during the distance test, these cases occurring only during accommodation at the near point.

Compensation by lens tilting must be extremely small, and is undoubtedly less in amount than compensation by partial contraction.

Partial contraction of the ciliary muscle was first pointed out by Dobrowolsky.[2] This view has been accepted by Landolt, Woinow, Pflüger, Mauthner, and others, while it has been opposed by no less distinguished observers than Hess, J. G. Bull, Sulzer, and Tscherning. The question is by no means settled, but it certainly seems as if the advocates of a dynamic lenticular astigmatism had a great deal in their favor, for the clinical facts and the voluntary control of the eye over astigmatism seems difficult to explain by any such fortuitous occurrence as dropping of the lens, tilting of the lens on the axis, or any of the other changes in the lens causing astigmatism, which, while they undoubtedly occur and have been demonstrated, certainly can not be the cause in the majority of cases.

The experiments of Hensen and Voelckers[3] are in the highest degree convincing, as showing that a meridional contraction of the ciliary muscle is possible, whatever may be its action on the shape of the crystalline lens. They found that irritation of the ciliary nerves by an electric current was followed by contraction in only that part of the iris and ciliary muscle supplied by that nerve. They also introduced needles through the sclerotic and cornea, and observed by the tilting forward of the needles which ones were acted on when a certain ciliary

2. Arch. f. Ophth., 1868, xviv, 3, 51.

3. Exper. Untersuchung ueber den Mechanismus der Accommodation, Kiel, 1868; also Arch. f. Ophth, 1873, xix, 1.

nerve was stimulated, proving that the chorioid is drawn forward in accommodation. They observed in the same manner changes in the curvature of the lens, by placing the ends of the needles in contact with the anterior and posterior surfaces of the lens. This was demonstrated in living animals—dogs, cats and monkeys—and also on a freshly enucleated human eye. The point of application of the electric current in the animals was near the ophthalmic ganglion.

CLINICAL DIFFERENTIATION.

From a clinical standpoint, we must distinguish carefully the static and the dynamic astigmatism of the lens. I think all will agree that the latter exists, no matter how it may be produced. It seems impossible otherwise to explain the vast number of persons whose corneal astigmatism is reduced 0.50 or 0.75 diopter, so that, having that amount of corneal astigmatism, no amount of refractive error can be demonstrated either with or without a mydriatic.

As Landolt[4] points out, "It may easily be demonstrated that the eye succeeds with a certain effort in overcoming weak cylindrical glasses. By what mechanism would it be possible to neutralize the inequality of refraction produced by the cylinder if not by the unequal contraction of this ciliary muscle, followed by a corresponding change in the form of the crystalline? This unusual and, for the non-astigmatic eye, unnatural muscular action reveals itself, moreover, by a rather disagreeable sensation, which from its resemblance to the one experienced during fixation of the punctum proximum leaves no doubt as to its origin. . . . The contraction of this muscle, limited to a single meridian, must cause unequal relaxation of the crystalline and make it assume a more convex form in one meridian only." It may easily be demonstrated, by putting a —0.50 cylinder before the eye (which is the utmost that I personally can overcome), that variations in the position of the head have no effect on the ease with which this cylinder can be overcome in the majority of cases, but only in the exceptional cases of "lens tilting" mentioned.

The dynamic astigmatism of the lens could hardly be expected to exceed a fraction of a diopter, and in prac-

4. Refraction and Accommodation of the Eye, p. 302.

tice this is found to be the case. The earlier text-books on refraction frequently led one to believe that a very considerable amount of astimatism might be uncovered by the use of atropin, but, as a matter of fact, we do not find this to be invariably the case, and even in those whose accommodation is young and vigorous any more than 0.50 diopter blurs distant vision. In practice, I find myself more and more inclined not to give cylindrical glasses, unless they improve the vision, and even if I have occasion to use myriaditic and develop what may be called a latent astigmatism I do not by any manner of means feel sure that such a glass can be worn after the effect of the mydriatic has passed off. However, the occurrence of these cases of latent astigmatism is a very strong point in favor of partial contraction of the ciliary muscle.

A dynamic astigmatism of the lens, which persists for a certain length of time, may lead to one of two secondary changes in the eye. The first of these is a greater development of the fibers of the ciliary muscle in the meridian of contraction. There seems no reason to doubt this in the face of the accumulated proof of the muscular development of the whole ciliary body in hyperopic cases (Iwanoff). The second change is in the shape of the lens. A lens in which a dynamic astigmatism persists for a certain length of time gradually becomes fixed in that shape, as the nuclear sclerosis advances. This is shown by those cases of corneal astigmatism of two or more diopters in which there is normal vision with only a fractional cylinder. Even with the aid of a mydriatic it is impossible to develop a greater lens astigmatism. Naturally we only meet with these cases in patients over 30 who have never worn glasses. These cases are, to my mind, a further proof of the existence of partial contraction of the ciliary muscle.

The cases above mentioned occur in astigmatism "with the rule." In astigmatism "against the rule" the dynamic astigmatism does not have the same tendency to become fixed. In presbyopic cases "against the rule" the lens astigmatism commonly disappears.

LATENT ASTIGMATISM.

At times we find cases in the transition stages between these changes; that is, with increased tonicity in the fibers of the ciliary muscle, but no permanent change in the shape of the lens. These cases belong to the class of so-called "latent astigmatism," and if a mydriatic is used a certain amount of lens astigmatism is manifest, though after the mydriatic has ceased its effect the tonicity of the fibers in the meridian of contraction may again compensate for the corneal astigmatism.

FACTORS IN TREATMENT.

In general, then, we have in the treatment of every case to consider the following factors, and, where absolute measurement fails us, to assign as nearly as possible a correct valuation in accordance with our judgment of the individual case: (1) Corneal astigmatism. (2) Lens astigmatism: (a) static, (b) dynamic. (3) The degree of compensation. (4) The factor in the error which is producing symptoms.

Obviously the last point is the end and aim of our efforts as practical ophthalmologists, and the relief of the irritative symptoms is the only question which greatly interests the patient.

TESTS EMPLOYED.

For determining the above mentioned points there are only two positive tests: (1) the ophthalmometer for the corneal astigmatism; (2) the shadow test for the total astigmatism. It may be urged against the ophthalmometer that the posterior surface of the cornea will modify its reading, but that this modification must be very slight indeed is shown by the well-substantiated assertions of Baker.[5] From a practical standpoint I never consider this factor. The shadow test, taken by itself, gives no idea of the proper proportions of the various factors to be considered, and, while undoubtedly of great value in association with other tests, is of limited value when taken alone. It must always be done with the aid of a mydriatic. Its most enthusiastic advocates lay great stress on the accurate determination (if not correction) of the total refractive error, and this point of view might be the correct one if we were dealing only with the eyes of the young in which the original error was not modified. In practice we find all sorts of modifying circumstances, with the changes in

5. Norris and Oliver's System, i, 138.

the ciliary muscle and lens above mentioned. In brief, the question must be approached from the standpoint of the physiologist and the pathologist (if one may use the term in this connection) rather than that of the anatomist.

As Hess says in his masterly paper read before this Section last year:[6] "Here" (i. e., under mydriasis)[4] "the optic conditions are so different from the normal that it is impossible to come to a conclusion as to the normal refraction of the patient's eye."

The subjective tests with the trial lenses I believe to be perhaps the most important in our list, when based on our other measurements, and the technic of applying them is very important. It hardly seems necessary at the present time to go into detail on this point, but I may say that the "fogging" method has been generally unsatisfactory in my hands, and I much prefer to test with cylindrical lenses in the axis of the corneal astigmatism, gradually increasing the strength of the lens and adding only enough spherical lens to bring up the visual acuity to the point where finer changes are more noticeable to the patient. I then vary the axis to find any modifications that may exist; if I am unable to find the correction which gives relief, I use a mydriatic and obtain a reading of the total error.

The actual lens prescribed depends on the judgment of the various questions above mentioned, taken in connection with the general muscular constitution (as bearing directly on the constitution of the ciliary muscle), the needs of the individual, and the existence of any local complications—as strabismus, heterophoria, etc., which need not be considered here. I do not underestimate the value of the ophthalmoscope in the treatment of refractive errors, but its bearing in the present question is only to give a close approximation to the total spherical error, which, of course, we must know, and it is of little value in the actual determination of the amount of astigmatism.

To obtain the lens astigmatism, we subtract the corneal astigmatism from the total, as obtained by either of the above mentioned methods. The proper appreciation of the true cause of the lens astigmatism and of the factors producing the visual disturbance will depend not so

6. The Journal A. M. A., July 20, 1907, p. 230.

much on mere figures as on the clinical conditions bearing on the case. To particularize, it is necessary to take up *seriatim* the different forms of astigmatism:

HYPEROPIC ASTIGMATISM.

The majority of cases of hyperopic astigmatism will fall under one of the following general classes:

1. *Low Degrees of Corneal Astigmatism, Completely Compensated by the Lens, Axis 90° or Thereabouts.*

These cases occur at any age, give no symptoms, and accept no cylindrical glasses with or without a mydriatic, and have normal vision with a corneal astigmatism of not more than one diopter, usual axis 90°, symmetrical in the two eyes. They form the largest class of cases. We see them only incidentally, in the course of treatment of other eye conditions—inflammations or presbyopia—and, of course, they require no correction. The compensating astigmatism of the lens is static, whatever it may have been originally. My own feeling is that a large proportion of such cases, perhaps the great majority, begin as a dynamic lens astigmatism, and that the efforts of the ciliary muscle are purposeful, and ultimately lead to full correction without the aid of cylindrical glasses.

2. *Higher Degrees of Corneal Astigmatism, with Partial Regular Compensation by the Lens, Axis 90° or Thereabouts.*

Under this heading we have the largest class of cases coming to us for treatment. The lens astigmatism occurs in the same axis—or very nearly the same axis—as the corneal astigmatism, and amounts to between 0.50 and 1 diopter. It is for this reason that we have the arbitrary rule of subtracting 0.50 diopter from the reading of the ophthalmometer in prescribing lenses, a rule which seems unfortunate as leading to a certain amount of misapprehension, though, in fact, our other tests usually give us approximately this result.

These cases, almost without exception, have a diminution of the visual acuity for distance (the amount depending on the degree of astigmatism) with asthenopia. Even small amounts of astigmatism are not properly to be called latent, though the meridional contraction occurs only at intervals when the patient is looking at the test card, and in most instances need not occur at all if the cylinders are carefully tried. By subtracting the total astigmatism (manifest with the trial lenses) from the corneal we have the lens astigmatism, and whether this be static or dynamic will depend on the severity of the asthenopia, the age of the patient, the length of time that the eyes have gone uncorrected, and the general muscular constitution of the individual.

After the age of 35 the compensating astigmatism is almost invariably static, and we may see even high degrees of compensation at this time; that is, 1.50 to 2 diopters, where glasses have never been worn and where the muscles have been allowed to develop gradually without undue forcing. In such cases, even under the influence of a mydriatic, the manifest astigmatism is not increased. Before 35, or thereabouts, the judgment of the character of the lens astigmatism is more difficult, and I have come to depend to a great extent on the finding of tender spots over the ciliary region, frequently in the meridian of contraction, when a dynamic astigmatism exists. If I find these tender spots, I suspect the astigmatism to be latent or dynamic, and I prescribe a mydriatic, both for accuracy in obtaining the test and for its physiologic action on the contracted fibers of the ciliary muscle. In most instances, the astigmatism will be found to be dynamic and needing partial or total correction, depending on the clinical features of the particular case, i. e., the amount of use of the eyes, the length of time since glasses have been worn, the age of the patient, and the general muscular constitution. One should be very careful in this connection not to overcorrect, for overcorrection is productive of much more irritation than undercorrection. Where no irritation of the ciliary muscle can be discovered, it seems unnecessary to use a mydriatic, and in practice I do not find that I am led into error through this line of procedure.

3. *Low Degrees of Corneal Astigmatism with Irregular Compensation by the Lens.*

This class is composed almost entirely of cases in which the corneal astigmatism is less than 0.75 diopter. It occurs most frequently in cases where the corneal astigmatism is not symmetrical; that is, one cornea may have a 0.50 diopter of astigmatism, the other none. In such cases the axis of the total manifest astigmatism represents a mean between the cornea and the lens, whose astigmatism, either from its original static condition or through faulty accommodative efforts, lies in an entirely different axis from the corneal. Such cases are much prone to vary. The astigmatism will appear and disappear, the axes will change from time to time, even where we use a mydriatic and endeavor to put them on more permanent bases.

In these cases, as in the former, I do not use a mydriatic, unless I have evidence of muscular cramp, as shown by tender spots over the ciliary muscle. I prefer to correct the manifest astigmatism after not less than two careful tests with the trial lenses. Unless there is a definite indication that the distance vision is accomplished through irritating accommodative effort, I prescribe the glasses only for the near work, and I often find that under this form of treatment the ciliary muscle adjusts itself, compensation is regained, and the glasses may be laid aside.

In this class of cases we frequently see the results of coordinated effort in the ciliary muscles of the two eyes; that is, where we have no corneal astigmatism in one eye and 0.50 diopter, axis 90° in the other eye, the same meridians will contract to such a degree that our final astigmatism will read axis 180° in each eye—say 0.50 diopter, axis 180°, in one eye, and 1 diopter, axis 180°, in the other eye, with 0.50 diopter or corneal astigmatism, axis 90°. In other words, the compensation in the eye with the 0.50 diopter of corneal astigmatism has overshot the mark and given us an excessive lens astigmatism.

4. *Corneal Astigmatism with the Axis at 180° or Thereabouts.*

In this class of cases, as is well known, the symptoms are very much more severe, compensation is much less apt to occur, and the lens astigmatism is frequently in excess of the corneal. Here we frequently find the lens astigmatism to be static, and the correction must be worn constantly. The reason for the increased difficulty of compensation in this class of cases over the preceding class is naturally to be looked for in a greater normal tonicity of certain fibers of the ciliary muscle over certain others, but so far we have no anatomic investigations to help us out on this point.

5. *Cases of Lens Astigmatism, Pure and Simple.*

In these cases the cornea shows no astigmatism, and the astigmatism is confined to the lens. It may be as high as a diopter, is accompanied by severe symptoms, and occurs most frequently below the presbyopic age. It is very desirable to use mydriasis in these cases, where even a small amount of muscular tenderness exists, as there is every evidence that the lens astigmatism is most frequently due to faulty ciliary contraction, and that if we keep our correcting lens a little under the full dynamic astigmatism with suitable management of the work done by the ciliary muscle, the astigmatism will ultimately disappear.

MYOPIC ASTIGMATISM.

In myopic astigmatism, we have, in general, a weaker ciliary muscle, and the compensating lens astigmatism is much less purposeful in its character than in hyperopic cases, as we should expect. While in the nature of the case there can be no constant correction of the astigmatism by the ciliary muscle, still in low degrees, unaccompanied by spherical error, we commonly find an attempt at correction or a contraction of the meridional fibers of the ciliary muscle, produced largely by certain habits in reading.

It must be remembered that within the far point of the meridian of greatest refraction (the most myopic), the only way the astigmatism can be reduced by the ciliary muscle is by correction in the opposite meridian, making both meridians myopic in the same degree, if the astigmatism is not too high; or reducing the astigmatism in the same way, if it is too great to be corrected entirely. We have, then, the same source of irritation as in hyperopic cases, but with a relatively weaker ciliary muscle, whose weakness depends on the amount of spherical myopia, etc. It is for this reason that we so frequently find severe asthenopic symptoms in myopic astigmatism, and that such cases so frequently simulate simple myopia in the distance test. Low degrees will almost always accept spherical lenses for distance, if the same be added until both meridians are corrected, which, of course, leaves one meridian overcorrected. For this reason, I always correct the astigmatism before I add the full spherical lens, and I find very few cases of plain spherical myopia, even where the error is as high as 10 diopters.

Myopic astigmatism occurs in the following general classes:

A. *Corneal Astigmatism, with Partial Regular Compensation by the Lens at the Near Point, Axis* 180° *or Therabouts.*

These cases have always marked diminution of distance vision with marked asthenopia for the near point on account of the meridional contraction of the ciliary muscle, as well as other factory, which we need not consider here. Low degrees may simulate a simple myopia, a patient may fail to notice an improvement in reading with cylindrical glasses, and, yet, they require full correction of the astigmatism, both far and near, if the ciliary muscle is to obtain its greatest power, and if the asthenopia is to be relieved entirely. On account of the difference in the constitution of the ciliary muscle and the fact that the dynamic astigmatism occurs only intermittently, compensation, as in hyperopic cases, does not occur, and full correction should be worn constantly.

If there is difficulty in inducing the patient to accept the cylindrical glasses called for by the corneal astigmatism, minus a certain amount for the lens (0.25 to 0.50 diopter), or if tenderness exists in the ciliary region, a mydriatic should be used, and the total static astigmatism be determined. It should never be forgotten that low degrees of this class may be due to overcontraction of the ciliary muscle in hyperopic astigmatism, simple or compound, but these cases have usually marked symptoms, and, moreover, are rather rare, errors of diagnosis in this connection being generally due to faulty technic with the trial case. The clock dial is of considerable value in the testing of these cases, for the lens astigmatism is apt to assume its static amount in the distance test, undisturbed by irregular ciliary contractions. It must be remembered, however, that where the eyes have been used without glasses for near work, especially in low degrees of spherical error, and where the muscular constitution is good, there may be some modification of the astigmatism at the distance, and we should be careful not to pay too much attention to any single test, but rather give weight to the preponderance of evidence in determining the full amount of astigmatism.

B. *Low Degrees of Corneal Astigmatism, with Irregular Modification by the Lens.*

These form a very large class, perhaps as large as the preceding. They show great variations in axes and amounts from the corneal astigmatism, which is usually "off axis," and not symmetrical in the two eyes. The principles that have already been discussed in the two previous classes of cases apply with equal force here, and it should especially be borne in mind that the lens astigmatism is so much less purposeful than in corresponding cases of hypermetropic astigmatism that the corneal reading, while important, is very little guide to the total astigmatism. I always try cylinders in the axis of the corneal astigmatism first, but if the indications are that the case belongs to the class under discussion, I do not hunt for the proper axis with the test lenses, but prefer to proceed at once to the clock dial test. This is apt to be of value, as dynamic astigmatism plays a relatively small part in such cases in the distance use of the eye, and the determination of the full static error is important.

C. *Lens Astigmatism Pure and Simple.*

In this class there is no corneal astigmatism, and the astigmatism is located entirely in the lens. It rarely exceeds 1 diopter, is static in character, has the same characteristics, and requires the same treatment as in the preceding class. It is very doubtful if a dynamic myopic astigmatism ever develops from a hypermetropic case, such changes being usually due to lengthening of the eyeball.

MIXED ASTIGMATISM.

These cases practically all belong to one class. The corneal astigmatism is high and "with the rule," in the vast majority of cases; in fact, mixed astigmatism "against the rule" has been with me one of the greatest of rarities. The distance vision is relatively good, when we consider the amount of the astigmatism, but asthenopia is severe. No complete lens compensation is possible, but almost invariably severe cramps of the fibers in the hypermetropic meridian exist, and are not at all readily overcome by any amount of care in testing with the trial lenses. Variations in the axis of the lens astigmatism from the corneal are uncommon, and when they do exist are of low degree, usually not more than 10° or 15°, and frequently less. Almost invariably we find a reduction of the hypermetropic meridian which is dynamic in character, and to my mind the only proper way to deal with such cases is to use a mydriatic, determine the full amount of astigmatism, and have the glasses put on before the effect of the mydriatic has passed off. We have here a condition of the ciliary muscle which may be considered a pathologic one, and the mydriatic is necessary, as much for a restoration of the fibers to the normal as it is for diagnostic purposes. Of course, this applies only to cases in which glasses have not been worn. Where the ciliary muscle is in better condition, it is frequently possible, by care in the technic of the trial case, to ascertain the astigmatism without a mydriatic. Where the full correction has been prescribed with the assistance of a mydriatic, the case should always be studied subsequently and the action of the ciliary muscle noted, and any irregularity in the focus met by an appropriate change of lens.

19 East Forty-fourth Street.

A STUDY OF ONE HUNDRED REFRACTION CASES IN INDIANS FRESH FROM THE PLAINS.*

CLARENCE PORTER JONES, M.D.

NEWPORT NEWS, VA.

Having had the good fortune to be able to study the refractive condition of the eyes in aborigines, and finding no literature whatever on the subject, I deem it not inappropriate to present a brief treatise on this subject.

The cases studied are confined wholly to pupils at the Hampton (Va.) Normal and Agricultural Institute, a school for negroes and Indians. This institution not being under government control, but, on the contrary, being a purely philanthropic enterprise, kindness, sympathy and individual application makes the stubbornness and distrust so inherent in the Indian melt away. The result is that he soon becomes an ideal student and is trained successfully to enter the realm of good citizenship.

Admissions to the school are made each month in the twelve, and several departments of instruction continue throughout the summer. This series of 100 cases covers exactly 289 admissions, the last being Nov. 24, 1907, four months before the compilation of the statistics. Therefore, I speak accurately when I state that the percentage having refractive errors necessitating the wearing of glasses to improve vision and to relieve symptoms of eyestrain is 34.6 per cent. The ages are from 14 to 22; Males, 127, in this series 44 cases, or about 35 per cent. Females, 162, in this series 56 cases, or about 34 per cent.

On admission a careful test of vision is made, and should it be below 20/20 in each eye, or should the usual symptoms of eyestrain develop subsequently, a

* This paper has been accepted by the Executive Committee of the Section on Ophthalmology of the American Medical Association, to be presented before the Section at the Chicago Session, June 2-5, 1908. Publication rights reserved by the American Medical Association.

thorough refractive test is made. In making this test I made careful and systematic use of the ophthalmometer, ophthalmoscope, retinoscope, phorometer and test lenses, employing a cycloplegic in every case. In these 100 cases—200 eyes—the refractive varieties found were as follows: Hyperopia, 38 eyes; simple hyperopic astigmatism, 26; compound hyperopic astigmatism, 60; myopia, 13 eyes; simple myopic astigmatism, 15; compound myopic astigmatism, 32; mixed astigmatism, 16.

The axis of hyperopic astigmatism was 90 degrees in 69 eyes, 180 degrees in 5, 45 or 135 degrees in 5, nearer vertical than horizontal in 13, and nearer horizontal than vertical in 6.

The myopic axis was 180 degrees in 38 eyes, 90 degrees in 4, 45 or 135 degrees in 4, nearer vertical than horizontal in 4, and nearer horizontal than vertical in 15.

Twenty states and territories are represented in the 289 admissions, 39 tribes, 26 in the series.

There are 3 cases of heterophoria amounting to as much as 2 degrees, no case being treated other than correcting the refractive error. No strabismus.

A marked tolerance for cycloplegics exists in the Indian. Scopolamin is not effective, being practically worthless. Homatropin 1/25 grain in each eye, applied by means of gelatin discs, is usually reliable; this dose was repeated in thirty minutes in about 10 per cent. of the cases. Atropin was necessary in 3 cases. A less than 2 per cent. solution of the latter was ineffective; also the strong solution of atropin was found necessary when its effect was desired in treating eye injuries of Indians occurring in the school work shops. In the series herewith charted, when no cycloplegic is mentioned, let it be understood that homatropin hydrobromate was used.

Fifty-one, or 17.65 per cent. of the whole number, had trachoma on entrance—16 cases in this series; the remaining 35 had normal vision. All trachoma patients are treated surgically, being promptly rolled by Knapp's forceps; and active after-treatment. In the 16 cases mentioned in the refractive series, the test was not made till the acute symptoms had subsided and the corneæ became clear. The care exercised by officers, physicians and nurses with these patients has prevented the spread of the disease at the institution.

Case number.	Vision Before Cycloplegia.	Vision During Cycloplegia.	Results of Examination, etc.	Lenses Accepted for Use. Spherical.	Lenses Accepted for Use. Cylindrical.	Tribe.	Remarks.
1.	20/70	20/40	20/20 w. +.75s. ⊂ +.50c. ax.90	+.50	[illegible]	[illegible]	....
	20/50	20/40	20/20 w. +.75s. ⊂ +.50c. ax.90	+.50	Same.		
2.	20/150	20/100	20/50 w. +.50c. ax.90 ⊂ — .75 ax.180	Same.	.....	Cherokee.	Scopolamin failed to produce cycloplegia; homatropin was successful.
	20/150	20/100	20/50 w. +.75c. ax.90 ⊂ —2.00c. ax.180	Same.			
3.	20/100	20/40	20/20 w. +.50s. ⊂ +.50c. ax.90	Same.	.....	Oneida.	....
	20/100	20/30	20/20 w. +.50s. ⊂ +.25c. ax.90	Same.			
4.	20/30	20/40	20/20 w. +.50c. at 90	Same.	.....	Chippewa	....
	20/30	20/30	20/20 w. +.25s. ⊂ +.50c. ax.90	Same.			
5.	20/70	20/150	20/50 w. +.75s	Same.	.....	Sioux	....
	20/70	20/150	20/50 w. +.75s	Same.			
6.	20/50	20/70	20/20 w. +.25s. ⊂ +.65c. ax.90	Same.	.....	[illegible]daga	....
	20/200	20/100	20/70 w. +.62c. ax.180	Same.			
7.	20/20	20/20	20/20 w. + .25c. ax.90	Same.	.....	[illegible]ha	Atropin 4 % sol., 5 instillations necessary to produce cycloplegia, scopolamin and homatropin having previously failed.
	20/100	20/200	20/20 w. +1.75c. ax.90 ⊂ —.50c. ax.180	Same.			
8.	20/30	20/30	20/20 w. +.50c. ax.90	Same.	.....	Seneca	Scopolamin failed to produce cycloplegia; atropin 2 % sol., 3 instillations necessary for success.
	20/30	20/50	20/30 w. +.50c. ax.90 ⊂ —1.00c. ax.180	Same.			
9.	20/200	20/200	20/20 w. +.75s. ⊂ +.25c. ax.180	Same.	.....	Chippewa	....
	20/70	20/100	20/20 w. +.75s. ⊂ +.25c. ax. 90	Same.			
10.	20/30	20/25	20/20 w. +.25s. ⊂ +.25c. ax.90	Same.	.....	Oneida.	....
	20/30	20/25	20/20 w. +.25s. ⊂ +.50c. ax.90	Same.			
11.	20/50	20/50	20/20 w. —.50s. ⊂ —.50c. ax.180	Same.	.....	Ponca	....
	20/50	20/50	20/20 w. —.50s	Same.			

Case. number.	Vision Before Cyclo-plegia.	Vision During Cyclo-plegia.	Results of Examination, etc.	rises for Spher-ical.	ckepted Use. ylin-drical.	Tribe.	Remarks.
12.	20/100	8/200	20/40 w. +1.50s. () +1.25c. ax.100	+.75	Same.	Chippewa	
	20/100	8/200	20/40 w. +1.50s. () +1.25c. ax. 80	+.75	Same.		
13.	20/40	20/150	20/20 w. +1.25s	Same.	.....	Chippewa	
	20/40	20/150	20/20 w. +1.50s	Same.			
14.	20/30	2 /40	20/20 w. +.50s	Same.	.....	Seneca	
	20/30	2 /40	20/20 w. +.50s	Same.			
15.	15/200	15/200	20/100 w. —1.75s. () —.25c ax. 180	Same.	.....	Navajo	
	20/30	20/35	20/20 w. + .50s	Same.			
16.	20/40	20/40	20/30 w. —1.12s	Same.	.....	Shawnee.	
	20/40	20/45	20/30 w. — .50s. () —.50c. ax.135	Same.			
17.	20/30	20/50	20/20 w. +1.00s. () +.50c. ax.90	+.75	Same.	Seneca	
	20/30	20/50	20/20 w. +1.00s. () +.50c. ax.90	+.75	Same.		
18.	20/30	20/40	20/20 w. +.75s	Same.	.....	Oneida.	
	20/30	20/40	20/20 w. +.75s	Same.			
19.	20/30	20/30	20/20 w. +1.00s	Same.	.....	Chippewa	
	20/30	20/30	20/20 w. +1.00s	Same.			
20.	20/40	20/45	20/20 w. +.50s. () +.50c. ax.90	Same.	.....	Oneida.	
	2 /40	20/45	20/20 w. +.50s. () +.50c. ax.90	Same.			
21.	20/200	20/200	20/20 w. —2.50s. () —25c. ax.180	Same.	.....	Assi ne.	
	20/200	20/200	20/20 w. —3.00s	Same.			
22.	20/100	20/200	20/30 w. +1.12s. () +.25c. ax.180	Sme.	.....	Chi pwya	
	20/100	20/200	20/20 w. +1.12s. () +.25c. ax. 90	Same.			

23.	20/70	20/70	20/20 w. —.25s. ⊂⊃ —.75c. ax.180	Same.	Seneca	
	20/70	20/70	20/20 w. —.25s ⊂⊃ —.75c. ax.180	Same.		
24.	20/30	20/40	20/20 w. —.62s. ⊂⊃ —.50c. ax.180	Same.	Oneida	
	20/30	20/40	20/20 w. —.25s. ⊂⊃ —.50c. ax.180	Same.		
25.	20/30	20/70	20/20 w. +1.00s. ⊂⊃ +.75c. ax.90	Same.	Winnebago	Trachoma: Lids rolled twice in one year, blue stick and bichlorid 1 to 500 ointment used alternately for period of 18 months. Refractive test made 20 months after entrance.
	20/30	20/50	20/20 w. + .75s. ⊂⊃ +.50c. ax.90	Same.		
26.	20/150	6/200	20/40 w. +1.25c. ax.90 ⊂⊃ —1.00c. ax.180	Same.	Pottawattomie	Trachoma: Lids rolled and blue stick used day for 3 months before refractive test.
	20/50	20/70	20/20 w. + .50s. ⊂⊃ +.75c. ax.90	Same.		
27.	20/70	20/100	20/30 w. +1.00c. ax.105 ⊂⊃ —1.50c. ax.15	Same.	Ponca	Trachoma: Lids rolled and bichlorid 1 to 500 ointment used daily for 5 months before refractive test.
	20/50	20/70	20/30 w. +1.50c. ax. 45 ⊂⊃ — .50c. ax.135	Same.		
28.	20/30	20/40	20/20 w. +.65c. ax.90	Same.	Chippewa	Trachoma: Lids rolled back and blue stick used twice a week for one month before refractive test.
	20/30	20/40	20/20 w. +.75c. ax.90	Same.		
29.	20/25	20/25	20/20 w. + .87s	Same.	Sioux	
	2 /30	20/30	20/20 w. +1.00s	Same.		
30.	20/100	20/150	20/30 w. —1.50c. ax.150	Same.	Pawnee	Trachoma: Lids rolled and blue stick used 3 times a week for 3 weeks prior to refractive test.
	20/70	20/100	20/20 w. + .75c. ax.135	Same.		
31.	20/100	20/100	20/20 w. +.87c. ax.90	Same.	Shawnee	
	20/70	20/70	/ 9 w. +.50c. ax.90	Same.		
32.	20/30	20/30	20/20 w. +.12c. ax.90	Same.	Oneida	Trachoma: Lids rolled and blue stick applied daily for 6 weeks prior to refractive test.
	20/200	20/200	20/20 w. —1.25s. ⊂⊃ —.87c. ax.180	Same.		
33.	20/100	20/70	20/30 w. —.37s. ⊂⊃ —.87c. ax.180	Same.	Seneca	
	20/70	20/50	20/20 w. —.37c. ⊂⊃ —.75c. ax.180	Same.		

Case number.	Vision Before Cycloplegia.	Vision During Cycloplegia.	Results of Examination, etc.	Lenses for Use. Spherical.	Lenses for Use. Cylindrical.	Tribe.	Remarks.
34.	20/30	20/30	20/20 w. +.50s.	Same.	.....	Pawnee.	....
	20/30	20/30	20/20 w. .50c. ax. 90	Same.			
35.	20/50	20/70	20/20 w. 1.25s. ⊃ +.50c. ax.90	+1.00	Same.	Chippewa.	Trachoma: Lids rolled, blue stick used 2 months prior to refractive test.
	20/50	20/70	20/20 w. + .75s. ⊃ +.75c. ax.90	+ .50	Same.		
36.	20/30	20/35	20/20 w. +.75s. ⊃ +.25c. 90	+.50	Same.	Sioux.	....
	20/30	20/35	20/20 w. +.75s.	+.50	Same.		
37.	20/40	20/45	20/20 w. +1.00s.	+.87	.....	Pima Sacaton.	Trachoma: Lids rolled twice in 4 months. Argyrol, 25 % sol., instilled daily for 6 months prior to test.
	20/40	20/45	20/20 w. +1.00s.	+.87			
38.	20/30	20/35	20/20 w. +.62s. ⊃ +.12c. ax.90	+.50	Same.	Chippewa.	Trachoma: Lids rolled, blue stick used 3 times a week for 2 months prior to test.
	20/30	20/35	20/20 w. +.62s. ⊃ +.12c. ax.90	+.50	Same.		
39.	20/20	20/25	20/20 w. +.25s. ⊃ +.12c. ax.90	Same.	.....	Sioux.	Headache. Test made 4 months after entrance.
	20/20	20/25	20/20 w. +.37s. ⊃ +.12c. ax.90	Same.			
40.	20/30	20/35	20/20 w. —.62s. ⊃ —.37c. ax.180	Same.	.....	Assinaboine.	Trachoma: Lids rolled, and blue stick applied twice a week for 2 months prior to test.
	20/30	20/35	20/20 w. —.62s. ⊃ —.37c. ax.180	Same.			
41.	20/50	20/100	20/20 w. 1.00s. ⊃ +.25c. ax.90	Same.	.....	Pottawattomie.	....
	20/50	20/100	20/20 w. +1.00s.	Same.			
42.	20/200	20/200	20/100 w. —6.00c. ax. 40	Same.	.....	Oneida.	Trachoma: Lids rolled 3 times, also blue stick and bichlorid ointment, 1 to 500. Test made 4 months after admission.
	20/100	20/100	20/70 w. —2.00c. ax.180	Same.			
43.	20/30	20/70	20/20 w. — .75s.	Same.	. .	Seneca	....
	20/30	20/75	20/20 w. —1.00s.	Same.			

44.	2 /70	20/70	20/20 w. —2.25s.	Sme.	.....	Sioux.	...	Trachoma: Lids rolled, bichlorid ointment 1 to 500 used 2 months prior to refractive test.
	20/50	20/50	20/20 w. —1.50s.	Same.				
45.	20/50	20/150	20/40 w. —1.75s. ⌒ —.25c. ax.180	Same.	.....	Sioux.	...	.....
	20/150	20/150	20/40 w. —1.75s. ⌒ —.25c. ax.180	[illegible]e.				
46.	20/150	20/150	20/30 w. —.50s. ⌒ —1.50c. ax.180	Same.	.....	Seneca	...	.....
	2 /150	20/150	20/30 w. —.62s. ⌒ — [illegible]. ax.180	Same.				
47.	20/150	20/150	20/20 w. +1.00s. ⌒ +.37c. ax.150	+.87	Same.	Omaha	...	.....
	20/150	20/150	20/20 w. + .87s. ⌒ +.25c. ax. 20	+.75	Same.			
48.	20/70	20/100	20/20 w. +.87s. ⌒ +.25c. [illegible]	+.75	Same.	Oneida	...	.....
	20/50	20/70	20/20 w. +.25s. ⌒ +.37c. ax.90	[illegible]				
49.	20/30	20/45	20/20 w. +1.00s.	Same.	.....	Shawnee.	...	.....
	20/30	20/45	20/20 w. +1.00s.	Same.				
50.	20/100	20/100	20/45 w. —1.25c. ax.55	Same.	.....	Arapahoe	...	.....
	20/100	20/100	20/45 w. —1.50c. ax.45	[illegible]				
51.	20/70	20/100	20/20 w. —1.50s. ⌒ —1.00c. ax.180	Sa me.	.....	Wi [illegible]go.	...	Exophoria 4°.
	20/70	20/100	20/20 w. —1.25s. ⌒ — .75c. ax.180	Same.				
52.	20/30	20/30	20/20 w. +.75s.	Same.	.....	Sioux.	...	Esophoria 2°.
	20/30	20/30	20/20 w. +.75s. ⌒ +.12c. ax.90	Same.				
53.	20/30	20/50	20/20 w. —1.25c. ax.90	[illegible]	.....	Sioux.	...	.....
	20/30	20/50	20/20 w. —1.25c. ax.90	Same.				
54.	20/100	20/75	20/30 w. +.62c. ax.180 ⌒ —.50c. ax.90	Same.	.....	[illegible]e.	...	.....
	20/100	20/75	20/25 w. +.50c. ax.180 ⌒ —.62c. ax.90	[illegible]				
55.	20/30	2 /40	20/20 w. +.87s.	Same.	.....	Shawnee.	...	.....
	2 /30	20/30	20/20 w. +.87s.	Same.				
56.	2 /40	20/50	20/25 w. +.50s. ⌒ + .37c. ax.90	Same.	.....	Chippewa	...	Trachoma: Lids rolled and 25 % sol. argyrol instilled t. i. d. for 2 months prior to refractive test.
	20/100	20/100	20/25 w. +.75s ⌒ +1.25c. ax.20	Same.				

Case number.	Vision Before Cycloplegia.	Vision During Cycloplegia.	Results of Examination, etc.	Lenses for Use. S[illegible]ical.	[illegible]cepted Use. Cylindrical.	Tribe.	Remarks.
57.	/ [illegible]	20/30	20/20 w. +.37c. ax.90	Same.	.....	Navajo	....
	20/100	20/100	20/45 w. +.50s. ⊂ +.37c. ax.90	[illegible]			
58.	20/100	20/100	20/30 w. +2.75 ax.105 ⊂ —1.50c. ax. 15.	Same.	.....	Oneida.	....
	20/100	20/100	20/30 w. +2.00c. ax. 60 ⊂ — .75c. ax.150.				
59.	20/30	20/30	20/20 w. +.62s	Same.	.....	Oneida.	....
	20/30	20/30	20/20 w. +.62s	Same.			
60.	20/20	20/50	20/20 w. +.25s. ⊂ +.50c. ax.90	Same.	.....	Cheyenne.	Eyestrain. Test made 3 months after entrance.
	20/20	20/50	20/20 w. +.25s. ⊂ +.50c. ax.90	Same.			
61.	20/35	2 /50	20/20 w. +.75s. ⊂ +.25c. ax. 110	Same.	.....	Pueblo	....
	20/35	20/50	20/20 w. +.75s. ⊂ +.25c. ax. 90	Same.			
62.	20/70	20/70	20/25 w. —2.50s. ⊂ — .50c. ax.180	Same.	.....	[illegible]ha	....
	20/70	20/100	20/30 w. — .50s. ⊂ —2.75c. ax.180	Same.			
63.	20/20	/ [illegible]	20/15 w. —1.00c. ax.180	Same.	.....	[illegible]he	Trachoma: Lids rolled, and blue stick used 3 times a week for 8 months before refractive test.
	2 /20	20/20	20/15 w. —1.00c. ax.180	Same.			
64.	20/150	20/200	20/100 w. —.50s. ⊂ —.75c. ax.135	Same.	.....	[illegible]minee.	....
	20/25	20/35	20/20 w. —.37c. ax. 135	Same.			
65.	20/25	20/30	20/20 w. +.25s. ⊂ +.25c. ax.30	Same.	.....	Arapahoe.	....
	20/25	20/30	20/20 w. +.75s. ⊂ +.25c. ax.30	Same.			
66.	20/150	20/150	20/30 w. — .50s. ⊂ —4.00c. ax. 15	Same.	.....	Pottawattomie.	....
	20/150	20/150	20/30 w. —1.50s. ⊂ —3.50c. ax.155	Same.			
67.	20/30	20/30	20/20 w. +.62s	Same.	.....	[illegible]e.	....
	2 /30	20/30	20/20 w. +.62s	Same.			

68.	20/75	20/100	20/30xw. +1.25s. ⊂⊃ + .75c. ax.90	Same.	.....	Chi ppwa	....
	20/75	20/100	20/30 w. + .87s. ⊂⊃ +1.00c. ax.90	Same.			
69.	20/150	18/200	20/30 w. —5.00s. ⊂⊃ —1.00c. ax.175	Same.	.....	Yuki	....
	20/150	18/200	20/30 w. —5.00s. ⊂⊃ — .62c. ax.5	Same.			
70.	20/200	20/200	20/20 w. +5.00s	+2.50	.....	Pawnee.	....
	20/200	20/200	20/20 w. +5.00s	+2.50			
71.	20/100	20/100	20/45 w. +.50c. ax.105 ⊂⊃ — .50c. ax.15	Same.	.....	Stockbridge	....
	20/100	20/100	20/45 w. +.62c. ax.100 ⊂⊃ —1.00c. ax.10	Same.			
72.	20/30	20/35	20/20 w. +.37c. ax.90	Same.	.....	Tuscaiora	....
	20/30	20/35	20/20 w. +.37c. ax.90	Same.			
73.	20/100	20/100	20/45 w. +1.25c. ax.90 ⊂⊃ —1.25c. ax.180	Same.	.....	Tuscarora	Atropin 3 % sol. to produce cycloplegia, scopolamin and homatropin having failed.
	20/70	20/100	20/40 w. + .37c. ax.90 ⊂⊃ —1.00c. ax.180	Same.			
74.	20/50	2 /50	20/20 w. —.50c. ax.15	Same.	.....	Sioux.	....
	20/50	20/50	20/20 w. +.50c. ax.75	Same.			
75.	20/30	20/40	20/20 w. —.75c. ax.180	Same.	.....	Oneida.	....
	/30	2 /40	20/20 w. +.50c. ax.180	Same.			
76.	20/50	20/75	20/20 w. +1.25c. ax.85	Same.	.....	Oneida.	....
	2 /40	20/60	20/20 w. +1.25c. ax.85	Same.			
77.	20/70	20/70	20/20 w. +.25s. ⊂⊃ +.87c. ax.90	Same.	.....	Winnebago.	Trachoma: Lids rolled, blue stick and argyrol 25 % used for 9 months prior to refractive test.
	20/50	20/50	20/20 w. +.25s. ⊂⊃ +.50c. ax.90	Same.			
78.	20/50	20/70	20/20 w. +.50c. ax.90	Same.	.....	Sei eca	....
	20/45	2 /40	20/20 w. +.37c. ax.90	Same.			
79.	20/30	20/35	20/20 w. + .50s. ⊂⊃ +.62c. ax.90	Same.	.....	Pawnee.	....
	20/30	20/35	20/20 w. +1.00s. ⊂⊃ +.75c. ax.90	+.87	Same.		
80.	20/40	20/45	20/20 w. +.37s. ⊂⊃ +.37c. ax.135	Same.	.....	Shawnee.	....
	20/40	20/45	20/20 w. +.25s. ⊂⊃ +.25c. ax. 70	Same.			

Case number.	Vision Before Cycloplegia.	Vision During Cycloplegia.	Results of Examination, etc.	Lenses for Spherical.	ccepted Use. Cylindrical.	Tribe.	Remarks.
81.	20/100	20/150	/ 2 w. —1.75s. ⌣ —1.00c. ax. 10	Same.	.....	Shawnee.	....
	20/70	20/100	/ 2 w. —.1.50s. ⌣ — .75c. ax.170	Same.			
82.	20/25	20/30	/ 2 w. +.50s	Same.	.....	Tuscarora	Headache. Test made one month after entrance.
	20/25	20/30	/ 2 w. +.50s	Same.			
83.	20/50	50/50	20/20 w. —1.50s	Same.	.....	Seneca	....
	20/50	20/50	20/20 w. —1.50s	Same.			
84.	20/150	20/150	20/20 w. —3.00s	Same.	.....	Seneca	....
	20/150	20/150	2 / 2 w. —3.00s. ⌣ —.50c. ax.65	Same.			
85.	20/150	20/200	20/20 w. —3.75s. ⌣ —1.00c. ax.180	Same.	.....	Sioux	....
	20/100	20/100	20/20 —3.00s	Same.			
86.	20/35	20/100	20/20 w. +.50s. ⌣ +.75c. ax.90	Same.	.....	Oneida	....
	20/35	20/100	20/20 w. +.25s. ⌣ +.75c. ax.90	Same.			
87.	20/150	20/150	20/20 w. +1.00s	Same.	.....	Seneca	....
	20/150	20/150	20/20 w. +1.25s	Same.			
88.	20/20	20/20	20/15 w. .37c. ax.90	+1.25	Same.	Oneida	Headache. Test made 3 months after entrance.
	20/20	20/20	0215 w. .25c. ax.90	+1.25	Same.		
89.	20/25	20/30	20/20 w. +.50c.ax.90	Same.	.....	Klamath	Symptoms of eyestrain.
	20/20	20/25	20/20 w. +.25s. ⌣ .12c. ax.90	Same.			
90.	20/30	2 /50	20/20 w. +.50c. ax.90	Same.	.....	Seneca	....
	/32	20/50	20/20 w. +.50c. ax.90	Same.			

91.	20/150	17/200	20/30	w. —2.50s ◯ — .50c. ax.180	Same.	.....	Seneca ...	....
	20/150	17/200	20/40	w. — .50s. ◯ —2.75c. ax.180	[illegible]			
92.	20/70	20/75	20/20	w. .25s.	+.100	.....	Oneida ...	....
	2 /70	20/100	20/30	w. 1.12c. ax.90 ◯ —.62c. ax.180 ...	Same.			
93.	20/20	20/25	20/15	w. +.50s	Same.	.....	Pima.	...Headache. Test made 3 weeks after entrance.
	20/20	20/25	20/15	w. +.5 0s	Same.			
94.	2 /40	20/40	20/20	w. +1.00c. ax.105	Same.	.....	Oneida. ..	...Trachoma: Lids rolled and argyrol 25 % sol. used daily for 2 months prior to test. Left hypophoria, 4°.
	20/40	20/40	2 /20	w. + .75c. ax. 75	Same.			
95.	20/40	20/45	20/20	w. +.87s. ◯ +.50c. ax.180	+.50	Same.	Pawnee. ...	....
	20/30	20/45	20/20	w. +.87s. ◯ +.50c. ax.180	+.50	Same.		
96.	2 /40	20/45	20/20	w. +1.12s.	+.87	Same.	Pottawattomie.	....
	2 /40	20/45	20/20	w. + .75s. ◯ +.62c. ax. 180	+.50	Same.		
97.	20/100	20/40	2 / 2	w. —1.25c. ax.180	Same.	.....	Apache	....
	20/100	20/40	20/20	w. —1.00c. ax.180	Same.			
98.	20/100	20/150	20/20	w. +1.00s. ◯ +.25c. ax.90	Same.	.....	[illegible]e. ..	....
	20/50	20/70	20/20	w. + .75s	Same.			
99.	20/30	20/100	20/20	w. +2.75s. ◯ +.62c. ax.90	+1.75	Same.	[illegible]a	....
	20/30	20/100	20/20	w. +2.25s	+1.50			
100.	20/30	2 /40	20/20	w. +.75s	Same.	.....	[illegible]nee....	....
	20/25	20/25	20/20	w. +.50s	Same.			

When cycloplegic is not stated, homatropin hydrobromate was the one used.

MEMORANDA

THE ASSOCIATION OF AGE AND INCIPIENT CATARACT WITH NORMAL AND PATHOLOGIC BLOOD PRESSURE.

A STUDY OF THESE CONDITIONS IN FOUR HUNDRED MEN ABOVE SIXTY YEARS OF AGE.*

D. W. GREENE, M.D.

DAYTON, OHIO.

As one studies the conditions of the eyes and blood vessels of elderly persons, especially of men above the age of 60 years, he becomes more and more convinced that certain changes are taking place in their tissues and organs with great uniformity. This uniformity is so pronounced as to suggest an inter-relation between these changes or the dependence of each on a common cause. These changes are incident to or at least associated with age, and are probably always degenerative.

The purpose is to show by statistics how uniform these changes are and their relation to each other, *if they have any.* It is desirable to emphasize the importance of age in its relation to cataract. The relation of age to blood pressure, *if any exists,* is not close and intimate. This will be shown later by statistics.

We are concerned at this time with the changes of age as we see them in the lens, and find them in the blood vessels by palpation and instrumental examination. It is difficult to estimate the influence of age in the etiology of blood pressure, since age is often associated with arterial sclerosis and high blood pressure, but not necessarily so, and can not be studied separate and apart from certain concomitant tissue changes or attributes which are believed to be pathologic

---

* This paper has been accepted by the Executive Committee of the Section on Ophthalmology of the American Medical Association, to be presented before the Section at the Chicago Session, June 2-5, 1908. Publication rights reserved by the American Medical Association.

themselves, and which those who indulge in excesses of any kind bring on prematurely.

The essential elements in the relation of age to cataract, close and intimate as they possibly are, have so far eluded demonstration, and statistics do not throw much light upon them. We know that the proportion of cataracts increases with each decade or half decade from fifty years upward, as shown by these and other statistics.[1] It is higher in the class of men with pathologic than in the class with normal blood pressure, but of the essential cause we know comparatively little. The works of Metchnikoff, "The Nature of Man," "Orthobiosis" and the "Prolongation of Life," give the best scientific exposition of age with which I am familiar.

Jackson,[2] of Denver, has given the statistics of 1,545 persons over 50 years of age, patients in Wills Eye Hospital, Philadelphia; 439, or 27.8 per cent., had some degree of lens opacity. Arranged in five-year periods, the per cent. showing such opacities was as follows: 15 per cent. between 50 and 55, 16.1 per cent. between 55 and 60, 30.2 per cent. between 60 and 65, and 77 per cent. between 65 and 75. Norris[3] has given statistics of 584 inmates of the poorhouse, between 50 and 60 years of age, in whom 264, or 45 per cent., had traces of cataract.

These statistics were compiled before the importance of blood pressure records were recognized, hence we lose whatever information such records might have furnished.

In the accompanying statistics age and incipient cataract have been considered at length and the result will be given further on, but the chief task I have assigned myself has been to show by abundant statistics what influence, *if any,* arterial sclerosis and high blood pressure have in the etiology of cataract. Theoretically there are many reasons why this influence should be great, and practically its importance seems not to have been overestimated. For example, with normal blood pressure I have found in 59 men, between 60 and 65 years of age, 37.3 per cent. of cataract; in 79 men, between 65 and

1. Oliver: A study of 3,436 cataracts operated by the staff of Wills Eye Hospital, Philadelphia, Trans. Am. Ophthal. Soc., xi, Part I.
2. Norris and Oliver's System of Diseases of the Eye, iv, 324.
3. Id., 289.

70, 41.8 per cent.; in 35 men, between 70 and 75, 54.3 per cent.; in 20 men, between 75 and 80, 70 per cent.; in 4 men, between 80 and 85, 75 per cent. A steady but not pronounced increase is observed up to the period between 85 and 95, in which the number of cases of cataract is too small to be of any statistical value.

With pathologic pressure I have found in 57 men, between 60 and 65 years of age, 42.1 per cent. of cataract; in 61 men, between 65 and 70, 54.1 per cent.; in 44 men, between 70 and 75 years, 55.8 per cent.; in 22 men, between 75 and 80, 68.2 per cent.; in 12 men, between 80 and 85, 83.33 per cent., and one man, 95 years old, one cataract, or 100 per cent., thus showing a steady rise in the per cent. of cataracts with age, which is greater in those with pathologic than in those with normal blood pressure.

These statistics further show that 79.5 per cent. of these 400 men had blood pressure between 130 and 180 mm. Hg, and the largest number of cataracts were found between these limits of pressure. For example, 79 men, between 65 and 70 years of age, had 33 cataracts, i. e., 41.8 per cent., with pressure under 160; 61 men, between the same ages, had 33 cataracts, or 54.1 per cent., with pressure above 160 mm. Hg. In other words, 61 men with pathologic pressure had the same number of cataracts that were found in 79 men with normal pressure, and the statistics also show that an increase in pressure of 41.4 mm. Hg in the pathologic over the normal class is accompanied by an increase of 17 cataracts, or 18.3 per cent. It is evident, therefore, that pathologic pressure, or the conditions which lead to it, have considerable influence in the etiology of cataract, and I can not agree with the statements of Frenkel and Garipuy that it does not.

In my service in the eye department of the hospital at the National Military Home, near this city, abundant opportunities are offered for observing the association of these conditions, and it has been my privilege to conduct the examinations which form the basis of this paper in that great field. It is believed that their value is greatly enhanced by the fact that they have been compiled by a single observer and his assistant, from men of the same class, of the same general age, living under uniform conditions as to diet, hours of sleep, amount of exercise, and surrounded by the same temptations as to drinking and other vices, but at the same time subject to parental military control.

More than 6,000 men, 60 years of age and over, with an average age of 67.72 years, have been available for the purpose.[4] Only such have been accepted, however, as have been able to walk to the clinic for eye and ear treatment and as I have been able to examine in the limited time at my disposal. No selection of cases has been made, but no one has been accepted for the examination unless a satisfactory view of the lens, blood vessels and details of the fundus could be had in one or both eyes. (This has excluded all mature and advanced immature cataracts of both eyes.)

To this end one or two instillations of a 1 per cent. solution of homatropin has been used in every case, and the examinations have taken a wider range than for cataract alone and have included all intraocular diseases and conditions. While it is well known that cataract does not necessarily start in both eyes at the same time, as a rule it does, and when present can be detected in the lower inner one-third or one-half of the periphery in more than 95 per cent. of all cortical cases, as spokes or striæ or as masses of opacity. Magnus[5] places the per cent. at 82.69, but in my experience it has been much higher, as I have only seen cortical opacity begin in the upper one-half of the lens in three of 600 cases examined, *with a dilated pupil.* The small percentage of all kinds of cataracts which mature is well known.

The statement of Walther,[6] that "Every one becomes cataractous who does not die prematurely," seems to have some statistical support. The plausibility of the statement is strengthened if we believe that the changes in the lens which lead to cataract are degenerative, and that the changes of age are also degenerative, or the statement of Roemer that cataract is the result of direct poisoning of the cells of the lens, and if we accept the teaching of Metchnikoff that "all deaths are accidental and premature under present conditions, because of auto-poisoning by the products of intestinal decomposi-

4. Annual Report of Board of Managers National Military Homes, 1907.

5. Norris and Oliver's System of Diseases of the Eye,, iv, 289.

6. Walther: Id., ii, 323.

tion. We reach a point where the inter-relation of all these conditions seems evident and their degenerative character apparent.

It seems to me that the essential, all important elements entering into the consideration of these subjects is wrapped up in their probably degenerative character, and their association together at a fairly definite period of life. When the effects of all of these influences are understood we shall know more of the etiology and pathology of age, cataract and blood pressure than we do at present.

The statement of M. J. Collins,[7] that "the cataractous process is not an exaggerated senile change, but due to disturbed nutrition of quite another nature, in so far as chemical and not morphologic changes are concerned," appeals to me as a fair statement at this time of the relation of age to cataract. The changes may be chemical or they may be morphological. They certainly amount to nutritive disturbances, and are closely related to the changes incident to age, if they are not one and the same thing. Roemer[8] has gone into the study of the subject from a different viewpoint, that of a direct poison acting on the cells of the lens, and attempts to show that cataract is probably due to the action of some cytotoxin on the protoplasm of the lens.

In relation to blood pressure itself, 200 men having so-called normal pressure, that is, under 160 mm. Hg, of the same general age, have been compared as to frequency of cataract with the same number of men having so-called pathologic pressure, that is, above 160 mm. Hg.

The examinations were made between 2 and 5 o'clock in the afternoon, with the patient in the sitting posture, the arm supported and on a level with the heart, perfect quiet of body and mind being enjoined. The Janeway sphygmomanometer was used, with 12 cm. cuff, above the elbow. Two or three tests were made in every case, and the reappearance of the radial pulse was the basis from which systolic pressure was read. As frequent reference has been made and will be made to pathologic blood pressure, it should be understood that its connection with arterial sclerosis is assumed.

---

7. Ophthalmic Review, November, 1889.
8. Ophthalmic Year-Book, 1906.

Many of the statistics have been compiled from the same material which was used in a previous paper.[9] Since that time 100 more examinations have been made along the same lines, so that for the statistics of the present paper 600 examinations and 555 blood pressure records are available. The paper contains the largest number of blood pressure statistics in association with age and incipient cataract with which I am familiar. Fundus blood vessel changes of arterial sclerosis have been extensively studied abroad by Gunn and many others; at home by Allaman, de Schweinitz and Reber of Philadelphia, Friedenwald, of Baltimore, Marple of New York, and many others, but the conditions of the lens, in association with age and blood pressure, I have found only briefly referred to in journals and at considerable length in an article by Frenkel and Garipuy.[10]

As my own studies have been along these same lines, and are so at variance with those they have presented in regard to blood pressure, it may be profitable to briefly state the conditions under which they examined 108 persons, with mature cataract, before and after operation, and compare the conclusions they reached concerning the influence of arterial tension in its etiology with those I have found in incipient cataract, but under a different standard of blood pressure, at a higher initial age and in men only. They used five standards of arterial tension as follows: (1) Very feeble tension below 101 mm., (2) feeble tension from 101 to 120 mm., (3) normal tension from 121 to 140 mm., (4) high tensions from 141 to 160 mm., (5) very high tensions above 160 mm. I have used only two standards for arterial tension, because I have not found such a refinement of tension necessary or even desirable. The whole subject is as elastic as the pressures themselves, and fine distinctions as to the exact amount of tension are not possible. We know, in a general way, that age, sex, occupation, general conditions, etc., influence blood pressure so greatly that we can speak only of certain upper and lower limits for the normal. There can be no fixed upper limit for pathologic pressure. for obvious reasons, and the lower limit must be arbitrarily fixed. However,

9. Ophthalmology, January, 1908.

10. Studies Concerning the Arterial Tension in Cataractous Individuals, Arch. d'ophth., October, 1906.

certain standards are sufficiently constant and desirable to recommend them for general use.

I have not met with a systolic pressure below 110 mm., and the average of these 400 records is 139.6 normal and 181 mm. Hg pathologic. Frenkel and Garipuy report that five of their elderly patients had pressure of 100 mm. and below, measured by a Laulaine's apparatus, which is similar to the Riva-Rocci. They do not so state, but a narrow cuff was probably used, which would give a higher reading than the actual pressure, which it is generally agreed can only be obtained with an armlet of 9 cm. or wider.

These authors state, "In plain figures the normal pressure never exceeds 130 mm., yet even in the normal a higher pressure may be found for a time." In my previous paper[9] I have reported the blood pressure records of 455 men above 60 years, with 130 mm. as the upper normal limit, and only had 17 cases under that standard, and only 125 cases with the upper normal limit fixed at 145 mm., and for the present paper it has been necessary to compile 555 records in order to find 200 men with blood pressure under 160 mm. Hg. It seems to me that a standard of 130 is too low for a class of elderly hospital and almshouse patients, many of whom must have been hard laborers at some period of life and sufferers from the deprivations and vices to which this class of persons are exposed, and that 160 mm. Hg is not too high an upper normal limit for them.

In reference to such a standard or upper normal limit for elderly persons, Janeway[11] says: "After 50 the average normal pressure varies from 130 to 145 mm. Hg (12 cm. cuff). Gumbrecht places it at 200 in old people, and Hansen at 170 mm. Hg (5 cm. cuff)." Other things being equal, blood pressure tends to rise higher in elderly persons than in those of middle life, just as it is higher in middle life than in childhood and youth. The reasons for this increase are self-evident if we accept the latest theories as to the pathology of arteriosclerosis and high blood pressure. They need not be considered in this connection. Frenkel and Garipuy say further: "We also find that age does not influence arterial tension; among the 80-year-old cataractous we have found two very high tensions (160 and 161 mm.), five normal ones and one very feeble one. The same figures are

---

11. Clinical Study of Blood Pressure, p. 109.

found in the different parts of life." I have not found so low tensions. In 16 men between 80 and 85 years I have found 13 incipient cataracts, 3 with normal pressures 130, 150 and 155 mm., and 10 with pathologic pressure from 167.5 to 235 mm.

Again, they state "that arterial hypertension is only exceptionally found in cases of senile cataract, based on their 108 cases. In 99 uncomplicated cases we have found 80 unelevated tensions, that is, 140 mm., 10 high tensions, not more than 150 mm., and only 9 with a very high tension." They state that these figures for arterial tensions are much lower than those found by them in glaucoma, and that Méo, in 13 old men, taken at random from the hospital with arteriosclerosis, found 177 mm. to be the lowest and 230 mm. to be the highest tension.

This does not seem to be a fair statement of the facts, as the pressures are used to affirm the contention that cataractous persons do not usually have arteriosclerosis and high tension. Without stating what the condition of the lenses was in these 13 men, it is certain that more than 50 per cent. of them had incipient cataracts, and that if they had been kept under observation, and had lived long enough, probably 25 per cent. would have developed mature cataracts.

They continue: "When referring to the properly so-called senile cataract which is not due to any lesion of the deeper membranes of the eye, nor to a general disease, among 99 individuals examined 5 had very feeble tension (100 mm. and below), 30 had feeble tension (101 to 120 mm.), 45 had normal tension (121 to 140 mm.), 10 had high tension (141 to 160 mm.), and 9 had very high tension (above 160 mm.)" I reported the blood pressure in 50 cases of mature cataract, which ranged from 130 mm. low to 210 mm. high and averaged 161.3 mm., their ages between 60 and 85 averaged 68.5 years. The urine was not examined for albumin and casts in the first 500 cases, but has been in the last 100. The examinations add nothing to our knowledge along these lines.

Finally, it is claimed by these authors, "In the foregoing pages we have reported on the results of our researches concerning the permanent arterial tension in 108 cataractous individuals examined by us; the object was to find whether the arterial tension in the cataract-

TABLE 1.—SHOWING AGE AND INCIPIENT CATARACT, IN 200 MEN WITH BLOOD PRESSURE UNDER 160 MM.

		Blood Pressure.			Cataracts.			
Age.	No. of Men.	Average.	Minimum.	Maximum.	Cortical. No.	Nuclear. No.	Cortico Nuclear. No.	Total. No.
60	7	142.8	130	150	..	..	..	..
61	9	142.2	115	150	2	2	..	4
62	14	139.6	115	155	3	..	1	4
63	13	139.2	110	150	7	..	1	8
64	16	139.4	125	155	5	..	1	6
	59				17	2	3	22
					28.8%	3.4%	5.1%	37.3%
65	22	138.2	110	155	8	..	3	11
66	20	137.5	115	150	4	1	3	8
67	16	144.4	110	155	4	..	..	4
68	8	140.6	130	150	5	..	..	5
69	13	138.8	125	155	3	2	..	5
	79				24	3	6	33
					30.4%	3.8%	7.6%	41.8%
70	12	137.1	115	155	7	..	..	7
71	4	136.2	130	140	..	1	..	1
72	6	142.5	130	150	1	1	..	2
73	8	137.5	120	150	2	1	2	5
74	5	135.0	120	150	3	..	1	4
	35				13	3	3	19
					37.1%	8.65%	8.65%	54.3%
75	3	135.0	130	140	1	1	..	2
76	5	145.0	135	155	2	..	..	2
77	5	133.0	120	145	3	..	..	3
78	4	143.8	135	155	1	1	2	4
79	3	138.3	130	145	3	..	..	3
	20				10	2	2	14
					50.0%	10.0%	10.0%	70.0%
80	2	140.0	130	150	1	..	1	2
81	..	....	...	...	..	..	..	..
82	..	....	...	...	..	..	..	..
83	2	142.5	135	150	1	..	..	1
84	..	....	...	...	..	..	..	..
	4				2	..	1	3
					50.0%		25.0%	75.0%
85	2	147.5	145	150	1	..	1	2
87	..	....	...	...	..	..	..	..
94	1	150.0	...	...	..	..	..	..
95	..	....	...	...	..	..	..	..
	3				1	..	1	2
					33⅓%		33⅓%	66⅔%
Averages..		139.6	125.8	150.4				
Total					67	10	16	93
								46.5%

Average age 68.51 years for 200 men.

ous was sufficiently high to consider these patients as arteriosclerotics." Later they say, "A senile cataract is not usually accompanied by arteriosclerosis." I am able, with a much higher standard, to confirm their statements that age does not materially influence arterial tension except in the general way just referred to, but I affirm, basing my opinion on these statistics, that there is a close and intimate association between arteriosclerosis and cataract, perhaps a relation to each other would not be too strong an expression.

And while the proportion of cases of cataract with pathologic pressure is not as great as might be expected.

In considering arterial sclerosis and high blood pressure as causes of cataract, we should not forget that the deleterious influences which these may have on the nutrition of the lens need not depend on high pressure alone, since in a certain proportion of cases high pressure is an incident in the course of and not a cause of arterial sclerosis. It is a common observation that extensive disease of the palpable vessels can exist without high pressure, and it is conceivable that the obstruction to the lumen of such vessels could seriously interfere with the nutrition of the lens in cases where arterial tension is not above the normal.

In comparing the statistics presented in Tables 1 to 4 with those given by these observers, it must be borne in mind that we have used a different instrument, a different standard for recording blood pressure, have studied different stages of cataract and different classes of persons. If the percentage of incipient cataract I have found with arteriosclerosis and hypertension is higher than that found by these observers, some of the discrepancy can be explained by assuming that old soldiers furnish a more favorable soil for the development of sclerotic or connective tissue processes. than the class examined by them, but a large part of the discrepancy can not be so explained, but must be charged to the process of reasoning which enables different observers to reach different conclusions from the same observed state of facts. These blood pressure statistics are in harmony with the observations of the best authorities along this line of study.

It may be of interest to state, in closing, and is germane to the subject, that I have in the past four months furnished about 250 cataractous lenses, from men above

TABLE 2.—SHOWING AGE AND INCIPIENT CATARACT IN 200 MEN WITH BLOOD PRESSURE OF 160 MM. AND OVER.

		Blood Pressure.			Cataracts.			
Age.	No. of Men.	Average.	Minimum.	Maximum.	Cortical. No.	Nuclear. No.	Cortico Nuclear. No.	Total. No.
60	8	183.8	165	220	1	..	..	1
61	7	174.3	160	190	3	..	..	3
62	17	172.9	160	210	6	1	2	9
63	13	182.3	160	250	6	..	..	6
64	12	170.8	160	200	2	2	1	5
	57				18	3	3	24
					31.6%	5.25%	5.25%	42.1%
65	16	175.3	160	240	8	..	2	10
66	7	180.7	160	210	1	1	1	3
67	17	190.9	160	300	6	..	2	8
68	13	178.8	160	200	6	1	..	7
69	8	178.8	160	250	1	4	..	5
	61				22	6	5	33
					36.1%	9.8%	8.2%	54.1%
70	18	180.0	160	220	6	..	2	8
71	6	190.0	160	255	1	1	1	3
72	10	184.5	160	230	4	1	..	5
73	5	188.0	160	215	2	2	..	4
74	5	210.0	170	260	3	1	..	4
	44				16	5	3	24
					37.2%	11.6%	7.0%	55.8%
75	8	191.3	160	280	3	..	..	3
76	3	183.3	160	200	3	..	..	3
77	6	173.3	160	210	2	2	..	4
78	3	173.3	160	180	..	2	1	3
79	2	175.0	170	180	2	..	..	2
	22				10	4	1	15
					45.4%	18.3%	4.5%	68.2%
80	4	185.0	160	220	1	1	1	3
81	1	180.0	...	...	1	..	..	1
82	2	207.5	180	235	1	..	1	2
83	4	167.5	160	175	1	..	3	4
84	1	165.0	...	...	..	..	..	..
	12				4	1	5	10
					33⅓	8⅓%	41.7%	83⅓%
85	2	172.5	170	175	..	1	1	2
87	1	170.0	...	...	..	..	1	1
94	..	....	...	...	..	...	...	..
95	1	200.0	...	...	..	..	1	1
	4				..	1	3	4
						25.0%	75.0%	100%
Averages..		181.0	162.1	215.0				
Total					70	20	20	110
								55.0%

Average age 68.55 years for 200 men.

TABLE 3.—SHOWING BLOOD PRESSURE WITH AGE AND CATARACT.

Blood Pressure.	No. of Men.	Age. Aver-age.	Age. Mini-mum.	Age. Maxi-mum.	Cataracts. Cor-tical. No.	Cataracts. Nu-clear. No.	Cataracts. Cort.-Nucl. No.	Cataracts. Total. No.
110	4	65.5	63	67	1	..	..	1
115	4	64.8	61	70	1	..	..	1
120	6	71.0	65	77	4	..	..	4
125	5	65.6	62	69	2	..	..	2
130	36	68.4	60	80	11	3	2	16
135	21	69.3	61	83	4	2	3	9
140	45	66.9	60	79	17	1	5	23
145	18	70.3	63	85	5	2	3	10
150	51	67.3	60	94	21	2	2	25
155	10	68.2	62	78	1	..	1	2
	200				67	10	16	93
160	43	68.9	61	83	16	7	3	26
165	10	68.8	60	84	4	1	1	6
170	38	68.1	60	87	10	6	6	22
175	13	68.8	60	85	7	1	2	10
180	32	69.3	61	82	9	2	2	13
185	4	67.2	61	73	..	1	..	1
190	21	70.5	60	76	7	1	2	10
195	1	71.0	..	..	..	..	..	..
200	13	71.8	64	95	6	..	3	9
205	3	70.0	63	75	1	..	..	1
210	5	68.6	62	77	2	..	1	3
215	2	71.5	70	73	2	..	..	2
220	5	70.2	60	80	1	..	..	1
225	..	...	..	..	..	..	..	..
230	2	69.5	67	72	1	..	..	1
235	1	82.0	..	..	1	..	..	1
240	1	65.0	..	..	..	..	..	..
245	..	...	..	..	..	..	..	..
250	2	66.0	63	69	1	1	..	2
255	1	71.0	..	..	..	..	..	..
260	1	74.0	..	..	..	..	..	..
280	1	75.0	..	..	1	..	..	1
300	1	67.0	..	..	1	..	..	1
	200				70	20	20	110

TABLE 4.—SHOWING CATARACT WITH AGE AND BLOOD PRESSURE.

Cataract. Kind.	No.	Age. Average.	Age. Min.	Age. Max.	Blood-Pressure Average.	Blood-Pressure Min.	Blood-Pressure Max.
Cortical	67	68.9	61	85	138.5	110	155
Nuclear	10	69.5	61	78	139.0	130	150
Cort.-Nucl.	16	70.2	62	85	140.9	130	155
	93						
Cortical	70	68.9	60	83	183.8	160	300
Nuclear	20	71.9	62	85	173.3	160	250
Cort.-Nucl.	20	74.3	62	95	178.3	160	210
	110						

60 years of age, to Prof. W. H. Howell of the Johns Hopkins physiologic laboratory, Baltimore, from the collection of such lenses in the National Military Home Hospital. Mr. Burge, working under the direction of Professor Howell, has found that "there is a marked decrease in the potassium and a corresponding increase in the calcium salts of the ash of such lenses." The work is not far enough advanced to reach any definite conclusion. I have Professor Howell's permission, however, to report this observation in advance of publication, for whatever it may prove to be worth. A full report will appear later in his laboratory bulletin. Mr. Burge's observation of the preponderance of the lime salts in such lenses suggests that the increase in these salts may be general throughout the body and may have some influence also in bringing about some of the processes which lead to aging and arteriosclerosis. The idea, I believe, has long been entertained that calcareous degeneration is one of the ultimate terminations of connective tissue proliferation in the arteries and perhaps in other tissues and organs.

My thanks are due to Col. W. E. Elwell of New York, inspector-general and chief surgeon of the National Military Homes for permission to use the material for the paper. I am under renewed obligations to Maj. F. W. Roush, surgeon, for his cooperation in the work, which is respectfully acknowledged. My assistant, Dr. A. W. Bartell, of the medical staff, has given me valuable aid and assistance in the last 100 cases examined. Dr. J. W. Millette of this city, my assistant in St. Elizabeth's Hospital, has compiled practically all of these statistical tables, and it is a pleasure to acknowledge that whatever of value they may have, in throwing light on the subjects of the paper, is due to the thorough manner in which he has presented the statistics by the above tables.

MEMORANDA

THE TREATMENT OF SOME FORMS OF LENS DISPLACEMENT OTHER THAN THOSE OF TRAUMATIC ORIGIN.*

L. D. BROSE, M.D.
EVANSVILLE, IND.

For a better comprehension as to the kind of cases to which reference is made in this paper I will enter on the subject by relating the following cases, classified under four groups. Group I embraces those cases of congenital lens displacement where treatment is sought, either to improve the existing vision, or because it is feared that at some future time the lens displacement may set up grave intraocular disease. Group II embraces those cases where the lens has become not only displaced but cataractous because of chronic intraocular disease. Group III includes those cases of congenital lens displacement complicated by acute glaucoma. Group IV includes those cases of displaced and cataractous lens that are the result of acute glaucoma.

GROUP I.

O. B., aged 14 years, consulted me May 18, 1898, because of poor vision, which on examination was found to be due to ectopia lentis, the lens in both eyes being displaced upward and slightly inward. Vision of right eye, 10/200, increased to 15/160 by minus D. 2.50 S. Vision of left eye, 6/200, increased to 15/70 with minus D. 2.00 S. The family of which he was a member consisted of father, mother and four brothers and sisters, all with poor eyesight, except the father, and due in each instance to upward congenital lens displacement. April 27, 1904, he again consulted me, and asked that a discission operation (suggested by me at the time of my first examination) be made on one eye. He was led into accepting the operation (1) because he was now teaching school and

* This paper has been accepted by the Executive Committee of the Section on Ophthalmology of the American Medical Association, to be presented before the Section at the Chicago Session, June 2-5, 1908. Publication rights reserved by the American Medical Association.

found his poor vision a decided handicap, and (2) by the circumstance that his mother had been rendered blind in one eye through an attack of acute glaucoma, and later had been obliged, during an attack of glaucomatous disease in the second eye, to undergo an emergency operation for the removal of the lens.

On July 19, 1904, he entered St. Mary's Hospital, where, on the following day, the left lens was needled. The operation was not followed by reaction, and he left the hospital at the expiration of one week. Dec. 24, 1904, and again April 15, 1905, the needle operation was repeated. By April 6, 1906, the lower portion of the lens had been absorbed, leaving a clear pupil and vision 15/40 with plus D. 13.00 S., and improved Nov. 24, 1906, to 15/20, with ability to read finest Snellen fluently with plus D. 15.00 S.

GROUP II.

E. S., a large and well developed man, 28 years of age, consulted me Jan. 13, 1902, with the complaint that he was losing his sight. The family consisted of father, mother and a brother, all with good sight, and he himself distinctly recalls that during school life there were seats in front for short-sighted pupils, but that his seat was always far back of these, and it was not until he was 18 years of age, and while sighting a gun, that he became aware of dimness in the right eye. Thereafter, in shooting he made use of the left eye, vision in which remained good until a few weeks before calling on me, when, after awaking one morning, he discovered it was likewise dim. He denies syphilis and does not recall an injury or previous eye disease.

Examination.—In both eyes there was downward displacement of the lens, tremulousness of the upper portion of the iris, which stood deeper than the lower portion. In the right eye, there was partial cloudiness of the lens, with vision 15/80, improved to 15/50 with minus D. 1.00 S., combined with plus D. 1.50 cylinder axis 90. In the left eye, there was a progressive cataract and vision 15/50, and not subject to improvement. By Oct. 4, 1902, there remained in the left eye only light perception while the cataract had matured, with distinct increase in the downward and forward displacement of the lens.

Jan. 29, 1903, he entered St. Mary's Hospital, where, on the following day, an extraction operation was undertaken under local anesthesia. An upward corneal section was made, followed by iridectomy. Immediately after the latter and before any other step in the operation was attempted, the four recti muscles were thrown into violent contraction, furrowing the eyeball and expelling particles of soft lens matter with considerable, very fluid, vitreous. The greater part of the lens, however, disappeared within the vitreous chamber and no effort at its recovery was attempted. The eye was bandaged and not disturbed until the third day, when the anterior chamber was found re-established and the corneal incision closed. On the seventh day, violent iridocyclitis set up, and a few days later a small hypopyon was seen on the floor of the anterior chamber.

Treatment.—Morphia subcutaneously, with hot local applications for pain, and large repeated doses of salicylate of soda. Eventually, the inflammation subsided, leaving a dense membrane occupying the original pupil. Fortunately, at the point where the iris had been excised, there remained in the dense secondary membrane a small round opening, so that vision 15/160 was gained by use of plus D. 10.00 S. Nov. 20, 1905, the sight in the right eye having sunk to the counting of fingers at two feet, and notwithstanding our poor success with the left eye and our telling him that the same unfavorable conditions existed in this eye as had existed in the other, so that the percentage of failure was necessarily greater than after ordinary cataract operation, he requested that I undertake an operation on it for sight restoration. This we did Jan. 3, 1907, making a small discission, albeit the patient was 33 years of age.

Within two hours after the operation the eye began to pain, and during the night the pain became so severe that it was attended by vomiting. Hypodermic injections of morphia brought only partial relief, and there being increased tension, with deep anterior chamber and semi-dilated pupil, an iridectomy was made. The choroido-ciliary inflammation gradually subsided, and at the expiration of eight weeks he had vision 15/200. April 8, and again September 18, the discission operation was repeated, and each time called forth more or less pain, soreness and intraocular inflammation, for the relief of which repeated paracentesis was successfully employed. After the last needling the lens rapidly underwent absorption, and our ultimate restoration of vision was 15/60, with the aid of plus D. 9.00 S., combined with plus D. 1.50 cylinder axis 120. However, in the vitreous humor many floating opacities remained.

GROUP III.

Case 1.—Mrs. J. B., aged 44 years, mother of the patient reported in Group 1, consulted me April 1, 1898. She stated she had always seen poorly in the distance, and four years ago completely lost the sight in the right eye through a violent attack of pain. At a glance, it was to be seen that the blindness was the result of an attack of glaucoma, the lens being pushed against the posterior surface of the cornea, with widely dilated pupil, atrophic iris tissue and equatorial staphyloma. With the left eye she counted fingers at fourteen feet, and read Snellen D. 1.50 at seven inches. The iris was tremulous below, and the lens was displaced upward and somewhat outward. Beyond a large crescent to the outer side of the optic disc, the fundus was without detectable lesion. On July 20, 1898, the eye began to pain and by the following day the pain became so violent that she had frequent attacks of vomiting while on her way to consult me.

Examination.—Intense circumcorneal injection; great increase of intraocular tension; pupil dilated and distorted by the transparent lens, which had partially escaped into the anterior chamber. Patient was directed to St. Mary's Hospital, where, under general anesthesia, a needle was passed through the outer side of the eye, from behind forward, and the lens secured so that it could not slip backward into the vitreous while attempting extraction. A downward corneal section was made, and the lens removed by a Weber scoop. No loss of vitreous occurred, and the eye rapidly healed, with vision 15/50, with plus D. 13.00 S.

Case 2.—Mrs. G. W., aged 38 years, and a sister to the preceding patient, consulted me June 7, 1898, when I found small maculæ corneæ in both eyes, due to measles in childhood, large posterior staphyloma, vitreous opacities, extensive disseminated choroiditis and double upward lens displacement. With the right eye she counted fingers at twelve feet, improved to 15/80, with plus D. 5.00 cylinder axis 90. With the left eye, fingers at eight feet, and improved to 8/200, with minus D. 11.00 S. The disseminated choroiditis and vitreous opacity was most pronounced in the right eye. Feb. 3, 1903, she again consulted me, when I found the right eye without light perception, the result of an untreated attack of glaucoma. She remained under observation during the following four months, receiving general treatment for the choroidal disease, then became discouraged over non-improvement, and I did not see her again until Nov. 21, 1905, when she came with an attack of glaucoma in the second eye. The disease had been permitted to exist five weeks without treatment and not even the perception of light remained in the eye. The severe pain she had suffered had almost disappeared and patient was told we were powerless to give her sight again.

Case 3.—J. W., the 43-year-old brother of the two preceding patients, consulted me May 28, 1898. He stated that about two years ago, the right eye pained him for a time and then in a day or two the sight, which had always been defective, became much more so.

Examination.—The transparent lens was seen occupying the floor of the posterior chamber, the iris below the pupil was pushed forward, while above it stood deeper and wobbled with every movement of the eyeball. The cornea and vitreous contained opacities, while vision in the eye was reduced to the counting of fingers at seven feet. By depressing the head and placing plus D. 10.00 S. in front of the eye he saw 15/200.

In the left eye the lens was displaced upward and outward, and he had vision 15/50, improved to 15/30 with minus 0.50 cylinder, axis 180.

On Nov. 24, 1900, he became aware that he was rapidly losing sight in the left eye and that he recognized the faces of those about him with difficulty. By the following day the eye pained him so violently that he had attacks of vomiting. I found the eye intensely injected, pupil dilated; the lens crowding the iris against the posterior surface of the cornea with great increase of intraocular tension. He still counted fingers with the eye at eight feet. Patient was forthwith sent to St. Mary's Hospital, where the anterior chamber was opened with a v. Graefe knife, and an iridectomy made. The operation was accomplished without wounding the lens or its capsule. After the second day, eserin was regularly instilled into the eye. Uninterrupted healing followed, with retraction of the lens into the lower part of the hyaloid fossa, and the recovery of vision 15/30 by the help of plus D. 16.00 S.

GROUP IV.

W. S., colored, 61 years of age, was admitted by Surgeon B. W. Brown to the U. S. Marine Hospital at this port, because of an attack of severe inflammation in the right eye, which had been treated without relief by a general practitioner some ten days, presumably for iritis. Surgeon Brown made the diagnosis of glaucoma and asked that I verify its correctness. I found the patient suffering great pain with tension in the eye greatly increased, and even light perception extinguished. An iridectomy forthwith executed relieved the pain, but did not restore sight.

Jan. 10, 1905, the left eye became hard and painful, and I was again invited to see the patient and do an iridectomy for glaucoma. This not only relieved his pain but restored sight.

Dec. 18, 1905, he again applied to the hospital because of failure of sight and was admitted by Surgeon J. B. Stoner, who in the interim had assumed command at this port, and it was through the kindness of Surgeon Stoner that I was again permitted to see the patient. I found the lens cataractous and slightly displaced downward and forward.

In October, 1906, the cataract having matured, I undertook its extraction. Notwithstanding a general atheromatous condition of the blood vessels and an irregular heart, we were obliged to operate under general anesthesia, because the patient was so excitable and nervous that mere contact of the hand with his face called forth violent starting up and excitation. On completion of the corneal section, made upward, the vitreous at once prolapsed into the wound so that the lens was extracted by aid of the Reisinger double hook. Uninterrupted healing followed, and, while there had been loss of considerable vitreous fluid, vision 15/50 resulted with plus D. 8.00 S., combined with plus D. 3.00 cylinder, axis 40.

In the treatment of cases embraced under Group I we have to consider, first, the amount of vision obtainable by means of correcting lenses and if it suffices for the person's calling in life. This being impossible of accomplishment, we may next consider operative interference, which may be iridectomy, discission or extraction. The age of the patient, the degree of displacement, the size of the lens and the amount of vision obtainable, either with or without correcting lenses, after complete mydriasis, enables us to decide for or against iridectomy.

Since congenital lens displacement is almost invariably upward, or upward and either to the nasal or temporal side, it follows that the point of election for iris excision would be below; hence, the possibility of the lens at some future time undergoing secondary downward displacement, either through elongation of its suspensory ligament or solution of its fibers must not be overlooked. Were this to take place, the benefit derived through the iridectomy would, for the greater part, be lost.

The family history of the forbears, as illustrated in Group III, may disclose this tendency, and I can not too strongly urge that it be carefully inquired into before the choice of iridectomy is finally made. Discission is proper when the patient is under 25 years of age and finds his vision insufficient for his needs. However, I have had the experience that discission was technically impossible of accomplishment, because the lens was so movable that it gave way under the needle without our being able to open its capsule. Extraction is naturally resorted to when it has been decided that operative interference is in place and that neither iridectomy nor discission is the thing to do. It is especially to be practiced in patients over 35 years of age.

Group II embraces a class of patients where the displaced lens is opaque and complicated by pathologic intraocular changes, so that in the choice of operative measures we must elect to do either discission or extraction. After the age of 25 my preference is for extraction, preceded by preliminary iridectomy. If the result is unsatisfactory and I am satisfied that the lens is capable of absorption through needling, I should elect to do this on the second eye rather than to extract. Before the age of 25 years, and provided the tendency to excitation of active intraocular inflammation is not too great, one may prefer the needle operation. A word of caution: Do not attempt to better a fair result through division of secondary membranous cataract when the vitreous contains opacities that in all likelihood will be increased thereby. The obtainable vision in this group will often leave much to be desired, and we must exercise care at the outset and not lead the patient to expect the impossible.

For the cases embraced under Group III, either iridectomy alone, or combined with extraction, must be considered. The position of the dislocated lens, whether it will likely be retracted again into the hyaloid fossa, whether one has wounded the lens or its capsule during the performance of the iridectomy, and whether the lens was previously, in part, opaque or not, must serve in deciding which operation it is best to make.

For the cases in Group IV, only extraction can be thought of in the restoration of sight, and since there is the added danger of the extraction being complicated by intraocular hemorrhage, the prognosis at the outset must be a guarded one. Preliminary iridectomy, if one has not already been made, is to be recommended, and if the intraocular tension is still suspiciously high, sclerotomy may be done ere attempting extraction of the cataractous lens.

MEMORANDA

A BETTER PROGNOSIS IN PENETRATING WOUNDS OF THE EYEBALL.*

JOHN A. DONOVAN, M.D.

BUTTE, MONT.

The title of this paper might well be "A Plea for the Injured Eye." Before this section a year ago a member said, in the course of some remarks, that he excluded all lacerated wounds and wounds of the ciliary body which everybody enucleated. With his extensive experience, this had a definite meaning in his own mind; to those less experienced it simply confirmed their already well-established ideas that all those eyes should be removed at once. At the same time Dr. A. E. Bulson[1] quoted a case in which, in his opinion, a probably useful eye was needlessly sacrificed by an ophthalmic surgeon without having given it the slightest possible chance to recover.

Important as it is that many eyes should be enucleated, and that done quickly, it does not obviate the fact that no eye should be enucleated till each side of its case has had a fair and impartial hearing.

In no other branch of ophthalmology is a practical knowledge so essential. In any other condition, there is time and opportunity for study, but in the case of severe injuries the patient's future depends on immediate resolution. Shall we enucleate or not; operate or wait; remove foreign bodies now or later? Immediate decision on some point is imperative. There are two or three weeks in which you may safely wait; then, why this rush to enucleate?

For some years I have been carefully investigating every case seen in which an eye has been enucleated, and

---

* This paper has been accepted by the Executive Committee of the Section on Ophthalmology of the American Medical Association, to be presented before the Section at the Chicago Session, June 2-5, 1908. Publication rights reserved by the American Medical Association.

1. Trans. Section on Ophthal., A. M. A., 1907, 363.

I am convinced, after making every allowance, that in at least one-half of these cases the eye was removed needlessly. In fact, I know of many very useful eyes that escaped because the patient refused enucleation. The most lamentable cases, as have on several occasions been emphasized before this Section,[2] are those eyes that have become lost or useless through meddlesome surgery. I have sometimes wondered whether if such interference had been avoided there would be so much sympathetic opthalmia. Consider in animals the number of eyes lost by injury, and recall, if you can, the blind ones through sympathetic ophthalmia. Most severely injured eyes are enucleated within the first few days; in fact, the sight of a lacerated or punctured wound of the eyeball, and especially wounds of the ciliary body, immediately brings to the mind of the average operator the thought of the necessity of enucleation as the only method of treatment, as surely as a case of malaria would to his mind suggest quinin.

This paper will not deal with treatment, except in a very general way to elucidate its idea, and for the same reason classifications will be avoided. In fact, the more injuries I see the more convinced I become that there is, and can be, no definite rule of treatment that can be applied to every case. For a thorough consideration of this entire subject in a brief practical manner I would suggest a careful study of that most excellent work of Ramsay's on Eye Injuries as one of the works in the line of conservatism, which I believe will be advanced still further.

I recall two locomotive engineers, now working, with normal vision (with glasses), who had extensive wounds, extending through cornea, ciliary body and sclera, with prolapsed iris and some escape of vitreous. Another patient, with similar injury, including the anterior capsule of the lens, more than a year ago, has now an opacity of about two-thirds of the capsule only, but this is slowly extending; still he has useful vision and otherwise a perfect eyeball. A later operation will probably restore sight.

In cases of prolapsed iris, unless it is very easily replaced, I prefer to cut it off, and, if possibility of infection exists, I invariably cauterize the edge of the wound

---

2. Trans. Section on Ophthal., A. M. A., 1907, 362; also Id., 1905, 83.

with the electric cautery or a probe heated by a spirit lamp. This, to many of you, will seem an unnecessary measure, but the results have been so uniformly good in so many cases that I believe it to be of a decided value.[3] Eserin, though universally advised, in my hands has proved useless.

In corneal and scleral wounds, a stitch is rarely necessary, though in scleral wounds the stitching of the conjunctiva to one side over the wound is often of value. Here, too, the cautery has a similar action, not only in producing a reaction which neutralizes or eliminates infection, but it forms an adhesive material, which seals the wound and hastens closure.

A much clearer conception of my position may be obtained by reading the history of one case.

History.—Mr. I., as the result of carelessness in blasting, had his face, upper portion of body, hands and arms filled with fine rock. The eyelids were much swollen but I could see much fine rock imbedded in both eyes.

Treatment.—They were washed repeatedly, and atropin and dionin was used. In five days the swelling had somewhat subsided. Cocain was used, and I removed from each eye as much rock as could easily be done; this was repeated every few days till the eyes were clean. Of course, the patient remained in bed. Some days later the ophthalmoscope showed but a faint reflex in the right eye; none in the left. Right eye continued to clear; left cleared some. It showed a detached retina. After four months, O. D. vision, with a cylinder, was 20/30, but there was a piece of rock imbedded in the iris. No irritation. Three weeks later lens began to become opaque. Used atropin and dionin constantly. Notwithstanding persistent and constant coaxing on his part, operation was postponed six months more. When active changes subsided the piece of rock was removed with a piece of the iris and the lens was extracted. Operation done two years ago; vision, with glass, is now normal. If our teachings were followed—all foreign bodies removed immediately—this man would long since have been blind.

Copper, brass and iron should be removed as early as a favorable opportunity will permit. Rock, glass and chemically inert matter at times seems to remain indefinitely, without reaction, but in every case must be carefully watched. Washing out the lens by opening its anterior capsule and introducing a syringe is the proper procedure when active symptoms do not soon

3. Am. Jour. Ophth., October, 1903.

subside, or at any time if a quiet eye becomes active and can not at once be controlled. In the majority of cases the foreign body will remain in the lens till all inflammation has subsided, when the lens can be removed with much less danger. Do not enucleate an eye, as I recently saw done by a well-known operator, because of a swollen lens.

In regard to magnet cases, which, unfortunately, in my experience, are the exception, extraction is so comparatively easy it should in every case be done at once. In these cases the eye should rarely be sacrificed. In one case, where I was obliged to make a cross-incision across the entire cornea and iris to extract a piece of steel imbedded in the posterior part of the eye, enucleation was refused. The patient was kept in bed, and now, after two years, he has a good, though blind, eyeball. In another case, a piece of steel entered the center of the cornea and partly passed through the eyeball. On removal it measured one-sixteenth less than one inch. Eye has light perception.

The use of saline solution, when required, should not be forgotten and usually the closed lids will hold it in.

Mr. J., aged 43. Extracted a dislocated cataract from bottom of a blind eye with Knapp's scoop. Lost three-fourths or more of vitreous. Filled eye with salt solution, injecting through the pupil. Result, normal eyeball.

In extracting foreign bodies from the eyeball, a T- or X-shaped incision is always preferable, and apparently closes just as readily as any other.

CONCLUSIONS.

1. Mild antiseptic cleansing—1-5,000 mercuric iodid (preferable), 1-2,000 mercuric cyanid or 1-5,000 mercuric bichlorid or saturated boric acid. Argyrol in special cases.

2. Remove all magnetic foreign bodies at once; also any or all that can be removed easier and safer now than later. Those remaining to be removed from time to time when the eye can most safely stand interference.

3. Enucleate at once only such eyes as have been totally destroyed. Even then it might often be better to wait till about the fourth day to avoid the possibility of any question arising later. All others should be cleaned, filled with salt solution if necessary, prolapsed

iris replaced or cut off and got in the best possible condition.

4. Cauterize infected wounds; stitch when lids will not hold edges in apposition; use atropin and dionin, as indicated. Hot applications are always safe and usually preferable to cold.

5. Keep patient in bed at least a few days, longer if possible, remembering that detachment of retina may have occurred.

6. Never interfere with an eye until you feel reasonably certain you are now doing the best thing, and that this is the best time to do it; otherwise always wait.

After ten years of active practice, constantly dealing with these injuries in the mines, smelters, railroads and shops, by carrying out the above suggestions, I have yet to enucleate my first eye that was not destroyed at once, or did not contain a foreign body, and so far, fortunately, I have never seen a case suggesting sympathetic ophthalmia where this line of treatment has been followed from the time of injury.

MEMORANDA

THE TREATMENT OF STRICTURES OF THE NASAL DUCT WITH LEAD STYLES.

H. MOULTON, B.S., M.D.
FORT SMITH, ARK.

The use of lead styles in the treatment of stricture of the nasal duct is not new. As early as 1867, Dr. John Green, of St. Louis, and, perhaps, others before him, pointed out the advantage of styles made of lead. But styles of this material, or any other, do not seem to have come into general use. Many text-books say nothing of styles. Some advocate gold or silver; a few mention lead; others condemn styles of any kind. My experience with lead styles during the past fifteen or sixteen years has been so favorable that it seems strange to me that they are not more generally used. It also seems justifiable to attempt to show why, when a style is to be used, lead may be entitled to preference.

I do not advocate the use of styles as a universal method of treatment of obstruction of the nasal duct. Many cases will yield to syringing, to syringing and probing, and to other methods; but there remain some cases in which even probing, faithfully carried out for a considerable time, in the most approved manner, fails to produce permanent results. Such cases are seen sometimes in chronic distension of the sac, with or without fistula, and even in simple stricture of the lower part of the duct without distension.

In such cases we are compelled to choose one of three procedures: (1) Leave the patient to his fate; (2) extirpate the sac; (3) adopt some means of permanent dilatation. In the old or feeble, in whom some operation on the globe is called for, and when time is an ob-

* This paper has been accepted by the Executive Committee of the Section on Ophthalmology of the American Medical Association, to be presented before the Section at the Chicago Session, June 2-5, 1908. Publication rights reserved by the American Medical Association.

ject, extirpation may be resorted to at once. But permanent dilatation has been so uniformly and happily successful in my hands, that it seems to me that it ought always to be employed first, when possible. Further, there are many patients who come from a distance, or who, for other reasons, find it impossible to submit to regular and frequent probings for the required length of time. To this class of patients some form of style is peculiarly applicable.

In selecting styles instead of canulas for permanent dilatation, one is influenced by the fact that experience has proved that canulas quickly become clogged with mucus and pus, becoming sources of infection, and at the same time, ceasing to act as drains. This can not be avoided, even by almost daily removal and cleansing, which process is even more irksome to both patient and surgeon than probing. Experience, on the other hand, proves that with a style properly inserted, secretions do not accumulate, the tears readily find their way along the sides of the style into the nose and the patient need not be seen oftener than once a month.

The reasons for preferring lead as the material out of which to make the styles are: (1) It is a pliable material; (2) it is easily cut, smoothed and adapted to each individual case by the surgeon himself; (3) it is comfortable to the patient; (4) it is not acted on by the secretions; (5) it is cheap and easily obtained. On the other hand the other materials available are all objectionable. Aluminum soon becomes corroded, silver also, in time. While this objection does not apply to gold, yet gold is expensive and hard to adjust on account of its rigidity.

I have found that the best lead wire from which to make these styles is probably the fuse wire used by electricians. It contains a little antimony, which in no way impairs its usefulness, but rather enhances it, as it renders it slightly firmer. It is kept in various sizes, according to the amperage it is expected to carry. The best sizes for styles are those of the 5, 10 and 15 ampere capacity, about 1 mm., 1.50 mm. and 2 mm. in diameter respectively; or the wire may be compared directly with the lachrymal probe.

The proper preparation and placing of the styles are essential to success, and close attention must be paid to this important, if simple, technic. After the canaliculus has been cut and the duct dilated, at one sitting or several, to Bowman's No. 5, or even to No. 8, if possible, the depth of the duct is measured on the probe, and a piece of lead wire is cut to the corresponding length, taking off about one-eighth of an inch from the lower end to prevent it from resting on the floor of the nose and allowing from one-fourth to three-eighths of an inch extra length on the upper end to be bent over at a little more than a right angle to prevent its slipping down out of reach. The main shaft of the style should be curved to fit the canal, as determined by the bend of the probe which has been passed. The shoulder or upper end should have a curve slightly down and forward so that it will lie in the slit canaliculus, out of view and without tension. The tip of this upper end must not turn backward toward the eyeball. If it does it will cause trouble by touching the eyeball or by compressing the tissues of the eyelid between it and the eyeball. There should be no tension. If the end sticks up a little, it may be bent down without withdrawing the style.

The style will partly adapt itself to the canal owing to its flexibility, but if the fit is not good, it must be withdrawn, remolded and reinserted till it occupies the proper position without tension. The size of the wire should be the size of, or slightly smaller than the largest probe which has previously been inserted. Before inserting the style, its ends may be smoothed with a fine file or a piece of hard wood. If too long it may be shortened and resmoothed; if too short a new one may readily be made. The making and inserting of the style after the duct is prepared and cocainized need not consume more than five or ten minutes.

After the first few hours, the patient will not be conscious of its presence. It may be worn almost indefinitely, unfelt and unseen. It is a good plan to feel for the lower end of the style with a probe passed along the under edge of the lower turbinate. It is a protection against the use of too short a style. The best instrument to use in inserting and withdrawing the style is a pair of dressing forceps or iris forceps without teeth or sharp edges. The insertion may often be accomplished with fingers alone.

It is best to see these patients once every three or four weeks to remove and replace the styles and to see that all is well. I have frequently allowed the style to remain for a month or longer without removal; in one case for six months and fourteen days. This happened in the case of a school teacher who went away in June, 1907, for her vacation and did not return when expected. However, the condition was good when she did return, late in December. There had been no irritation, the tear passage was clean and the style was neither corroded nor incrusted. So far, the case promises to remain a permanent cure of a very chronic dacryocystitis with acute exacerbations. From choice, I would not leave a style in place so long; but this case shows how harmless the procedure may be during the time which a style is being worn. In every case there is perfect drainage of tears and never any inflammation; hence patients find it agreeable.

The cure may be effected in some cases in a month, in others a much longer time will be required. In one case, that of a woman of 35, I was forced to continue its use for a year and a half, before finally and permanently removing it. In this case the cessation of all treatment was in September, 1900. During seven and a half years since then, I have frequently seen the patient. There is an open duct, no epiphora, and no distension of the sac. This was an especially difficult case. It had lasted for many years, with much secretion and great distension of the sac, and the stricture was almost impervious. Probing had been tried for several months before resorting to the style.

On June 1, 1906, I inserted a lead style into a nasal duct which I had been probing with only temporary improvement for six months. On July 1, 1906, I removed the style which had thus been in the duct one month. Now two years have passed without a relapse. As a rule, after a style has been worn a month or two, I leave it out for a week. Then, if syringing is in any way difficult, I reinsert it for another month. The very old cases of very tight strictures require the longer time.

In no case is appropriate nasal, or other treatment that may be called for to be neglected. I could report many more cases but hope I have said enough to induce every ophthalmologist to try a method which, in my hands, has been uniformly successful.

IMPERFORATION OF THE LACHRYMONASAL DUCT IN THE NEWBORN, AND ITS CLINICAL MANIFESTATIONS.*

WILLIAM ZENTMAYER, M.D.
PHILADELPHIA.

The common clinical manifestation of obstruction to the lachrymonasal duct in the newborn has been usually described under the term "congenital dacryocystitis," a very unsatisfactory one as a cystitis is not usually present, and when present is of secondary origin. Jackson[1] has recently written on the subject under the title of "Delayed Development of the Lachrymal-nasal Duct," an entirely proper term, in a restricted sense, but not intended to cover all the conditions which may give rise to the symptoms of so-called congenital dacryocystitis.

Until the appearance of the paper of Peters[2] but little consideration had been given this interesting and important subject and it is only within the past decade that frequent references to it are to be found in literature. Few of these are by American authors, and these mostly within the past three or four years. Historically, it is of interest to note that in the first edition of the Graefe-Sämisch Handbuch, Schirmer states that until Critchett published his cases, infants at the breast were considered exempt from dacryocystitis (Kipp). Kipp[3] says his statistics show that 10 per cent. of all cases of dacryocystitis, among which were several cases of phlegmon of the sac, occurred in children, under 1 year of age. But it was not until the appearance of the paper of

---

* This paper has been accepted by the Executive Committee of the Section on Ophthalmology of the American Medical Association, to be presented before the Section at the Chicago Session, June 2-5, 1908. Publication rights reserved by the American Medical Association.

1. Ophth. Rec., July, 1907.
2. Klin. Monatsbl. f. Augenheilk.; also Ztschr. f. Augenheilk., 1899.
3. Trans. Am. Ophth. Soc., N. Y., 1879.

Peters that the subject was broadly considered, and a causal relationship established between the clinical phenomena and the developmental peculiarities of the lachrymal passages. The investigations of Rochon-Duvigneaud,[4] Vlacovitch,[5] Stanculeanu,[6] and others, established from anatomic research the existence of structural abnormalities as well as delayed development as causes.

As it is the author's purpose to present principally the clinical side of the subject and to emphasize the method of treatment which he considers best meets the indications, no extended account of the embryology of the tear passages will be given.

EMBRYOLOGY.

The accepted view of the development of the lachrymonasal canal is that in the young fetus there exists a groove between the external nasal, the fronto-nasal and the maxillary processes, extending from the eye to the outer border of the nasal opening. The nasal duct arises as a thickening of the epidermis along the line of the lachrymonasal groove. This forms a solid ridge, which separates, except at each end, and forms a solid cord (Ryder). This cord becomes converted into a canal by a separation of the epithelial cells. The resulting débris, up until the seventh month or later, fills the canal with a gelatinous mass.

ETIOLOGY.

The possible causes of the condition manifesting itself as a discharge from the puncti, a distension of the sac or an abscess in the newborn are sixfold: (1) Delayed separation and necrosis of the epithelial cells forming the cord from which the canal is formed. (2) Retention of the separated cells through imperforation of the septum between the lachrymonasal duct and the nasal chamber. (3) Through obstruction due to annular folds of the mucous membrane which may form at any point within the duct, Huschke's and Hasner's valves. (4) Faulty development of the cartilages (D. Gunn[7]). (5) Partial occlusion by pressure of inferior turbinate. (6) Stenosis from pressure exerted on the bones of the

4. Arch. d'ophth., February, 1899; February, 1900.
5. Beitr. z. Augenh., 1892 (Nagel's Jahresb., ii).
6. Arch. d'ophth., February, 1900.
7. Ophth. Rev., February, 1900.

face during instrumental labor. (The last group is a suppositional one, suggested by Peters' observation that in one of his cases there were marks of the forceps over nose on the side corresponding to the discharge from the punctum.)

The majority of the cases doubtless fall under the second group, as here the cause is one for which the anatomic possibility exists in every fetus. It would seem probable that this affection might be found proportionately more frequently in the prematurely born as the septum is usually present until shortly before birth, but Stanculeanu[6] found the condition of so-called congenital dacryocystitis present only four times in twenty embryos at the seventh month, the period previous to which, according to this writer, the lachrymonasal duct is never patulous. He believes that this observation overthrows the classical theory as to the pathogenesis of this condition. He was, however, unable to demonstrate an infection to explain the cases that he did observe; but Rochon-Duvigneaud[4] holds that to produce this condition there must be an exaggerated proliferation of the epithelium of the canal. Morax believes that infection first takes place after the birth of the child, and therefore considers the term "congenital dacryocystitis" incorrect.

COMPLICATIONS.

A distension forming a diverticulum at the lower part of the sac is an associated condition, the presence of which, often suspected from the clinical phenomena (Vossius,[8] D. Gunn,[7], Addario) has now been demonstrated in section by more than one investigator (Rochon-Duvigneaud,[4] Vossius[8]). This abnormality may be due to a faulty development, or as is more often the case, by distension of the duct by retained epithelial débris and mucous secretion. The latter, as pointed out by Bochdalek, forming a consistent mass, may, in itself, obstruct the lumen of the canal and hinder egress to the nose. Mayou[9] has shown that throughout development the lower end of the lachrymal duct is extremely small and remains so at birth, being partially occluded by pressure of the inferior turbinated bone. That a catarrhal or even purulent conjunctivitis may be excited by the contents of the lachrymal sac was demon-

8. Beitr. z. Augenh., i, 1891.
9. Roy. London Ophth. Hosp. Rep., xvii, 246, January, 1908.

strated by Ollendorff's[10] cases and by the cases of Gunn,[7] where the inflammation of this membrane at once subsided when the duct was made patulous.

Lachrymal abscess figures as a sequel to atresia of the duct. D. Gunn[7] has seen five cases of this nature in infants ranging in age from nine days to six months, in which the method and result of treatment left no doubt as to their origin. Mayou[9] has treated 8 cases occurring in the first few weeks of life the result of secondary infection from ophthalmia neonatorum or from organisms which may gain entrance to the lachrymal sac. Van Duyse,[11] Selenkowsky[12] and others record like cases.

SYMPTOMATOLOGY.

It needs but a brief chapter wherein to describe the symptoms by which congenital obstruction of the lachrymonasal duct presents itself. Immediately, or within a few days after the birth of the child, a small amount of white or yellowish-white discharge is noticeable at the inner angle of the eye. The conjunctiva is usually normal, or but slightly injected. There may or may not be fulness over the sac. Pressure applied over this region may cause a gelatinous white fluid to exude from the punctum. If there has been distension, the pressure may cause the fulness to disappear, accompanied or not by a discharge from the puncti or from the nose. In some instances there is associated a catarrhal conjunctivitis, which occasionally takes on a purulent type.

If proper treatment is withheld, under the influence of winking, the conjunctival secretions penetrate and infect the gelatinous contents of the sac and excite an inflammation which may continue as a subacute condition or kindle an acute process.

The affection is very rarely bilateral.

BACTERIOLOGY.

As might well be expected from the circumstances, a great variety of micro-organisms have been found in the secretion. Merconti[13] saw a bacillus resembling the coli communis. The gonococcus of Neisser was found by

10. Ophth. Klin., Jan. 20, 1907.
11. Ann. Soc. de méd. de Gand., 1892, lxxi, 11-19.
12. Vestnik oftalmol., xix, No. 1.
13. Atti. d. r. Accad. d. fisiocrit. di Siena, 1892.

Antonelli[14] and Mayou,[9] the pneumococcus by Hirsch[15] and the *Staphylococcus pyogenes aureus* by Selenkowsky,[12] and the Morax-Axenfeld bacillus by Mayou. Ball[16] states that the xerosis bacillus, the pneumobacillus and the *Bacillus fetidus ozena* have all been found.

PROGNOSIS.

This is undoubtedly good in a great majority of instances, as it has been shown that in those cases where there is either an incompletion of the cleaning up process or an imperforation of the thin diaphragm at the inferior meatus, Nature, in time, corrects the trouble; but at any stage in the process, infection of the contents of the canal may determine an inflammatory process, leading to abscess formation, if immediate drainage into the nose is not secured. An injury to the cornea, or a marasmic ulceration of the cornea, might endanger the safety of the eye, as evidenced by Selenkowsky's case of phlegmon of the tear sac in the newborn in which the *Staphylococcus pyogenes aureus,* of a highly virulent type, was present in large numbers. Purulent conjunctivitis may be set up by infection.

Considering that one careful observer has found that 25 per cent. of his cases of dacryocystitis occurred before the tenth year, it is likely that chronic dacryocystitis in the child may be looked on as a possible sequel to the congenital obstruction.

DIAGNOSIS.

To those familiar with the occurrence of the affection, its diagnosis presents no difficulties; but to the general practitioner, alert to possible occurrence of gonococcal conjunctivitis, the presence of a white secretion in the eye, just after birth, is a disturbing symptom. The absence of inflammatory phenomena, with puffiness of the lids, the benignity of the course, the usual monolateral development, and the scantiness of the discharge, should ease his mind, and if it does not, a microscopic examination of the discharge would.

Terson[17] has seen in a prematurely born, but well de-

14. Quoted by Vossius, Ann. de méd. et chir. inf., 1905.
15. Arch. Ophth., 1907, xxxvii, 61.
16. Modern Ophthalmology.
17. Arch. med. de Toulouse, 1904, 306-310.

veloped female child, a hemispherical fluctuating tumor, of about the size of a hazelnut, overlying the right lachrymal sac. It was absolutely irreducible and unattached to the skin. The nature of the cyst was problematic. According to Terson, the possibility of such a tumor being a meningocele, an encephalocele, or of the nature of a true prelachrymal serous or fatty cyst, must be borne in mind. The elder Terson removed from an adult the anterior portion of a prelachrymal cyst which was entirely independent of the healthy lachrymal passages, yet proved, histologically, to be made up of tissue normal to the lachrymal sac.

According to Terson the differential diagnosis between prelachrymal cysts of various kinds, and so-called congenital dacryocystitis is extremely difficult. In certain cases it must rest entirely on the irreducibility of the tumor.

TREATMENT.

Varied opinions are held concerning the proper management of these cases. Some surgeons (Weeks,[18] Jackson,[1] Peters,[2] Panas, Terson,[17] Valude[19] and others), believing that as the condition is one which, in the vast majority of instances, will correct itself in time, presumably without exciting any secondary disturbance, advise a simple collyrium, the use of solutions of silver, of pressure, and massage, until Nature has asserted herself, or for several months before employing operative procedures, Ollendorff,[10] Koster,[20] Cutler,[21] Rochon-Duvigneaud,[4], Parsons,[22] Bochdalek and others[23] employ probing or syringing. Peters has, at times used Mayou probes. Parsons, who holds a decided opinion as to the injurious effect of probing in the adult, apparently makes an exception in treating this affection in the young, as he states that a single probing usually brings about a cure. Mayou[9] believes that aspiration fails to clear the duct when there is congenital narrowing, and says that this view is further borne out by the clinical fact that, if one of these patients "is seen before an ab-

18. THE JOURNAL A. M. A., Dec. 10, 1904, p. 1760.
19. Bull. Soc. de pédiat. de Paris, 1899, i.
20. Graefe's Arch., Nov. 5, 1905.
21. Arch. of Ophth., May, 1903.
22. Brit. Med. Jour., Feb. 23, 1907.
23. Fejer: Arch. f. Augenheilk., February, 1907; Rabinovich: Russk. Vrach., St. Petersb., 1902, i, 1206-1208; Kamneff: Vrach. Gaz., St. Petersb., 1902, ix, 29; Levy: Paris Thesis; Jemsolinski: Vestnik oftalmol., 1903, xx; Pechin: Arch. d'ophth., 1905.

scess forms, one careful passage of a probe is generally sufficient to effect a cure." Jackson, in quoting Weeks'[18] advice simply to cleanse the conjunctival sac and protect the parts until Nature has had a fair opportunity to establish a passage, and that if this has not occurred at the end of two months to slit the canaliculus slightly and pass a small Bowman probe, states that he would not limit to two months, or even six months, the period in which it is proper to try milder measures, provided the symptoms are controlled by such treatment.

A successful method, not recommended by any writer, was witnessed by Copez. According to Van Duyse,[11] this author saw a lachrymal tumor rapidly cured by the nurse applying mouth suction to the nose of the infant.

As the possible results of delayed opening of the tear passages may be the occurrence of infection, with its usual sequelæ and dangers, it does not seem to the author a wise procedure to wait on Nature an indefinite period to eliminate this menace; especially as the therapeutic measures advised in the palliative treatment include the continued use of organic salts of silver at home, thus adding to the former dangers the one of argyrosis, the use of massage, a measure to which Ollendorff[10] ascribes the blame for the occurrence of necrosis in one of his cases; also, seemingly, disturbance of the nutrition of the infant (Cutler[21]).

No doubt the danger of allowing Nature to effect the cure would be slight if the patient could be kept under constant supervision, but this is rarely possible, especially when the treatment may be giving no results.

As it seems to be the practice of some of these clinicians to use probes to overcome the obstruction when the expectant treatment has failed, it would appear to me that some such procedure is indicated at once, when simple pressure over the sac fails to give permanent relief. Maternal pride shrinks from displaying a pussy-eyed infant to the critical public, and the author has received from no one more grateful thanks than he did from a mother whose infant had been treated expectantly for weeks.

The result secured by probing in the first case of my series was so brilliant that I pursued the same course in my subsequent cases, and, with one exception, with the same success, namely, disappearance of the trouble after a single probing. In the exceptional instance it was necessary to repeat the probing three times.

Doubtless, for those unaccustomed to passing probes, it would be wiser to counsel measures requiring less skill. For this reason, syringing has been recommended by some, and while it is possible in some cases to force a passage in this way, it does not seem to me to be less difficult than probing, unless the baby be etherized, a measure which I have found unnecessary in passing probes. Probing here is done under different circumstances than in lachrymal obstruction in the adult. As a rule, no resistance is met with, and the probe readily follows the natural passage, which, according to Mayou,[9] is inclined much more backward than it is in the adult, a probe making an angle of about 45 degrees with the forehead when passed through the duct.

PRINCIPLES UNDERLYING THE OPERATIVE TREATMENT OF STRABISMUS.*

EDWARD JACKSON, M.D.

DENVER.

It seems profitable to discuss here chiefly principles that are but partly recognized, forgotten or ignored, rather than those regarding which there is full recognition and agreement. We never forget that the normal contraction of a muscle brings its origin and insertion closer together. But it often seems to be forgotten that such normal contraction does not arise in the muscle itself, but is absolutely dependent on the nerve impulses coming to the muscle from the motor centers. Functionally the muscle has no existence apart from the nerve supply. Even its anatomic integrity depends on receiving the proper nerve impulses. If these are cut off permanently the muscle atrophies completely. If they are seriously interfered with degenerative changes set in. If they are diminished the muscle shrinks; if they are increased it hypertrophies. No operative readjustment of the ocular muscles can be permanent that is opposed by these nerve impulses; none can be completely successful that is not supplemented by them.

Our so-called "muscle operations," done on tendons of insertion, are attempts to modify the final mechanical results of nerve impulses. The position of an eye at any instant, or its habitual position, depends on nerve impulses. Only when we can not alter such impulses are we justified in attempting to change their mechanical effects by operation. The size, strength and habitual contraction of the different ocular muscles depend as

*This paper has been accepted by the Executive Committee of the Section on Ophthalmology of the American Medical Association, to be presented before the Section at the Chicago Session, June 2-5, 1908. Publication rights reserved by the American Medical Association.

much on the nerve impulses going to them, and as little on congenital peculiarities of the muscles themselves, as do the size, strength and habitual contraction of the muscles that give the soldier his erect carriage or the musician his perfect technic.

Normal binocular vision, as developed in man, rests on highly complex, exact reflex movements. The normal binocular movements are continuously guided by the sense of diplopia and the desire to avoid it. Between the seeing of the two eyes and the movements of the two eyes there is the most minute and comprehensive co-ordination, and the reflex to diplopia, the "fusion sense," dominates every normal ocular movement.

Strabismus is a fault of binocular movement. Somewhere in the co-ordinating mechanism, or the structure it controls, there is a break, a defect. The mechanism of co-ordination is still functionally active, although in some respects crippled and imperfect. The investigation of the particular kind of fault in the co-ordinating mechanism must, in each individual case of squint, precede the selection or planning of any rational operation for its correction.

TWO CLASSES OF OPERATIVE CASES.

The peculiarities of each particular case must be considered, but, in a general way, all cases may be placed in two groups: (A) Those in which the co-ordinated movements of the two eyes are to be guided by the visual impressions made on both, cases capable of true binocular vision, more or less completely developed; (B) cases in which the binocular movements must be guided by the visual impressions of one eye, the eye which "fixes." In the former class the problem is much more complex, the operation is to be an adjuvant, carefully planned to give assistance to the development of and utilization of nerve impulses. In the latter class the nerve impulses have been developed, and, in a sense, fixed, and the operation merely adapts the parts to secure from these impulses the best mechanical results.

In the past, operative success has been most frequently achieved in this latter class, because the nerve impulses to be dealt with, those of fixation with a single eye, were best understood. Normal binocular fixation is still an obscure subject, and of imperfect and abnormal types of binocular vision, such as exist in many cases of squint, we know very little. The nerve impulses connected with such anomalous use of the eyes are pretty certain to overcome and nullify attempts at operative correction, planned without attention to their influence. When, however, we come to understand better the abnormal, but definite and sometimes very persistent co-ordinations that exist between the perceptions and the movements of the two eyes in established strabismus, operative measures more in harmony with the real need of the case may yield good results. In Class A operation can disturb the existing co-ordination, giving opportunity for a new one to be formed under more favorable conditions, as with correcting lenses. With this in view it may well be repeated; its aim should be, not so much exact adjustment, as to establish mechanical relations that nerve impulses will tend to carry forward to complete the cure. In Class B the object of operation is rather the direct, accurate mechanical adjustment of parts, making due allowance for the temporary effects of operation, the modifications produced by cicatrization, and the degenerative and regenerative changes that occur in the muscles.

ASSOCIATED ACTIONS OF OCULAR MUSCLES.

Of the infinite number of movements of which each eye is capable, not more than six at most can be brought about by the contraction of single muscles, and only two of these, convergence and divergence in the horizontal plane, are movements frequently performed. Convergence above or below the horizontal plane, like elevation or depression with the eyes directed forward, require the cooperation of two or more muscles.

While, theoretically, a few movements might be made by single muscles, it is not certain or probable that even these motions are thus produced. For the sake of smoothness, exactness and certainty of movement it is likely that changes of innervation occur in two or more muscles for every movement made. Conversely, each muscle takes part in the execution of many different movements, and even of movements in quite different or opposite directions. To operate on a certain muscle, to increase or diminish its effect on a single movement or group of movements, without any consideration of the effects that will be produced on other movements, is to invite disaster, or to trust to nature for a general readjustment, of muscular actions which the surgeon has never even thought of.

The direction in which the cornea is turned by contraction of a certain extraocular muscle depends on the relation of its point of insertion to the center of rotation of the eyeball. As the eye moves this direction changes, and a corresponding change occurs in the influence of the particular muscle. For instance, the superior rectus, inserted above the cornea and acting on a line passing to the nasal side of the center of rotation, when the eye is in the primary position, tends to turn the cornea upward and inward. When, however, the cornea is turned outward, so that the vertical axis lies in the same vertical plane as the line in which the superior rectus acts, this muscle turns the eye directly upward. If the eye is directed still further toward the temple, so that the line on which the superior rectus acts passes to the temporal side of the center of rotation, this same muscle tends to turn the eye up and out.

Only when the eye is in a certain position can the superior rectus act simply as an elevator. The more the eye turns inward from this position the more it becomes an adductor of the eyeball. The more it turns outward from the same position the more it becomes an abductor. The same is true of the inferior rectus, which in one position may act simply as a depressor, but in all others acts also as an adductor or abductor.

In the adduction of the eye the internal rectus takes part in all positions of the eyeball. It may be called the primary adductor. In most positions it is assisted by the superior and the inferior recti, which may be called secondary adductors. The power of the primary adductor progressively diminishes as the eye turns in and the muscle shortens. The adductive effect of the secondary adductors progressively increases as the eye turns in; that is, the power of these muscles thus becomes more and more devoted to turning the eye in.[1]

In abduction the external rectus always takes part. It is the primary abductor. The obliques assist it, but least when the eye is turned in most strongly, so that the visual axis is nearly parallel to the plane of action of the superior and inferior obliques. As the eye turns outward the obliques become more and more effective as

1. Trans. Section on Ophthalmology, A. M. A., 1906, p. 237.

secondary abductors, until in extreme divergence they become the more important factor in abduction.

The superior rectus may be called the primary elevator. Such it is when the eye is turned outward, the inferior oblique acting rather to produce torsion. But when the cornea is turned toward the nose the inferior oblique becomes the elevator and the superior rectus has more influence in producing torsion. If, however, the eye is turned strongly up the internus and externus come to the assistance of the primary elevator and help to turn the cornea up. Their insertions being brought above the center of rotation, they become secondary elevators.

Similarly, the inferior rectus may be called the primary depressor of the eye, its tendency being always to turn the eye down, though least effective in this way when the eye is turned strongly in, and the inferior rectus tends to produce torsion, while the superior oblique becomes a more efficient depressor. But when the eye turns down, so that the insertions of the internus and externus are below the center of rotation, these muscles become secondary depressors. The importance of their function as secondary depressors increases as the eye is turned down.

The obliques may be called the primary muscles of torsion. When the visual axis is turned to the temporal side, and level, so that it makes equal angles with the directions of the four recti muscles, torsion is entirely effected by the obliques. But in other positions the recti muscles take part in torsion; the vertical recti, as the eye turns in from this position; the lateral recti, to a less extent, as the eye is turned up or down.

SECONDARY ROTATORS IN STRABISMUS.

In all cases in the execution of a particular movement the further that movement is carried the greater the share that the secondary rotators take in producing it. In strabismus the position of the deviating eye has departed from the normal. The relative importance of the primary and secondary rotators in determining its position correspondingly varies from the normal. The higher the degree of squint the greater this departure, and the greater the share of the secondary muscles in producing and maintaining the deformity.

Consider the bearing of this on particular operations.

In a case of high convergent strabismus the eye is held in its abnormal position by the excessive contraction of a whole group of muscles, the internal, superior and inferior recti. Tenotomy of the internal muscle alone is but a partial tenotomy, as regards the muscles concerned. The indication is clear for extending the tenotomy to the superior and inferior tendons, and on them graduating it to the needs of the case. Without such extension tenotomy is absolutely ineffective in high convergent squint.

A superiority of advancement lies in the fact that it changes the position of the eyeball, and so lessens the power of the secondary rotators, whose influence is so large a factor in the maintenance of the squint, and renders more efficient the action of the secondary rotators that oppose the deviation. For example, in convergent strabismus advancement of the internus, actually turning the eye out, diminishes the power of the superior and inferior recti to turn it in, and increases the efficiency of the superior and inferior obliques in turning it out.

There is another difference between the actions of primary and secondary rotators, of great importance with reference to strabismus operations. The primary rotators tend to equilibrium with the eyeball in a median position. The secondary rotators tend indefinitely to increase the deviation. Thus, in convergent strabismus, the greater the squint the less the influence of the internus, and the greater the influence of the externus, tending to turn the eye to a normal position. But the greater the squint the greater the influence of the secondary adductors in perpetuating it and increasing it, while the influence of the obliques as secondary abductors is correspondingly lessened. Tenotomy, confined to the primary adductor, the internus, lessens the relative power of that muscle, leaves convergence more a function of the secondary adductors, and, therefore, more likely to be extreme. Or, if excessive convergence is overcome, it leaves the eye with a weakened primary adductor to oppose the abductors, and, therefore, especially liable to turn out.

The primary rotators have a peculiar importance in opposing extreme movements in the opposite direction. The secondary muscles have very little value in this direction. Crippling of the primary rotators leaves the eye in a condition of unstable equilibrium, more liable to deviate under slight influences. Nor is this crippling confined to the muscle operated on. Tenotomy of the internus is followed by retraction of that muscle, but it is also followed by retraction of the externus. It is the retraction of the externus and consequent turning of the cornea outward that produces the desired correction of the convergence, for which the tenotomy of the internus is done. This shortening of the externus diminishes somewhat its power of rotating the eyeball outward. Hence, by the one operation of tenotomy done on the internus, both internus and externus have their power lessened, and the rotation of the eyeball is left more under the control of the secondary adductors, the superior and the inferior recti, and the secondary abductors, the superior and inferior obliques. The eyeball is left in the condition of unstable equilibrium, where the mutually opposing forces that tend to bring it toward a central position are weakened, and those which tend to carry it away from this position and hold it away from the central position are left relatively stronger.

LATERAL DISPLACEMENT OF TENDONS.

Another principle that must come to be more generally recognized in the operative treatment of strabismus is that the effect of a muscle on the eyeball can be altered by displacing its insertion laterally. I have previously pointed out that the recti muscles, all having practically the same origin at the apex of the orbit, come to exert different influences on the eyeball through the different positions of their insertions.[2]

If it were possible to shift the insertion of one rectus to the site of the insertion of one of the others its function would be correspondingly altered. Thus, if we could attach the superior rectus to the eyeball at the nasal side, where the internus is inserted, it would have very much the effect on the ocular movements normally produced by the internus. Such complete shifting of insertion is, of course, impossible, and any shifting brings a bending of the muscle that tends rather to produce torsion. But it is practicable to shift the tendons laterally in such a way as to cause an important change

---

2. Trans. Section on Ophthalmology, A. M. A., 1905, p. 73.

in the effects produced by the muscles acting through them.

One method of producing lateral displacement is by the extended tenotomy, which I described in 1905. This method was probably practiced and its good effects reported, without much theorizing on the subject, by some of the earlier operators for squint. Another method of securing lateral displacement I described as practiced on the superior rectus for paralysis of the superior oblique.[3]

A third method was brought to the attention of the last Heidelberg Ophthalmological Congress by Hummelsheim. He experimented first on the ape. He removed as much as possible of its internal rectus to destroy the function of that muscle. He then split the tendon of the inferior and superior recti, and transplanted the nasal half of each tendon to where the internus had been inserted. The animal was still able to execute movements of convergence and lateral movements toward the side of the excised muscle. Hummelsheim then performed a similar operation on a case of congenital abducens paralysis, in which the eye was unable to turn beyond the median line. He split the tendons of the superior and inferior recti and transplanted the temporal portions to the point of insertion of the externus. The result, reported five weeks after the operation, was an ability to abduct this eye thirty degrees beyond the median line.

At the French Ophthalmological Congress, in 1907, Dransart presented a case of injury to the superior oblique, in which by grafting its tendon on the upper part of the external rectus he obtained a good result. As to the best method of securing lateral displacement, to enable one muscle to take up the function of another, considerable experience will be required to decide. The point here emphasized is the importance of this principle in the operative treatment of strabismus and the need for its more general recognition.

The question of re-education of nerve centers, so that they can execute desired movements with unaccustomed means, is a large one. Only experience can settle the limits of possible achievement in this direction. But

---

3. Ophthal. Rev., March, 1903.

we know that after Motais' operation the patient can learn to close the eyes firmly, without the lifting of the upper lid, that at first occurs from contraction of the superior rectus, and tendon transplantations in other parts of the body seem to show that the possibilities of alteration in the function of muscles are quite extensive. But in the case of the superior and inferior recti we have muscles that normally aid in convergence, and probably to a slight extent in divergence, when convergence and divergence are extreme. There is every reason to expect that they can largely take up these functions in cases of disability of the lateral muscle.

EQUILIBRIUM OF LIMITED MOVEMENT.

When extreme and permanent strabismus is brought about by complete loss of power in a certain group of muscles, leaving their physiologic opponents in unresisted control of the position of the eyeball, it should be possible to greatly lessen deformity, either by destroying the influence of the dominant muscles or, better, by neutralizing it through transference. Strabismus of this kind most commonly follows oculo-motor paralysis, because such paralysis acts on a whole group of muscles. Paralysis of the sixth nerve leaves the obliques still able to oppose convergence. Paralysis of the fourth nerve leaves the inferior rectus and the superior rectus and the externus to take up the different functions of the superior oblique. But oculo-motor paralysis destroys all the adductors, and leaves, unopposed, the externus and the superior oblique to turn the eye away from its normal region of fixation.

Some very good results from the operative crippling of unopposed muscles have been reported, notably by Prince.[4] But I would suggest that it may be possible to so operate on the superior oblique as to make it something of a substitute for the internal rectus by a readjustment through which most of the belly of this muscle is attached to the tendon of insertion of the internus. Such an operation I have done on the cadaver. Vertical deviation can be prevented by fibrous attachments, and by adding any necessary readjustment of the

4. THE JOURNAL A. M. A., Oct. 13, 1888, also Am. Jour. Ophthalmol., September, 1902.

external rectus it may be possible to bring about equilibrium and limited movement near the center of the field of fixation.

In cases of this kind we may be confronted with the difficulties connected with binocular vision. Where binocular vision is absent readjustment for cosmetic effect may not be very difficult. But with the liability to annoyance from binocular diplopia the difficulties of the case are enormously increased. Even here, however, re-education, with aid by blurring of the sight with lenses, may render relief possible.

SUMMARY.

Let us bring together the principles underlying the operative treatment of strabismus that have been here discussed and those that have more commonly received discussion. The ocular movements are executed and controlled by nerve impulses, originated and guided by visual impressions. When these nerve impulses are faulty and can not otherwise be sufficiently modified to produce normal movements, readjustment by operative treatment may be resorted to. This readjustment may be accomplished: (1) By giving greater effect to certain impulses, advancing the insertion of a muscle; (2) by diminishing the effect of certain impulses through tenotomy, setting back the insertion of a muscle; (3) by transferring the impulses so that they will produce results different from those to which they were originally directed, lateral displacement of insertions; (4) by combining two or all of these changes.

Tenotomy allows retraction of the tenotomized muscle and also retraction of its opponent which is no longer resisted. The increase of power secured by muscular advancement may be temporary or illusory. Only modified nerve impulses are required to increase or diminish the power of any muscle. All muscle operations, temporarily suspending function, are followed by degenerative changes in the muscle substance.

Operation on a muscle should be undertaken only after careful consideration of all the movements in which it takes part, either as a primary or secondary rotator of the eyeball. The more important object in the treatment of strabismus is to bring about a muscular equilibrium. Static equilibrium so that muscular rest will leave the two eyes fixing the same point in a central position, and dynamic equilibrium, balanced movements, easy binocular fixation of greatest usefulness around this central point. A less important object is to secure movements, from this central point, of greatest range and with the least expenditure of effort. Where these objects are not attainable by increasing the power of a certain muscle or muscles they are to be sought by diminishing the power of opposing muscles or by transference of muscular power from one movement to another.

MEMORANDA

THE MOTAIS OPERATION FOR PTOSIS.*

HENRY DICKSON BRUNS, M.D.

NEW ORLEANS.

This operation seems to have been practised but little by American ophthalmologists, and this brief contribution is submitted in the hope of awakening interest and of inciting my colleagues to give the operation a trial. The experience of a single operator must count for little, as, in the first place, ptosis is uncommon, and, in the second, not all cases are suitable for this operation. Of some 27,000 cases seen in my clinic at the Eye, Ear, Nose and Throat Hospital, of New Orleans, only twenty-two were cases of uncomplicated ptosis. Three cases were of traumatic origin. Cases in which the eye is otherwise seriously diseased are, of course, unsuitable for the Motais operation, as are recent cases of paralysis, often amenable to treatment. "If other branches of the third nerve are paralyzed, it may be inexpedient to cure the ptosis, because the patient will be subjected to the distressing annoyance of double vision."[1]

Unfortunately, the patients who seek hospitals for relief usually apply so late that no thought of therapeutic rescue can be entertained. Congenital ptosis depends on absence or ill-development of the levator palpebral superioris, or in some instances, it is believed, of the center belonging to the nerve branch supplying the muscle. In these cases, surgery alone holds out a hope.

The operation proposed by von Graefe, excision of a lanceolate portion of the skin and orbicularis of the

---

* This paper has been accepted by the Executive Committee of the Section on Ophthalmology of the American Medical Association, to be presented before the Section at the Chicago Session, June 2-5, 1908. Publication rights reserved by the American Medical Association.

1. Noyes, 1890, p. 264. (Two of the tabulated cases referred to recovered under treatment.)

affected lid, gives but slight relief. The well-known operation of Panas, in which a tongue formed from the skin of the lid is sewed under another undermined portion of skin between the upper end of the tongue and the upper margin of the eyebrow, gives relief, but is objectionable for more than one reason. First, uncovering of the pupil is only to be effected by the same hyperelevation of the brow, by action of the occipitofrontalis, that has already disfigured the patient. It is an awkward substitution of the physiologic action of one muscle for another. Second, the grafting of one portion of skin, still covered with its epithelium, beneath the raw surface of another, is unsurgical, and occasionally leads to unpleasant results. All operations which connect the tarsus with the frontalis by means of buried sutures, or by shortening the tarso-orbital fascia, accomplish their purpose in the same way. While they may be free from the objection of passing an epithelium-covered flap beneath the skin, they attain this only at the expense of leaving silver wire (Mules) or sutures of other material buried in the wound.[2]

The operations of Everbusch and Hugo Wolff, for advancement of the levator, are much more physiologic, but it is evident that it would be useless to advance the completely paralyzed muscle of a long-standing acquired ptosis, or the ill-developed or unenervated one of a congenital ptosis. Certainly it would be embarrassing to attempt such a procedure only to find that the muscle was entirely absent. Nevertheless, I do not doubt that, under such circumstances, these operations may have been of benefit, not by accomplishing the purpose originally intended, but by shortening the tarso-orbital fascia, and so giving to the frontalis better control of the lid. Such an advancement should, however, be the operation preferred in cases of recent traumatic ptosis, where there is reason to believe that the muscle or its tendon had been cut or torn from its attachment.[3]

The unphysiologic nature of these procedures, and the objections and difficulties often in the way of obtaining a satisfactory result, long caused me to hesitate. Therefore, when I first read[4] Motais' description of his operation, its bold conception, its physiologic nature and

2. Wilder: Ann. Ophth., viii, 1898.

3. Oliver: Resection and Advancement of the levator p. muscle in traumatic-ptosis, Univ. Med. Mag., October, 1897.

4. Rev. d'Ophth., 1899.

delicacy of technic appealed to me strongly. The essential feature of this method consists in the grafting of a slip from the tendon of the superior rectus into the lid between the skin and tarsus. I understand that some surgeons have made certain modifications in the manner of accomplishing this, and have permitted the modified operation to be called by their names. This seems to me entirely reprehensible and I agree with a confrère of Motais', who has well said: "Be the procedure what it may, the moment it is a question of grafting a slip from the superior rectus into the paralyzed lid, the operation is that of Motais."

The plan of operation is simple. The usual aseptic precautions having been taken, and the eye having been well bathed with a 4 per cent. solution of cocain and a 1 to 1,000 solution of adrenalin, with the eyeball drawn forcibly down, a short distance above the upper margin of the cornea, over the insertion of the superior rectus (7.7 mm. Fuchs), an incision, entirely through the conjunctiva, is extended upward as far as possible, an assistant holding the lid back and away from the ball with his fingers; the lid is then everted and the incision continued through the cul-de-sac to the very margin of the tarsus. The conjunctiva is dissected up at each side of the incision, and then well retracted, so as to expose the tendon of the superior rectus thoroughly. A strabismus hook is passed beneath the tendon, a snip of the scissors on its end allowing it to pass freely from side to side, until the tendon lies on its shank. It is then pulled forward to the insertion on the sclera, and backward toward the equator of the eyeball, so as to rip up the tendon as completely as possible. A fine but strong silk ligature, armed at each end with a small curved needle, is then passed through the tendon held on the strabismus hook, from without toward the sclera and then out again, in such a manner as to embrace the middle third of the tendon as close to its insertion as possible. The ligature is immediately firmly tied down. With fine scissors the bit encircled by the ligature is now dissected out of the insertion of the tendon and the incisions prolonged upward until a narrow slip, or tongue, comprising about the middle third of the tendon in width, and as long as possible without cutting into the belly of the muscle, is isolated. This is held at the free end by the double-needled ligature, and unless the hold is firm and not likely to slip, the success of the whole operation is imperiled. If there be any risk of this, the tip of the slip had better be doubled back on itself a short distance, and the ligature tied once more around the doubled portion.

The lid being once again everted by the surgeon, the tip of his left forefinger upon the skin overlying the tarsus, with a blunt pointed scissors a dissection is freely made between the skin and tarsus, beginning at the point where the original incision through the conjunctiva met the superior margin of the tarsus, and continuing down to the free edge of the lid at its central point. With the lid still held everted on the surgeon's finger, one of the needles carrying the ligature made fast to the tendon slip is now passed between the tarsus and skin and is made to emerge through the skin of the lid at about 1/16 of an inch from its free margin; the second needle is passed in the same way and emerges through the skin at the same distance from the free lid-edge as the first, but about ⅛ of an inch away, nearer the outer or inner canthus, as the case may be. By pulling on the two threads and pushing the lid upward and backward, the tendinous slip is made to leave the plane of the levator and pass between the tarsus and the skin, until its tip lies under the skin just above and near the center of the free lid-margin. The slip is then made fast by tying the two threads over a tiny roll of gauze. The end of the gauze and the eyelashes had better be cut close to the lid-edge to prevent their rubbing against the exposed cornea.

If the operation has been performed properly the lid is now much puckered and drawn up at its central portion; as would be a drop curtain with a draw string run through the middle of its width. The pupil is disclosed and the patient is hardly able to cover the cornea by his own effort. In this, as in all operations on the lids, the immediate effect must be exaggerated, if we wish the final result to be efficient and satisfactory.

The lid being now well drawn away from the eyeball, and not everted, the conjunctival wound is closed by three or four sutures, equally distributed between the corneal margin and the margin of the tarsus. The last suture, passing through the loose conjunctiva of the cul-de-sac should be applied with special care, and should take a rather deep, wide hold in the membrane on each side of the wound; indeed, two sutures should be applied if good approximation can not be had with one, for one of the accidents described by foreign operators is prolapse of the fornix conjunctivae.[5] Care must be taken not to involve the grafted tendon slip in these conjunctival stitches; at the same time, it must be neatly covered over.

I dress by instilling argyrol solution, covering the closed eye with a disc of gauze soaked in the argyrol solution and holding all snugly in place with a pad of

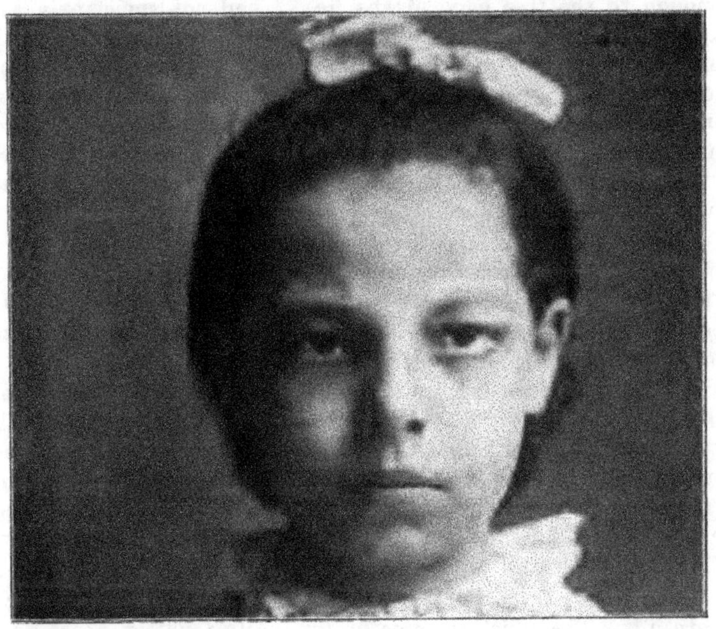

Fig. 1.—Patient in Case 4. Result of operation for congenital ptosis.

absorbent cotton and a flannel bandage. Whatever dressing may be applied should be removed cautiously on the following day, and the eye inspected, to guard against ulceration of the cornea caused by contact with the dressings. After two or three days, if the patient is of an age and temperament to be trusted not to interfere with his eye, the dressing is discontinued, except at night, or a cataract cage may be substituted. On the

5. See Oliver's Case of Traumatic ptosis, loc. cit.

fifth or seventh day the ligature is clipped, and if this is done carefully at one point it may often be drawn away entirely.

Case 1.—In my first case I tied the ligature on the conjunctival surface of the lid, and kept the eye bandaged several days, following the original directions of Motais. To my chagrin, I found, on removing the dressing, a deep ulcer near the center of the cornea. When the ulcer healed, a dense central leucoma remained, and the eye was quite useless.

Case 2.—In my second case I tied the ligature on the skin surface of the lid; a practice, as I see from a later publication, to which Motais, too, had soon been driven. Healing was uneventful, but I had not drawn down the end of the slip close enough to the free edge of the lid. I had not sufficiently exaggerated the immediate results, and not more than one-sixth of the normal pupil was uncovered. The paralysis was of long standing, and there was much redundant, puckered skin in the upper lid. I believe the result of the operation could have been made perfect, by the excision of a properly proportioned, leaf-shaped bit of skin, and I proposed this to the patient, but she declined.

Case 3.—This patient was a comparatively young negro man, with acquired ptosis, and the operation seemed to be entirely successful, but as he ran away before the end of the second week, the case can not be recorded either as a success or as a failure.

Case 4.—G. S., a quadroon child of 8 years, with congenital ptosis of the right lid, was operated on under chloroform, with the immediate result of lifting the lid three-fourths as much as its fellow. Healing was uneventful; the dressing was discontinued after twenty-four hours and argyrol solution instilled every hour. The ligature was removed about the sixth day. The ultimate result was eminently successful (Fig. 1).

Case 5.—J. G., a light mulatto woman, aged 62. Ptosis of both lids. The affliction came on gradually fourteen years ago. She was operated on under cocain and adrenalin anesthesia. On the day following the operation the dressings were renewed, and in two days they were discarded altogether and argyrol solution was instilled every half hour. On the eighth day the ligature was removed, and the conjunctival sutures came away. The result of the operation was permanent during the time that the patient was under observation. Later, at her request, the operation was done successfully on the other eye; but owing, doubtless, to a slight difference in the degree of tension exerted on the two superior recti, there was vertical diplopia, which persisted during the few weeks she continued to visit the clinic. This is a complication to be remembered where it is proposed to operate on the lids of both eyes (Fig. 2).

Case 6.—The patient was an old man, with heavy puffy eyelids, and the result of the operation was very poor. Afterward a lanceolate piece was removed from the redundant skin of the lid, but the effect was still unflattering.

The foreign literature on the subject I have not attempted to review and have been unable to find anything by an American author,[6] except the paper read by Dr. William T. Shoemaker,[7] of Philadelphia, before the Section on Ophthalmology of the College of Physicians of that city. It is an interesting contribution, containing the report of three cases, one successful, one partially so and one a failure. The failure was due to

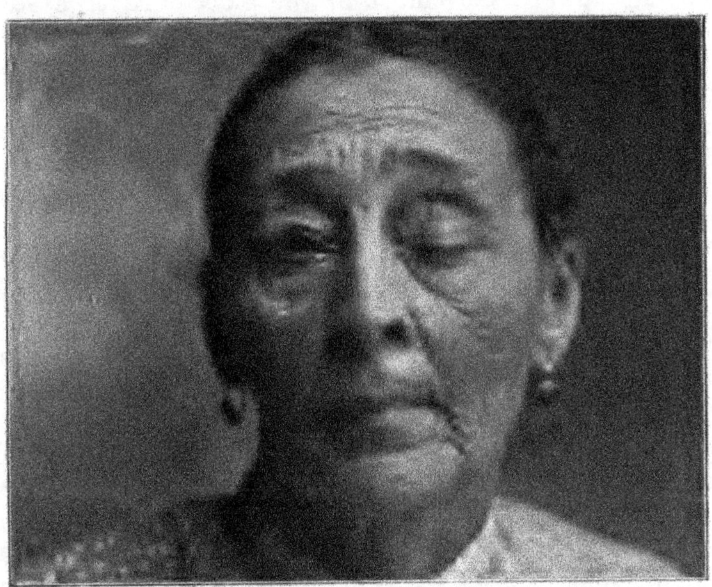

Fig. 2.—Patient in Case 5. Result of operation on right lid for ptosis. Later an operation was performed on left lid.

extending the incisions marking out the slip for transplantation into the belly of the rectus muscle. The muscle proved friable and the slip broke off, vitiating the attempt. We are certainly indebted to Dr. Shoemaker for recording what is, so far as I know, an hitherto unnoted danger. I agree with Dr. Shoemaker that the operation is simple only in plan or conception; the technic, owing to the minutiæ, is difficult. It is true, also, that the operation is not perfectly physiologic, but

6. I acknowledge with thanks the assistance of Drs. de Schweinitz and Edward Jackson.

7. Ann. Ophth., October, 1907.

it is certainly a far nearer approach to normal conditions to connect the powerless lid with a muscle so close to its proper one, as the superior rectus, than to make use of the frontalis. The increased elevation of the lid on turning up the eyeball, wholly wanting in all the other operations, is surely a great gain and approximates the physiologic condition. I doubt that Motais meant more than this in claiming a physiologic nature for his operation, and it seems quite inconceivable that he should have expected the transplanted slip to acquire an independent innervation and, therefore, power to lift the lid without contraction of the whole superior rectus and an upward movement of the globe. After a successful Motais operation the eye can be closed; the orbicularis being relaxed, the lid flies back to a fixed position above the pupil, and when the eyeball is turned up the lid is still further retracted. Can any operation, with the exception of nerve grafting, bring about a nearer return to physiologic conditions in a paralyzed part?

Dr. Shoemaker is right when he maintains that paralysis of the superior rectus is not a contraindication to the operation. I used this overstrong expression in my former paper;[8] the dominant idea in my mind, and doubtless in the minds of others who have fallen into this error, is the loss, under such circumstances, of the supreme advantage of increased elevation of the lid when the glance is directed upward.

I cannot agree, however, that the operation is no more than a fastening of the lid to the eyeball, such as the further modification of Cannas' modification by Dr. Shoemaker would bring about. In concluding his "six steps in the Motais operation" Dr. Shoemaker says: "No conjunctival stitches are required." It may easily be seen, that if the conjunctival stitches are omitted, obliteration of the cul-de-sac and mere fastening of the lid to the globe might occur; but something more than this is obtained when the conjunctival stitches are used and, following the injunctions of Motais, those closing the wound in the folds of the fornix are placed with special care. Then the upper cul-de-sac is maintained and no true symblepharon occurs. Besides, as already noted,

8. This paper having peen published in a general and not a special journal, has doubtless escaped Dr. Shoemaker's attention, as he does not refer to it.

the European operators warn us that two sutures should be put through the membrane of the cul-de-sac if one fails to close the incision neatly, lest prolapse of the fornix should occur. Of this accident, I have no personal experience, having always used the conjunctival stitches.

As to Dr. Shoemaker's proposal to expose the upper margin of the tarsus, by an incision through the skin, and to stitch the tendon directly to it I have only to say that experience would lead me to fear an insufficient result. In all cases in which I have met with but partial success, it has seemed to be due to failure to attach the tendon slip near enough to the free edge of the lid. For the present, further criticism of procedures which have as yet not been put in practice would seem superfluous.

One other practical point deserves consideration. Step four of Dr. Shoemaker's description reads: "Through the free end of this tongue, the needles of a double armed thread are passed from within out." The tendons of the recti muscles being composed of dense longitudinal strands, held together by an exceedingly fine connective tissue, sutures passed through these tendons and drawn on, have, as we have all experienced, a great tendency to cut through the interfibrillar tissue and come away. If this is true of the whole tendon, in which, as in certain advancement operations, we may place the sutures quite a distance from the cut end, how much greater the danger must be in a narrow tongue, one-third the width of the tendon, and much frayed by the passage through it of two threaded needles. It will be noted that in my description of the operation, freely translated from the French of Motais, I have specially cautioned the operator to secure the slip by tying the ligature firmly down before the tongue is separated from the body of the tendon. I believe we should be very firmly convinced of the security of our hold on the slip before abandoning this precaution. Finally, it would seem that as the merits or demerits of the operation are not yet absolutely determined, it would be well for American ophthalmologists to take part in the determination.

MEMORANDA

THE TREATMENT OF RECURRENT PTERYGIUM.*

H. GIFFORD, M.D.

OMAHA.

Knapp,[1] speaking of the treatment of pterygium, says: "I have seen, in my consultation room, a few patients with unusually bad relapses, patients that had been operated on both in America and in Europe. The hard fleshy mass was very disfiguring and so tightly stretched and unyielding that the eye could not be moved beyond the median plane, and diplopia existed in more than half of the field of vision. It gave me the impression of a keloid scar. I advised some patients against a further operation. The result was they took the first transatlantic steamer, were operated on and came back, to put it mildly, unimproved." Later, under conclusions he says: "Pterygia that have relapsed after one or several operations and have the aspect of a keloid scar should not be meddled with."

The condition of this class of patients is so deplorable that it would be unfortunate if this verdict of so high an authority (the only distinct reference to this condition that I have come across) should be considered final. I have seen several of these cases, and, as my experience has led me to an entirely different opinion, I feel called on to relate some of it.

CASE 1.—*History.*—The first patient was a man, 33 years of age, who had a pterygium removed from the left eye four times before coming to me. Each time it had returned, producing a condition somewhat worse than he had had before.

Examination.—When I saw him, a broad tense fold of conjunctiva extended from the caruncle nearly to the center of

---

* This paper has been accepted by the Executive Committee of the Section on Ophthalmology of the American Medical Association, to be presented before the Section at the Chicago Session, June 2-5, 1908. Publication rights reserved by the American Medical Association.

1. Norris and Oliver's System, iii, 839.

the left cornea. The eye was turned in about one line when he looked straight ahead and it was impossible for him to turn it out beyond the median line. He had distressing diplopia, headaches, dizziness and a train of nervous symptoms which had brought him into a nearly suicidal frame of mind.

Treatment.—I first operated by dissecting the growth off the cornea and the adjacent portion of the globe, without excising any of it, and covered the defect by a small lip flap. The growth returned promptly, and I made a second attempt, covering the defect with a large pedicled flap of conjunctiva, twisted down from above the cornea. This operation was also a failure, the immediate good result being followed by a recurrence of the growth on the cornea and a return of the diplopia. The third time I dissected back an unusually large amount of conjunctiva without excising any of it, leaving the globe bare all around the inner two-fifths of the cornea, for a space from one-fourth to nearly one-half inch in width. This was covered with a large Thiersch flap from the forearm, the eye then being held in a position of abduction by a suture passed through the tendon of the external rectus, and the skin of the outer canthus; both eyes being bandaged for forty-eight hours after the operation. The result was a perfect success. The operation was done thirteen years ago and there has been no relapse since; the abduction of the eye is not absolutely normal, but it is free enough to avoid any inconvenience under all ordinary conditions.

CASE 2.—*History.*—This patient, a man, aged 56, came to me for a primary operation for a good-sized pterygium on the inner side of the left cornea.

Treatment.—I first operated by the ordinary lozenge shaped excision; then by sliding flap without excision; then by the application of a small Thiersch flap, which I found after about two months carried well on the cornea by the returning pterygium. By this time the patient had marked decrease in abduction, with diplopia in the outer half of the field. I then dissected back the conjunctiva, much as in Case 1, and covered the defect with a large epithelial[2] flap, taken with a razor, from the inner side of the lower lip. This produced a permanent cure, no relapse having occurred in the succeeding ten years.

CASE 3.—*History.*—The patient, a man, aged 33 years, had been operated on four times by other oculists before coming to me. The conditions were much the same as in Case 1, but

---

2. For some years I thought that the communication which I made on the subject of epithelial lip flaps, in 1897, contained the first suggestion of applying the Thiersch method of getting grafts to mucous membranes. Not long ago, however, I came across an article by Wölfler, in Langenbeck's Archiv, published in the 80's, in which he described the use of flaps taken with a razor from mucous membranes for some plastic work about the eye.

the diplopia and distress were not so pronounced. A free dissection with the application of a large epithelial lip flap effected a cure with the first operation; no relapse after eight years.

Case 4.—*History.*—This patient (Fig. 1), a man, aged 54 years, had had a pterygium removed from the left cornea at least seven times before coming to me. He had to some extent lost track of the number of his operations; he thought it was ten, but was sure of at least seven.

Examination.—When I first saw him, he had a broad, red, deep-seated pterygium reaching nearly to the center of the left

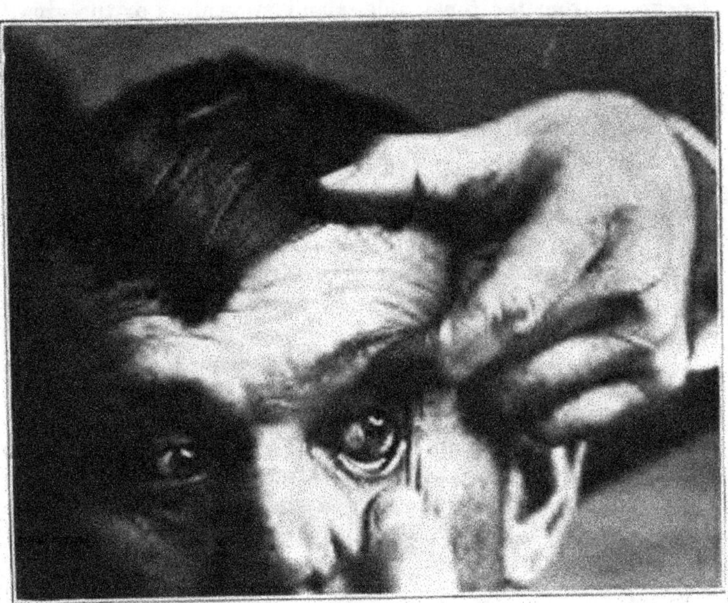

Fig. 1.—Result in Case 1 about ten years after the last operation. In this, as in all of these cases, the flap grew back on the cornea for about 1 mm. within the first month after the operation, but made no further progress after that.

cornea, the greater part being above the middle line. The eye could not be moved out beyond the center, and he had diplopia in all the left half of the field.

Treatment.—I operated by putting on a large skin flap, as in Case 1, but made the mistake of injecting cocain solution under the conjunctiva. This gave perfect anesthesia, but made the membrane so swollen that it was difficult to arrange the skin flap as accurately as usual. The immediate result was good, but (either because of the faulty application of the flap, or, more probably, on account of the deep groove in the cornea, which the repeated operations had made it necessary to make in removing the growth), in six weeks the man came back with the Thiersch flap growing over on the cornea at a comparatively rapid rate, about one-half the space between the margin and the center being covered by it. Then, under chloroform, the flap and the conjunctiva were dissected off and slid back toward the nose, and the bare space on the globe nearly covered with a still larger flap. This gave an excellent result, and as the man promised to let me know if he had any farther trouble, and I have heard no complaint for the fifteen months since the operation, I judge the effect to be permanent.

Case 5.—*History.*—In this case, the patient, a girl, aged 15, had a broad pseudo-pterygium following a burn in early childhood, reaching two-thirds of the way to the center of the cornea from the inner side, about two-thirds of the growth being below the median line.

Treatment.—I dissected this back and covered the defect on the globe with a Thiersch flap. This flap grew back over the corneal edge about one-sixteenth of an inch, but as it stopped there and the motility of the eye was perfect, I considered the result good. But I either forgot to give the girl instructions about keeping the flap wiped off, or else she forgot to carry them out, and the resulting deformity and irritation, which always occur when the toilet of a large Thiersch flap on the eyeball is neglected, caused her to seek advice elsewhere. The result was that in the course of the next six years she had the eye operated on seven times by three oculists in different cities. These operations included the application of two grafts of rabbit's conjunctiva and two lip grafts.

When I saw her again, eight years after her first visit to me, the appearance of the eye was much as it had been before my first operation. There was a decided difference for the worse, however, inasmuch as while, at first, she had practically no subjective symptoms and no appreciable reduction of motility, she now was unable to turn the eye outward more than two lines beyond the median line, and she suffered greatly from headaches and diplopia. She admitted that my first operation had done her more good than anything else, but she still had such a prejudice against the Thiersch flap treatment, that at the next operation I tried an epithelial lip flap. This healed perfectly and showed no tendency to grow back on the cornea. However, the abduction was still deficient, and after two weeks I added another lip flap at the nasal side of the first. For a time, the result was excellent, but gradually, without any return of the growth on the cornea, the lip flaps shrank laterally, so that after six weeks the restriction of motility and the headaches were giving decided trouble again.

Then, without disturbing the lip flaps, I dissected back the conjunctiva and put on a Thiersch flap about 3/16 by 3/5 inch in extent. The immediate result of this operation was excellent, and when she returned eight months later there was no further extension of the growth on the cornea, the headaches

had practically disappeared, and she could produce diplopia only by looking far to the left. This gave her almost no inconvenience, but as her heart was set on getting as nearly perfect a result as possible, I put in another skin flap about one-eighth inch wide, along the nasal border of the flap put on at the preceding operation. This gave perfect motility to the eye, and as she wipes the flaps every day, there is no irritation, and the eye looks almost normal. And so, after twelve operations, five of them charged to my account, the girl is, I think, cured. A tiresome record, surely, which I give for the benefit of the easily discouraged; but will any one deny that, to a young woman, the result is worth the trouble produced by my five operations?

My experience, then, indicates that all of these bad cases of recurrent pterygium can be cured if a large enough Thiersch flap or epithelial lip-flap is put on. Figures 2 and 3 indicate relative size of the flap to be used. In doing the operation it is important, in dissecting back the conjunctiva, to clean the cornea and sclera very thoroughly and to be sure that the flap is

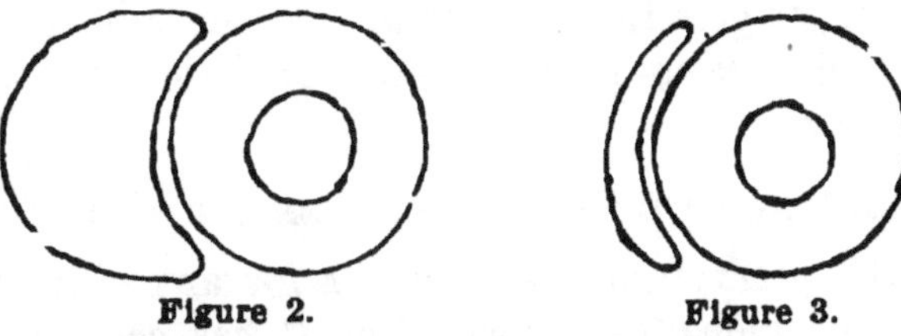

Figure 2. **Figure 3.**

Fig. 2.—Relative size and position of flap used in severe cases.
Fig. 3.—Size and position of flap used in simple recurrences.

well attached to the globe before the lids are allowed to close. The device which I have adopted in Case 1, of fixing the globe in a position of abduction to prevent displacement of the flap, may be necessary in some extreme cases, but if the flap is pressed down firmly with an absorbent cotton toothpick swab, slightly moistened, so as to bring its entire under surface into close contact with the globe, and the lids are held open for three to five minutes thereafter, then both eyes kept closed with a rather firm bandage, with plenty of cotton, for 48 hours, failures from displacement of the flap will be rare.

In applying the latter, it is sometimes necessary to tuck the edges in under the loosened conjunctiva. and I have once or twice protected the well-applied flap by temporarily drawing the conjunctiva partly over it with a suture. The flap should be slid directly from the razor to the globe. It should be cut large enough, and, after covering the defect on the globe, the excess on the temporal side is trimmed off so as to leave bare the cornea and a strip of sclera about 1/16 inch wide between it and the flap.

Skin flaps should be very thin. The best surface from which to cut them is the inner forearm. In obtaining epithelial lip flaps, the clamp which I have invented for this purpose and described eleven years ago is unnecessary and I have practically discarded it. If the operator, with the thumb of the left hand protected from slipping by cotton, turns out the left side of the patient's lower lip, while an assisant turns out the other side, the operator can, with a sharp razor, get as large a flap as is necessary from the space between the thumbs. The assistant should have a moist swab ready, against which the razor can be pressed in cutting the flap loose. These delicate lip flaps should be spread out carefully on the razor, and then slid at once to the globe. If, in manipulating one, it gets turned over so that there is any doubt as to which side is up, it is better to throw it away and get another.

REGARDING THE CHOICE BETWEEN LIP AND SKIN.

For the pterygium operation, or for any other operation on the globe, each sort of graft has certain disadvantages. The chief objection to the skin flap is that it remains skin. The statement to the contrary, which is not infrequently met, can only be explained by supposing that the writers, without personal experience, are copying the statement from others, or that when they have used skin for filling defects in mucous membranes their grafts have not healed on, but have merely acted as a protective under which the epithelial cells have filled in the defects. As the result of hundreds of operations and experiments bearing on the subject, I am certain that a piece of skin, when once established on a mucous surface, shows absolutely no tendency to change either in character or size.

I have just removed a skin flap from a conjunctival sac into which I implanted it fourteen years ago. During this period it had shown absolutely no tendency to lose its epidermal characteristics. On account of not being subject to the friction which skin generally gets, these flaps can not clean themselves on the eyeball and the epidermis collects on the surface and not only looks very unpleasant, but, probably from a certain amount of decomposition, it sets up considérable irritation. On the other hand, if the surface is wiped carefully every day or two, these flaps look first-rate and cause no trouble.

Lip flaps have the disadvantage that, no matter how thin they are cut, they have, on the eyeball, a slight reddish color. Moreover, in some cases they show more tendency to shrink, after apparently perfect healing, than the skin flaps do. Of this I am sure, in spite of the fact that I have cured some cases with lip flaps when skin flaps (not large enough) have been tried without success. In practice I choose the lip flaps when, on account of the age or disposition, a slight redness of the eyeball is of no importance, or when I have reason to think that the instructions about wiping a skin flap would not be carried out. When the patient prefers a slight advantage in appearance at the expense of the regular and indefinitely to-be-continued trouble of wiping the flap, I use skin; also in extra bad cases of recurrence, such as Cases 4 and 5. In such cases, having once stopped the tendency to recurrence with a skin flap, if the bother of wiping it becomes too irksome, or, if in spite of some care, it still causes trouble, it can be excised later and replaced by lip. I have had to do this in two cases.

TREATMENT OF LESS SERIOUS RECURRENCES.

The slight recurrences in which the conjunctiva grows back on the cornea for a millimeter or two and there stops, require no treatment, but when a pterygium returns for the first time and apparently is progressing steadily, without any reduction of motility, a cure can probably be effected in most cases by the application of a narrow circumcorneal skin flap, as originally proposed by Dr. F. C. Hotz, to whom we owe the introduction of the Thiersch flap in the treatment of pterygium. In general, however, I believe we can more surely prevent a second recurrence by using a somewhat larger flap, applied as in Figure 3. Whether to use skin or thin lip flaps for this purpose can be determined by the considerations indicated above.

THE PREVENTION OF RECURRENCES.

In discussing the prophylactic treatment of recurrent pterygium, one might legally drag in all the various operations that have been tried as primary measures, but on this point I will merely say that, after trying a number of different operations, I have settled on the McReynolds operation as that which gives the smallest proportion of recurrences. I operate on about sixty cases every year, and, as I always tell patients that there is no hurry about an operation unless the growth is at least half way to the center, I do not operate on more than two-thirds of the cases that I see. Recurrences with McReynolds' operation have amounted to about 2 per cent.

I have made some very slight deviations from McReynolds' original plan; first, in using a single needle instead of a double needle thread. By passing the needle first through the conjunctiva at the bottom of the pocket, then up through the point of the pterygium, then back down to the bottom of the pocket again, one gets exactly the same result without the bother of a double needle. I also think it worth while to cut off part of the covering of the pocket in some cases where, after drawing the tip of the pterygium down under the conjunctiva, quite a redundant flap is left above it. This serves no useful purpose, as the surface is covered entirely without it; it merely makes a somewhat unsightly lump which I believe has favored the recurrences in the few cases in which I have seen the growth come back.

Other points to be considered in a primary operation are the use of a very sharp knife in dissecting off the growth from the cornea, so as to leave practically nothing of the growth and yet to take off as little as possible of the corneal tissue. It is also important to scrape the exposed sclera very clean, and where, within a day or two after the operation, a margin of fibrin can be seen extending for one or two mm. over the corneal edge, I believe it is well to scrape this off once or twice until the corneal epithelium has a chance to cover the defect.

RESTORATION OF THE CONJUNCTIVAL CUL-DE-SAC FOR THE INSERTION OF AN ARTIFICIAL EYE.*

M. WIENER, M.D.

ST. LOUIS.

Wherever great difficulty is encountered in combating a certain disease or condition, we also find numerous methods for its relief. Thus when we have an orbital socket contracted by scars from burns or otherwise, we have the choice of many modes of procedure for restoring its depth so that it may retain a glass eye. Knapp[1] states that of the numerous attempts in the past twenty-five years which have been made to remedy this unfortunate condition he has not seen a single case either of his own or of others where there had been more than temporary improvement; this, too, including cases where the only object was to fit a stump for the prothesis of an artificial eye. Fuchs says cases of extensive symblepharon are incurable.

Czermak[2] says there are many devices for relief of symblepharon, but few are successful. Nine years ago May[3] reported the restoration of the conjunctival cul-de-sac by means of Thiersch's skin grafts, in which he used a porcelain shell covered with grafts from the arm or thigh, the shell being held in place by three stitches in the lid. Hotz[4] and Woodruf[5] have employed similar means, using a lead plate covered with skin grafts; while Wilder[6] found paraffin plates most advantageous in keeping the grafts immovable.

---

* This paper has been accepted by the Executive Committee of the Section on Ophthalmology of the American Medical Association, to be presented before the Section at the Chicago Session, June 2-5, 1908. Publication rights reserved by the American Medical Association.

1. Norris and Oliver, System Diseases of Eye.
2. Augenärztlichen Operationen, 1893.
3. Arch. Ophth., 1899, 182.
4. Ann. Ophth., 1905.
5. Ann. Ophth., April, 1903.
6. THE JOURNAL A. M. A., 1906, xlvii.

Leslie Paton[7] successfully relieved a case of symblepharon by sewing a piece of mucous membrane from the roof of a frog's mouth. Maxwell[8] uses skin flaps from the lid with good results, but there remains a scar on the cheek and some objectionable puckering. There

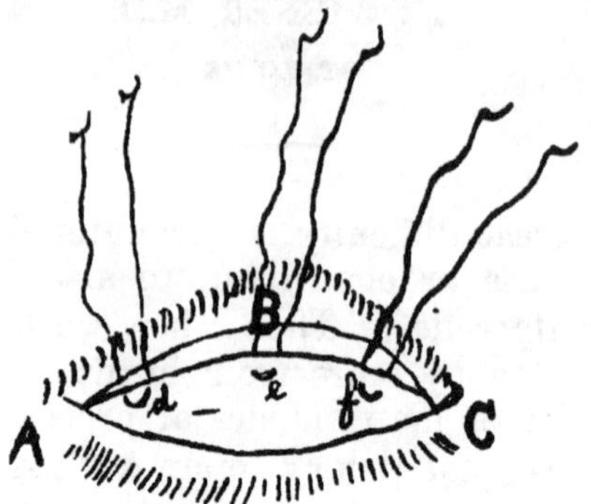

Figure 1.

have been methods similar to these devised by Pravosud, LaGrange,[9] Wicherkiewicz, Bruch, Gidney,[10] and others, but all along the same lines.

My method has its use where the socket, while shrunken, has still a small amount of conjunctiva left. An incision (A, B, C, Fig. 1) is made through the conjunctiva and a flap, including only the conjunctiva, is carefully dissected down to the lid margin (A C, Fig. 1). This dissection after being started with a knife can

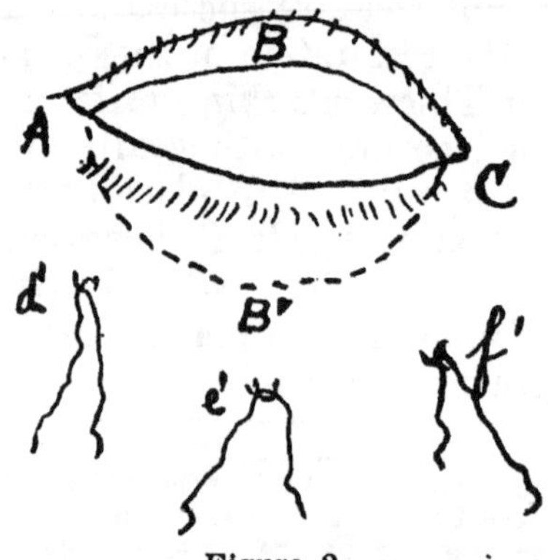

Figure 2.

7. Lancet, April 23, 1904.
8. Ophth. Rev., 1903.
9. Arch. d'Ophth., 1905.
10. Indian Med. Gaz., 1904.

easily and quickly be finished with a small curved blunt scissors. The dissection is then continued with the scissors so as to loosen the skin below the lid margin (A C to B, Fig. 2), leaving a raw surface toward the bulbar side extended from B to B′ and A to C (Fig. 2), and on the palpebral side A B C (Fig. 2). Then sutures with a needle on either end are introduced at the points d, e, f (Fig. 1), and passing them through the bottom of the newly made sulcus are brought through the skin at d′ e′ f′ (Fig. 2) and tied over a button. This gives a conjunctival covering for the lower lid and leaves the bulbar surface A B C B′ (Fig. 2) to be covered. This is done by covering a lead plate, previously shaped, with grafts from the thigh and placing carefully in position. A dressing is then applied and both eyes bandaged, the patient remaining undisturbed in bed for four days, when the outside dressings are replaced by clean ones without disturbing the plate. On about the eighth day the plate may be removed, cleaned and replaced. The glass eye can usually be worn by the tenth or fourteenth day. The stitches at d′ e′ f′ (Fig. 2) are not removed, but are tightened each day after the fourth day until they pull through. This is an additional help to holding the lower sulcus intact, as the internal scars resulting tend constantly to pull on the bottom of the sulcus and thus heighten the effect. It is important that these stitches should be allowed to pull through and not be removed before, for one is tempted to remove them after a week when the lower sulcus may appear too deep. I have made this mistake, thinking I had secured a lower sulcus of exaggerated depth, when, on removing the stitches, it rose too high and became almost obliterated, so that the stitches had to be replaced. The following cases are of patients treated in the above manner:

Case 1.—*Patient.*—Miss H. P., aged 28, of Helena, Mont.

History.—Lost left eye, when 8 years of age, following measles. Evisceration performed by a prominent ophthalmologist in Kansas City. She was able to wear an artificial eye for six years, when the socket became inflamed, contracted, and expelled the eye. Was treated until inflammation subsided, and then, being unable to wear a glass eye, was operated on three successive times by one ophthalmologist, and once by another, without success. Since then she had been told by several others that nothing could be done and that further operative procedure would be useless. She was compelled to wear dark glasses to hide the deformity, which was very embarrassing.

Examination.—Patient came to me for examination Oct. 8, 1904, and examination showed a much shrunken socket, traversed by scars, with no lower sulcus and a very shallow upper one.

Operation.—On Oct. 11, 1904, the above described operation was performed at Washington University Hospital under local anesthesia, skin for the grafts being taken from the arms. Both eyes were bandaged and not disturbed until the fourth day, when the outside dressing was removed, stitches tightened, and fresh dressing applied. October 24 the dressings were entirely removed, lead plate taken out, and a reform eye inserted. This was worn continuously for three days, being taken out only to be cleaned; and on October 27 the eye was worn

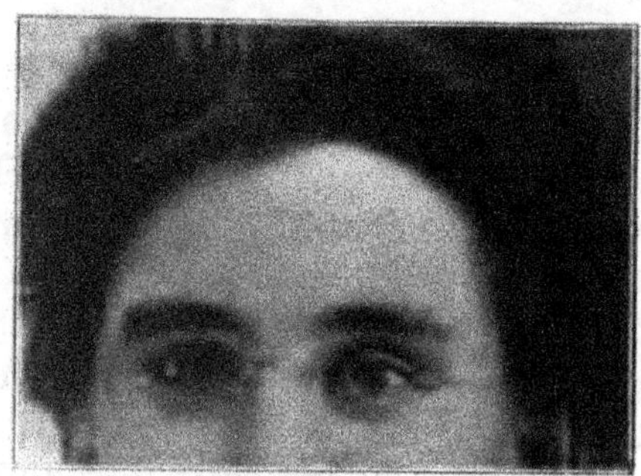

Figure 3.

all day and taken out at night. Two of the stitches were pulled out on the eleventh day and the inner one pulled out on the fifteenth. The photograph (Fig. 3), shows the appearance of patient wearing a Snellen reform artificial eye three years after the operation. As will be seen, there is practically no sinking of the upper lid, while the eye has good movement.

CASE 2.—*Patient.*—Miss N. S., aged 17, Macedonia, Ill., came to Washington University Hospital Feb. 5, 1907.

History.—The patient had an atresic left eye due to a wound from a 22-caliber bullet, which had gone through the lower lid and lodged in the globe. There was a gap in the center of the lower lid margin and almost complete symblepharon of lower lid.

Operation.—The eye was enucleated the following day, at the same time the edges of the lower lid were approximated. On February 27 the above described operation was done and the patient treated in much the same manner as in Case 1. She is now able to wear a well-fitting artificial eye.

Cases 3 and 4.—Two other patients also were operated on at the Jewish Hospital, one on Nov. 26, 1907, and the other on Dec. 27, 1907. The immediate results in these cases have been good, but I have not thought it wise to report them in detail as they are of too recent date.

My reason for presenting this method is that my greatest difficulty heretofore, and also of my friends whom I have questioned, has been to establish a sufficiently deep lower sulcus. This operation has seemed to have overcome this difficulty.

MEMORANDA

A FURTHER CONTRIBUTION TO PALLIATIVE OPERATIONS FOR BRAIN TUMOR.*

WILLIAM G. SPILLER, M.D.

Professor of Neuropathology and Associate Professor of Neurology in the University of Pennsylvania.

PHILADELPHIA.

Since the publication of the paper by Dr. Charles H. Frazier and myself,[1] some articles of much interest bearing on decompressive operations have appeared. It is the author's intention to refer briefly to the more important of these, to report some cases not included in the former paper with Dr. Frazier, to discuss palliative operation where choked disc is the only important sign of intracranial disease, and to report cases of this character, to speak of rapid increase of blindness under certain conditions as a result of decompression, and of palliative operation performed when the respiration has ceased, but the heart is continuing to beat; and to give the present condition of some of the patients described in the previous paper.

Recurrence of choked discs may occur after decompression, as described by de Schweinitz and Thomson.[2] Their patient was trephined for the relief of the symptoms of a tumor, believed to be situated in the right motor area. The tumor was not removed. Three and one-half months after operation the double optic neuritis had subsided and there was postneuritic atrophy. One year later the patient returned with all the symptoms of brain tumor re-established, from which he had

* This paper has been accepted by the Executive Committee of the Section on Ophthalmology of the American Medical Association, to be presented before the Section at the Chicago Session, June 2-5, 1908. Publication rights reserved by the American Medical Association.

* From the Department of Neurology and the Laboratory of Neuropathology of the University of Pennsylvania.

1. The Journal A. M. A., Sept. 1, 1906, p. 679.
2. Arch. Ophth., 1905, xxiv.

been entirely free, totally blind and with double optic neuritis, the apex of each swelling being 6 D., or as high as it had been before the original operation.

De Schweinitz[3] states that his experience has been somewhat as follows: Usually there is no marked change in the swollen nerve head after trephining in which the dura has been opened, or after the removal of a tumor, until the tenth to the fourteenth day. He has not seen decided subsidence of engorgement edema at the end of forty-eight hours, except in one instance, when within that period, following the removal of a cerebellar cyst, there was a decline of several diopters in the height of the swollen papilla. It is not uncommon to find within the first thirty-six hours, and even earlier, a diminution in the congestion of the retinal vessels. After the tenth to the fourteenth day there is gradual subsidence of the neuritis, from six weeks to two months being required for its complete disappearance. The ultimate vision may be (a) better than that which existed prior to the operation; (b) equal to that which existed prior to the operation; (c) worse than that which existed prior to the operation. Sometimes total blindness results.

In the cases with preservation of vision, either as good as or better than that which the patient possessed before the operation, the sight may be better in one eye than in the other, or exceedingly defective in one eye and good in the other, or one eye may be blind and the other retain or regain excellent vision. The most satisfactory results follow the reduction of great intracranial pressure, provided the papillitis or choked disc has not so long existed that it has already destroyed the optic nerve fibers. He gives the results in three cases.

In a certain number of cases de Schweinitz found that during the first day or two after trephining there may be a slight increase in the neuritis, or a slight increase in edema, associated with fresh hemorrhages. This is apparently of no importance, as the added edema and fresh hemorrhages disappear in the subsequent general subsidence of the swelling. In some of these cases there are marked degenerative changes in the retinal vessels. De Schweinitz, on several occasions, noticed a temporary depreciation of vision within the first week

3. Univ. Penn. Med. Bull., April and May, 1906, and personal communication.

after the operation, probably due to shock or hemorrhage, and which, apparently, is of no importance in the subsequent preservation of vision, provided the primary vision has been good and the neuritis of comparatively short duration. Where little vision exists prior to trephining, this may rapidly disappear after trephining, especially if there has been much hemorrhage.

Bruns,[4] in his excellent work on tumors of the nervous system, puts the matter of decompression in this manner: "Shall one refuse this possibility [palliative operation] of considerable relief from the disorder to those in whom a localizing diagnosis is not possible even after longer observation, or removal is unattainable? I think we are not justified in so doing." In speaking of saving sight by decompression, Bruns mentions that many persons with brain tumor may live long, and that all the symptoms of tumor may disappear spontaneously, except that blindness may become complete. Such a case seems to be Case 5 of the paper by Dr. Frazier and myself, which is referred to further on in this article. In cases of this character, decompression would probably have saved the sight.

The danger of blindness is great when vision begins to fail with choked discs, and flecks of fatty degeneration in the retina are always serious. If the tumor implicates the basal visual tracts, decompression can not prevent blindness. Usually, this may be recognized by typical contraction of the visual field, and then decompression is not to be recommended.

Some have held that it would be well to rest content with decompression when the tumor is in the posterior cranial fossa, and not to attempt its removal because of the danger in so doing; this opinion Bruns does not share. I must confess that I am partly persuaded that in many cases decompression is the best procedure, as the attempt to remove a tumor of the posterior cranial fossa usually terminates fatally, or the condition of the patient after the removal of a tumor from the cerebellopontile angle is so pitiable that death is welcomed as a release. It is true that a few brilliant cases are on record, but many failures are recorded. Further improvement in technic may make these operations on the posterior cranial fossa more successful. I am referring

4. Die Geschwülste des Nervensystems, 2d edition, p. 282.

especially to the cases in which the tumor is in the cerebello-pontile angle.

Relief of pressure is not obtained in all cases by trephining and opening the dura to allow escape of fluid, and the decompression is not without danger. Bruns advises against it when the patient is in deep stupor, and, at the same time, the symptoms indicate that the tumor is very large; palliative operation could only serve to restore a consciousness which mercifully has been lost. He is not referring to decompression in the sudden attacks of syncope in cases of brain tumor; such as I have seen repeatedly. Bruns thinks the dura must be opened in palliative operations, and this view I fully share. In one of his cases, Bruns recommended operation over the left parietal lobe, the prolapse of the brain that followed caused ataxia and optic aphasia, so that under some conditions the results of decompression may be serious. A less important region should be chosen for decompression.

When the cerebrospinal fluid does not escape after trephining, and relief of pressure is not obtained, Bruns recommends puncture of the ventricle, following the teaching of Wernicke, Sahli, Kocher, and von Bergmann. Continuous drainage may be employed. Lumbar puncture Bruns regards as dangerous in brain tumor, as the medulla oblongata may be crowded into the foramen magnum and obstruct it so as to prevent the escape of fluid. This opinion experience has fully confirmed.

It is necessary to mention that some authors speak of trephining as synonymous with decompression. The opening in the skull should be larger than that made by a trephine when relief of pressure is sought.

Alfred Saenger[5] reports 19 cases of brain tumor with palliative operation. In two cases, improvement occurred after the trephine opening was enlarged so that more cerebrospinal fluid could escape. In two cases trephining had no beneficial results as the tumor was too large. The condition was made worse only in one case, and in this the tumor was at the base. In all the other cases beneficial results were evident. Saenger states that Finkh, in 1904, collected 31 cases from the literature; in 30 of these the choked disc disappeared; in one case the symptoms increased. According to his

5. Klin. Monatsbl. f. Augenheilk., 1907, p. 145.

statistics, palliative operation causes improvement of vision in 73 per cent. of the cases.

Saenger chooses as the time for operation the commencement of diminished visual acuity. He selects the region where the tumor is supposed to be, but when this is impracticable he recommends the decompression to be done over the right parietal region.

Lumbar puncture, or puncture of the lateral ventricle, is not to be compared with decompression, as either method is much less effective than decompression.

The dura was always opened in von Krüdener's[6] cases. Only those patients were operated on who were in danger of complete blindness and were in a late stage, otherwise the author thinks the results probably would have been better. He states as certain that trephining causes altered conditions of the circulation and brings about a reduction of the choked discs, which is noticed in the first twenty-four hours following a diminution in the congestion of the blood vessels. The diminution in the swelling begins, however, on the second or third day, and the swelling does not completely disappear after two or three weeks, as the papillæ are still somewhat elevated. If the trephine opening grows together in such a way as to cause a continuance of the intracranial pressure, the papillæ soon attain their former prominence.

He does not hold a very positive opinion regarding the effect of trephining on inflammation of the optic nerve, as he had only one case in which probably basal meningitis was present, although the result seemed to be good. He has not observed a sudden reduction in the papilla immediately after the operation, although he has observed the eyegrounds during and immediately after the opening of the cranium. The change was always very gradual, and not until the evening following the operation or the next day could he say positively that the veins were somewhat smaller and the papilla and adjacent retina somewhat paler, although the arteries were not wider. Changes in the hemorrhages, in degenerative foci in the macula, or in the edema of the retina when present were always slight.

Subjective disturbance, unconsciousness, especially from brain tumor, disappear at times entirely, and he thinks trephining is proper when pain and the feeling as

---

6. v. Graefe's Arch., 1907, lxv, 69.

though the head would burst are present and blindness threatens, although he believes that a tumor grows more rapidly after the cranium is opened. The pressure of the distended third ventricle and of the distended floor of this ventricle on the chiasm can be removed at times by trephining. After we learn to distinguish between increased intracranial pressure of inflammatory origin and that of non-inflammatory origin, trephining will be more advantageous. There is more danger of prolapse of the brain with hydrocephalus in children. In hydrocephalus of childhood he found that the protruding brain so closed the opening in the skull in some instances that no liquid escaped and the bandages remained dry; in other cases the bandages were soaked the day following the operation.

Single or repeated lumbar puncture in twelve cases of brain tumor produced no effect on the choked discs. Also in cerebral tuberculosis lumbar puncture produced no improvement in the condition of the eyegrounds. Division of the dura of the optic nerve, recommended by de Wecker, was useless, and some stretching of the nerve occurred because of the small field of operation. In a case of cerebral tuberculous meningitis, in which an exudate was found in the sheaths of the optic nerves. lumbar puncture produced no visible change in the eyegrounds. Lumbar puncture has been believed by quite a large number of writers to aid in recovery from meningitis, and where this occurs it may affect the optic nerves, and it should be employed in syphilitic meningitis with papillitis. The effect is not to be determined by the ophthalmoscope, and consists probably in slight relief of pressure from the papillæ and brain, so that more blood may reach the diseased parts.

von Krüdener observed in one case that after removal of the brain pressure meningitis developed on the brain and optic nerves, and notwithstanding the intense inflammation the choked disc gradually and constantly diminished. This would seem to me to indicate that decompression may be useful in inflammatory conditions. but in a case of purulent meningitis, that Dr. Frazier and I recently have had, palliative operation was followed by death within a few days. von Krüdener and others (Brüns) have observed that after trephining in hydrocephalus choked disc disappeared, although no liquid escaped on account of the prolapse of the brain.

It is not necessary to assume the existence of phlogogenous substances in the cerebrospinal fluid to explain the choked disc of brain tumor and of hydrocephalus, and the inflammatory appearances so often present are a result of stagnation of lymph and of edema. In local brain pressure von Krüdener accepts the opinion of von Graefe, and explains them as the result of compression of the cavernous sinus and congestion in its venous tributaries. He thinks the future must decide whether it would be advisable to remove the bone about the cmasm under certain conditions to relieve choked discs. He has done puncture of the ventricle twice with the drill, according to Kocher's idea; the cases were not very suitable and the choking was not affected thereby. Wilbrand and Saenger[7] believe that when the pressure is lowered in the spinal canal the medulla oblongata is pressed downward, and until the pressure is restored the circulation of fluid from the cranium to the spinal column is prevented.

Lumbar puncture has usually little effect on choked disc for several reasons, the pressure is not always the same in the vertebral cavity and the cranial cavity, and probably is higher in the cerebral ventricles than in the sheath of the optic nerve. After lumbar puncture the pressure on the brain is relieved and the circulation of blood is improved, and thereby poisonous products are removed; and probably it is useful in syphilitic choked disc. Lumbar puncture has been recommended by many as a therapeutic and diagnostic means for syphilitic choked disc.

von Krüdener speaks of two other forms of choked discs, viz., from aneurism of the carotid artery and after operations on the ear. The former may be unilateral one or two years, and later become bilateral. and may be accompanied by very high swelling. The latter occurs. with abducens paralysis. Gradenigo assumes that a meningitis occurs at the point of the petrous portion of the temporal bone and extends to the optic nerve; other authors speak of edema and compression of the wall of the sinus from an edematous brain.

Risien Russell[8] recognizes that it is useless to trephine for the relief of intracranial pressure when the patient is deeply comatose or the heart has failed, but he thinks

7. Die Neurologie des Auges, III.
8. Brit. Med. Jour., Oct. 27, 1907.

it should always be attempted when the respiration alone has ceased and the heart is continuing to beat, even though the chances of saving the patient's life may be remote. He believes that some reported cases seem to show that by removal of a part of a tumor the growth of what is left may be retarded. This has always seemed to me very doubtful. He says he is strongly impressed with the value of trephining for the relief of optic neuritis in order to preserve sight, that he recommends that no patient suffering from intracranial tumor should be allowed to become blind when in this operative measure we have a means of preventing it, provided the operation is undertaken early enough. He does not believe that trephining will relieve every form of optic neuritis, whether due to increase of intracranial pressure or not. It would be worse than useless, he thinks, to trephine when the optic neuritis is of toxic origin. It seems to me, however, that this question is open to discussion.

Lumbar puncture can only be regarded as a temporary measure and can not be expected to relieve symptoms in the permanent way that trephining does. In lumbar puncture he thinks we have a means of relieving urgent symptoms of pressure, when to wait for a surgeon to trephine would be to allow the patient to die; or it is valuable when the patient's condition is too serious to permit the major operation, even when a surgeon is available. In both these classes of cases relief by lumbar puncture may be sufficient to permit of the major operation of trephining later. Lumbar puncture, in his opinion, is valuable for diagnosis and for the relief of urgent symptoms in cases of intracranial tumor, but is not likely to permanently relieve symptoms and prolong life or to effect a cure.

J. Mitchell Clarke[8] recommends that when no localizing signs are present the trephining should be done at the site of a persisting tender area, and in one of his cases a large tumor of the upper parietal lobe was found in this way. Dependence on a tender area in one of my cases, Case 2 of the paper by Dr. Frazier and myself, proved unreliable. Clarke thinks a palliative trephining makes a later diagnosis of location more difficult.

Mr. Marcus Gunn[8] states that when the papilla becomes more opaque and sometimes more prominent, the hemorrhages increase in size and number, there are inflammatory exudations on the disc and surrounding retina and vision has become impaired; the prognosis regarding the saving of vision is bad after relief of intracranial tension, although he has known useful vision obtained even in such unfavorable circumstances. Palliative operation to save vision is useless in the stage of gradually decreasing vascularity of the papilla, when parts of its surface become even paler than normal, while the prominence either persists or slowly subsides and the branches of the central artery become diminished in breadth.

Certain conditions Mr. Gunn emphasizes as important, viz.: The degree of swelling of the papilla in itself is not an accurate indication of the visual prognosis, and all the ophthalmoscopic appearances must be considered. The presence of retinal hemorrhages does not contraindicate surgical intervention, nor is retention of normal vision before operation a safe guide, though it is more favorable. Vision previously normal may be lost after operation. Visual improvement may ultimately be very satisfactory, even though long delayed. In one of his cases very slight improvement in vision was observed after two months, yet two months later the result was most satisfactory, one eye having regained 6/5 from 6/18, and the other 6/6 partly, from mere hand reflex. Some of the most striking results in vision he has observed after operation were in cases of cerebellar tumor. So far as vision is concerned he has found that it makes little difference whether the tumor is removed or whether the dura is merely freely opened.

Mr. Gunn has had no experience regarding the relief of tumor papillitis by lumbar puncture; he believes it would not afford so thorough a relief as the cranial operation, and would need to be frequently repeated. He does not favor opening the optic nerve sheath immediately behind the globe. We may well, I think, ask why it should be recommended, as it does not relieve the other distressing symptoms. It would have to be performed on both optic nerves, and the opening is liable to soon close up.

Mr. Gunn mentions that tumor papillitis is commonly associated with hypermetropia and is relatively rare in myopia. It appears as if in myopia an increased pressure within the sheath space is less likely to affect the optic nerve and more likely to be relieved by filtration or absorption of the excess of fluid.

H. C. Thomson[9] reports a case of tumor supposed to be in the temporal lobe in which palliative trephining caused gradual subsidence of the optic neuritis, and in a few weeks the discs showed only an insignificant trace of infiltration. During the six months following the operation the symptoms did not increase, but later did so. He refers to a case of cerebellar tumor in which palliative operation also was effective.

Merz[10] has studied the causation of optic neuritis. He states that in his experiments, in which he produced increased intracranial pressure by injecting fluid, changes in the rabbit, consisting of venous hyperemia and arterial anemia of the retina and the appearance of vessels in and about the disc which usually are not visible in the healthy eye, can be brought about almost instantly. In dogs a longer time is required for the development of the venous hyperemia; the difference is owing to the different arrangement of the vessels in the eyes, that in the dog more nearly resembles the condition in man. The further changes in the fundus of the dog appear two or three hours after the beginning of the increase in tension. The papilla becomes gradually edematous, loses its sharp outlines, projects forward and acquires a rosy hue. After eight or ten hours the arteries and veins arch perceptibly in passing from the papilla to the retina, and they appear blurred, veiled or even in places interrupted from the edema and cloudiness of the tissues in which they run. Further observation is usually impossible because the animal dies.

In every case, dog or rabbit, the subvaginal space about the optic nerve was found to be dilated. The cerebrospinal fluid passes between the dural and pial sheaths to the bulbar end of the space which ends in a blind sac. Since the intracranial tension does not diminish the liquid distends the subvaginal space, and more excessively at its bulbar end. Thus arises the ampulla-formed dilatation described by Manz, Schultén and others. Frequently a round-cell infiltration is found in the sheaths of the nerve and the surrounding connective tissue and the subvaginal space suggesting a perineuritis.

No one doubts the possibility of a choked disc arising in certain cases after the introduction of various poi-

---

9. Brit. Med. Jour., Dec. 21, 1907, p. 1761.
10. Arch. Ophth., 1901, xxx, p. 349.

sons into the body. Experimental and clinical observations teach us that undoubtedly choked disc develops at times in consequence of local irritation of the papilla and optic nerve from toxins and various poisons. Solowieff found that the introduction of the *Staphylococcus aureus* into the vitreous was in most cases followed by papillitis and choked disc. Selenkowski made similar observations. Hallermann saw choked disc in a case of erysipelas of the face, Adamück in a case of retention of urine. The inflammation theory is admissible for some cases of choked disc but not for the majority of cases. No one has determined the presence of phlogogenous substances in cases of brain tumor, and it is in these cases that choked disc most frequently appears. For the unprejudiced investigator the mechanical theory has more points of plausibility than the inflammatory. Twenty hours of slightly increased intracranial tension is sufficient in dogs to cause edema of the optic nerve.

White blood corpuscles emigrate in large numbers from the vessels and form the round cell infiltrations, especially in the parts most exposed to pressure, such as the outer sheath and the neighboring tissues. Thus increased intracranial tension suffices to cause symptoms of stasis and even of inflammation in the optic nerve and papilla.

Increased intracranial tension alone is sufficient to produce choked disc. There is similarity in anatomic construction between the eye of the dog and that of man.

Brudenell Carter, in three cases of choked disc, made an incision through the outer sheath of the optic nerve, and in each case vision improved and the symptoms of papillitis decreased and all the other symptoms of increased intracranial tension vanished.

Other important papers on cerebral decompression that have appeared since our former paper[1] are those by Starr,[11] Chance[12] and Stieren.[13]

It is sometimes extremely difficult to decide what is best to be done when choked discs are the only sign of intracranial disease. The patient may otherwise appear to be in perfect health, and the physician hesitates to recommend the opening of the skull. It may be difficult to convince the patient and his relatives that a neoplasm

11. The Journal A. M. A., Sept. 22, 1906, p. 926.
12. Penn. Med. Jour., August, 1907, p. 877.
13. Ophth. Rec., March, 1908, p. 139.

probably is present, especially if the physician also be in some doubt about the diagnosis, and he is likely to be if choked disc is the only sign. There is the possibility that the swelling may be caused by nephritis or some form of meningitis, and as yet we are uncertain as to whether the choked disc of meningitis is improved by decompression.

Antisyphilitic treatment may be beneficial and cause great improvement for a time, as in Case 1, but such treatment is known to be useful occasionally in glioma or other form of cerebral neoplasm. Valuable time may be lost by attempting to relieve the symptoms by mercury and iodid, and yet a too hasty operation is to be deprecated. The suggestion of decompression seems so terrifying to the patient, and so unnecessary in view of what appear to him as insufficient symptoms, that he is likely to be driven to consult some other physician, and possibly he may be assured in this consultation that he need have no fear and that recovery without operation will occur. When the patient finally consents to decompressive operation, valuable time often has been lost, and it may be too late to save the eyesight. The following case illustrates these statements:

Case 1.—Miss K., aged 20 years, was referred to me Nov. 15, 1906, by Drs. Ferguson and Schneiderman.

Examination.—Dr. Schneiderman first examined her eyes Sept. 29, 1906, simply because she complained of headache. He found slight optic neuritis and a flame-shaped hemorrhage in each eye, more marked in the right eye. An increase of optic neuritis was observed October 6, and by November 15 the swelling was 4 or 5 D. in each eye, and more in the right eye. Central vision was full, but the fields were contracted. Headache had been severe since June, and was both frontal and occipital. She had not had vertigo, but she felt as though she staggered, and yet her mother had not seen any ataxia. Nausea was felt November 14. Menses were always late, and were more delayed during the past few months. She had complained of numbness occasionally for more than a year, from the back of the head, down the neck into the left shoulder, and down the left arm. It was a sensation of pressure, not of pain. She had not had convulsions. Dr. Schneiderman found the pupils normal and no paralysis of ocular muscles.

In my examination the left corner of the mouth did not seem to be drawn up quite so well as the right, possibly the left lids were not closed so forcibly. The right patellar reflex was weak, the left was uncertain. There may have been a slight Romberg's sign, but it was not positive. In walking she had the sensation of going toward the right, but she did not stagger. The Achilles reflexes were about normal. The urine showed only a trace of albumin and no casts.

Dr. de Schweinitz reported Nov. 22, 1906: Central visual acuity normal. Visual fields and accommodative power normal. No diplopia and no paresis of any external ocular muscle. Double choked discs, with many hemorrhages, the elevation of the discs being 5 D. The ocular symptoms, he thought, were those of brain tumor.

Treatment.—Syphilis seemed very improbable, but my advice was to try antisyphilitic treatment, pushed rapidly, with careful observation of the eyegrounds, and with the understanding that a palliative operation should be performed if any further destructive changes were observed. Decompression would not have been considered at that time by the patient or her relatives, but I warned them earnestly of the danger of blindness they were incurring in delaying it. I did not see the patient again until June 15, 1907. She had improved under iodid and mercury. The headache had disappeared. Dr. Schneiderman found the fields better, the contraction was slight, vision was normal, and the swelling of the discs was slight, not over 1 or 2 D. The left disc was a little pale. The patellar reflex was present on each side, but was diminished.

She consulted me again Oct. 5, 1907. She had disobeyed instructions and had not visited Dr. Schneiderman for three months, and her eyes were worse. She had now about 6 D. of swelling, more in the left eye. She had not taken mercury and iodid properly. Vision was 5/4 in the right eye and 5/5 in the left. She had had much vertigo, and at times lost her sight temporarily. My examination failed to reveal other important symptoms. It seemed too risky to delay decompression by attempting further treatment with mercury and iodid, and I advised her to submit to operation. She was unwilling to do so, and consulted Dr. Van Pelt, who later referred her to Dr. Mills, from whom she received the same advice which now she accepted. I am indebted to Dr. Mills for the notes taken after the patient came under his care.

Dr. de Schweinitz made an examination of the eyes Jan. 14, 1908, and reported as follows: The vision of the right eye is reduced to the ability to distinguish hand movements; of the left eye the largest letter on the type card, that is, Snellen 200, could be distinguished uncertainly at about 2 feet. Both discs showed the decided changes of beginning postpapillitic atrophy. The right disc is swollen still about 3 or 3.50 D., the left disc somewhat higher, between 4 and 5 D. It was difficult to make these measurements exactly as she was lying in bed.

Dr. C. H. Frazier performed a palliative operation Jan. 10, 1908.

The report of Dr. Van Pelt, who has had the patient under observation since the operation, is as follows: Jan. 30, 1908. In the right eye the swelling of the optic disc has decreased from 5 to 2½ D. since the operation. In the left eye the swelling has decreased from 3½ to 2 D. The optic nerve shows evidence of increasing atrophy, and the retinal arteries are becoming more attenuated. These atrophic changes are more decided in the left eye. The vision has markedly decreased in each eye in the last ten days.

CASE 2.—*History.*—Miss F., 19 years of age, was referred to me from the service of Dr. John H. Musser, Sept. 5, 1907. She had had headache since April, 1907, nearly every morning. The pain was back of the right ear and was sharp. This area of the head was not tender to touch. The headache disappeared almost every day about 11 o'clock, although occasionally it persisted all day. It was more severe in April or May, 1907, and at that time she had much nausea. She vomited often when she had the pain, and sometimes when the pain was not severe. She had some diplopia in looking toward the right, but she thinks it was formerly in looking toward the left. She was of fragile build, weighed 85 pounds, and appeared anemic. The patient's mother died of tuberculosis, though she herself had never had any distinct pulmonary trouble, and yet Dr. A. Fife found some suspicious signs at the right apex, but he was not positive of their value.

Examination.—A report of Dr. Fife from Dr. Musser's office stated that the urinary examination was practically negative, but the specific gravity was low, 1007, with the faintest possible trace of albumin. The microscopic examination was negative. There was no indican, no urobilin and no sugar.

Dr. T. B. Holloway reported Aug. 21, 1907:

Vision, O. D., with plus .75 ax. 90 (now wearing) = 5/12.

Vision, O. S., with plus .75 ax. 90 (now wearing) = 5/12.

Pupils are 7 mm. in diameter, each reacts slightly to light, accommodation and convergence. When eyes are rotated laterally to the right and to the left a nystagmoid movement develops at the outer limits of rotation, probably slightly more marked on the right side. There is a slight limitation of outward rotation of the right eye, questionable on the left. The diplopia fields show a paresis of the right external rectus. In each eye the media are clear and the fundus shows a choked disc, the height of the swelling being 4 to 4.50 D. There is no demonstrable ocular lesion of tuberculosis.

Sept. 2, 1907. Fundus condition unchanged. Fields show moderate contraction. Direct light reflex practically abolished in the left eye; with condensed light a feeble attempt at iris contraction can be noted at the lower pupillary margin. I examined this patient repeatedly at intervals of several weeks, but was unable to find any other signs of organic disease.

Dr. de Schweinitz wrote on Sept. 23, 1907: "She has very decided choked discs, a little greater on the right than on the left side, and somewhat greater now than when you received the report from Dr. Holloway on August 15. There is no hemianopsia, but there is a paresis of the right external rectus."

An examination of the blood gave: hemoglobin, 72 per cent.; red blood corpuscles, 4,960,000; white blood corpuscles, 10,000. Differential blood count: polymorphonuclears, 66 per cent.; large mononuclears, 5 per cent.; lymphocytes, 25 per cent.; transitional, 2 per cent.; eosinophiles, 2 per cent.

It seemed to Drs. Musser, de Schweinitz, Frazier and me advisable to have a decompressive operation in order to save vision. Dr. de Schweinitz wrote Nov. 20, 1907: "I examined Miss F. yesterday and found the vision very much reduced as compared with what it was when Dr. Holloway first examined her on August 15, when it was 5/12, while to-day it is only 5/30, and that not quite perfectly. There has been very little change in the appearance of the optic nerves. They are swollen moderately, not more than 2 or 2½ D., possibly 3, while at that time they were swollen to 4 or 4½ D. Somehow the discs do not impress me as very surely dependent on increased intracranial pressure. I presume, however, that a simple trephining could do no harm, although I should think it very desirable to make it as nearly a bloodless operation as possible, because a very little additional drain would surely very greatly depreciate the vision. The results of trephining, however, I am inclined to think are very problematical." This latter view we all shared.

Operation.—A decompressive operation was done by Dr. C. H. Frazier Dec. 3, 1907. A small hernia formed at the site of operation. It was painful to touch.

Dr. de Schweinitz reported December 10. There is absolutely no change, the neuritis being exactly of the same height that it was before the trephining and the visual acuity also is unchanged. December 23. There is marked improvement in the vision of the left eye, with stationary improvement in the neuritis, possibly a little subsidence; stationary vision in the right eye with marked increase in the swelling of the disc.

Notes made by me Jan. 14, 1908, stated that the patient had been in the hospital about a week after the operation, and during that time and the week following the return to her home she was entirely free from headache. When the headache returned it was not so severe as it had been before the operation. She had had very severe headache during the past two or three weeks. A careful examination failed to reveal any localizing signs of disease. Lumbar puncture was performed by Dr. Frazier; this was followed by severe headache, a flush over head and neck, feeble respiration, and very slow pulse; from this condition she soon rallied. She was discharged, January 22, in much better condition.

In the following case the question of decompression was considered, but the operation was not performed:

CASE 3.—C., a boy, aged 14 years, was sent to me Dec. 19, 1907, by Dr. G. E. de Schweinitz, with the following report: Double optic neuritis is subsiding, with every indication of rapid atrophy beginning. The swelling of the disc is now about 4 D.; apparently no paralysis of any external ocular muscles exists; very curious symmetrical defects are seen in the nasal field of each eye. Such defects, however, I think are now universally conceded to be due, not to lesion around the chiasm, but to lesion of the optic nerve itself, and I have seen them before with optic neuritis when there evidently was no chiasm lesion.

History.—The boy had scarlet fever at the age of 3 years, which left a discharging ear. In March, 1904, he was operated on for mastoiditis. He had very severe nephritis at that time, and was in a serious condition after the operation. The discharge of the left ear continued after the operation. Optic neuritis was discovered in October, 1906. He had not had headache, dizziness, nausea or vomiting.

Examination.—I found that the left pupil was a little larger than the right, both irides responded to light, the left iris not so promptly as the right. He was partially deaf in the left ear. A careful examination failed to reveal other signs of disease. The case seemed to Dr. de Schweinitz and to me unsuitable for a palliative operation. A cerebral abscess might be present, and if this were the cause of the optic neuritis decompression might be of benefit. Rapid optic atrophy was present, and the report of the urinary examination was: one-fifth of 1 per cent. of albumin; no sugar; hyaline casts and cylindroids; and a specific gravity of 1016. It seemed probable, in the absence of all other cerebral symptoms, that nephritis was the cause of the atrophy, and a palliative operation was not performed.

The increase in the blindness which follows relief of intense intracranial pressure, and possibly the hemorrhage into the retina which occurs in some instances, as in Cases 4 and 5, may be explained by the sudden relief of the extracerebral pressure, with persisting intradural pressure. Cushing[14] remarks: "It must be remembered, however, that the sudden removal of pressure from the brain when the blood pressure has been forced to considerable heights, may be followed by a paralysis instead of a release from the major compression symptoms. The

14. Am. Jour. Med. Sciences, September, 1902.

occasion of this is readily brought out by postmortem examinations, which, under such circumstances, oftentimes discloses a brain and medulla of a uniform cherry-red color, from the widespread extravasation of blood, due to the multiple rupture of the minute blood vessels. The external supporting pressure of the high intracranial tension has been suddenly removed, leaving the internal or intravascular pressure too great for the strength of the vessel walls."

De Schweinitz thinks the increase in blindness which occurs in advanced cases is caused by the loss of blood in the operation (personal communication).

The following two cases illustrate the occasional occurrence of retinal hemorrhage after palliative operation:

CASE 4.—This was a case of cerebellar cyst, in the service of Dr. Wharton Sinkler. Dr. de Schweinitz stated that there was exceedingly rapid subsidence of the optic neuritis, but, in spite of it, rapid loss of vision occurred. There were symptoms of cerebellar tumor, and the operation, in two stages, was performed by Dr. Wm. J. Taylor. A cyst protruded when the skull was opened on the left side, ruptured spontaneously, and a stream of clear, straw-colored fluid squirted at least a yard. Considerable hemorrhage occurred at the first operation. The boy improved after the operation, except that immediately following it a hemorrhage developed in the right eye, and resulted in complete loss of vision.

Examination.—The notes as obtained from Dr. de Schweinitz and Dr. Holloway are as follows:

Oct. 1, 1907.—O. D., one letter on 6/30, one letter on 6/22; Snellen. O. S., 4 letters on 6/6, Snellen. Pupils 4½ mm., react to direct and indirect light, accommodation and convergence. Media clear; each eye shows a pronounced choked disc, height 6 to 7 D. One rather marked hemorrhage at the lower edge of swelling in O. S. No macular stellate figure. Convergence exceedingly poor, O. S. usually deviating. No hemianopsia. Will attempt fields later. T. B. H., fields taken October 4.

Oct. 8, 1907.—Optic neuritis (choked disc) O. D. + 8 D.; O. S. + 7 D. deS.

October 18.—O. D., height of swelling about 7 D.

October 25.—O. D., no change. O. S. shows beginning stellate figure in macula. T. B. H.

November 5.—O. D., disc + 3-4 D.; O. S., + 5-6 D. deS.

November 10.—Vision, O. D., doubtful light perception. O. S., 4/20 and one letter on 4/15. O. D., disc 3-4 D.; O. S., 4-5 D. Vessels in each eye 1-1½ D. higher. deS.

November 15.—O. D., blind; O. S., 5/15; O. D., no light reflex, in O. S. prompt. Indirect light reflex absent in O. S., present in O. D. Both react to convergence and accommodation. O. D., 4 D.; O. S., 5 D. T. B. H.

November 19.—Disc swelling about 3. Edges of disc beginning to appear. deS.

December 3.—O. D., + 4 D.; O. S., + 5 D. deS.

December 6.—O. D., blind; O. S. = 6/30. Fundus as when last seen. T. B. H.

In the macular region is a faint delicate, almost complete stellate figure, the striæ showing as milky lines rather than pure white. Within this area are several short white striations. At the outer limits of the stellate figure are several linear hemorrhages. One fresh hemorrhage on temporal slope of swelling. O. S. still some evidence of hemorrhage below disc. Height of swelling 7 D. In the macular region a number of fine yellowish spots, associated with several punctate hemorrhages. (T. B. H.)

Jan. 10, 1908.—Seen in out-patient department. Discharged from house Dec. 31, 1907. O. D. blind; O. S. 6/60. O. D. media clear, disc shows picture of subsiding neuritis, outline of disc distinctly seen, pale, edges blurred, arteries contracted, moderate perivasculitis; granular macula. O. S. media clear, fundus as in O. D. except in immediate region about disc, especially on temporal side, are a few punctate exudates. No hemorrhages in either eye. Height of filled-in discs, 2.50 D.

Case 5.—W. R., 43 years of age, white, house painter, was a patient of Dr. C. S. Potts, with whom I saw the patient, and to whom I am indebted for the notes.

History.—Family history negative. He has used considerable alcohol, has had much family trouble of late. Syphilis denied. He was struck in the right temporal region with brass knuckles one year before admission (Nov. 6, 1907). Symptoms of present trouble began about September, 1906. with headache and dizziness. On admission he complained of severe constant headache, worse at night, situated in right parieto-occipital region; of vertigo and excessive vomiting, not dependent on taking food. He had cerebellar gait, usually, but not always, fell toward the right. Slight ataxia in the right arm was present when finger to nose test was attempted, but there was no weakness of cranial or spinal nerves. The reflexes were about normal, except that the patellar reflex was slightly exaggerated on the right side. No Babinski sign was obtained. He had diplopia at times. Nystagmus was seen in both eyes when he looked either to the right or to the left.

Examination.—Ocular examination was made by Dr. Fox Nov. 9, 1907. O. D. optic nerve decidedly red and vessels have pinched appearance as of optic neuritis. O. S., optic neuritis, slight hemorrhage just above optic nerve; slight paresis of left third nerve.

November 16.—Optic neuritis has greatly increased in both eyes. Veins exceedingly tortuous; apex of swelling, 7 D.

Treatment.—Operation by Dr. S. C. Burns Nov. 27, 1907. An opening was made in the occipital region, and the right lobe of the cerebellum was exposed, but nothing abnormal was found. The brain did not bulge unduly into the opening.

November 29.—Examination by Dr. L. Webster Fox. No change in the conditions found at examination on November 16. December 15: O. D., still pronounced swelling of nerve, with slight hemorrhages in striated form, showing through the outer halo of the circle, veins pronounced, arteries almost obliterated. Head of nerve intensely red.. Probable change for the better. O. S., nerve still shows pronounced swelling. Hemorrhage of retina, down and out from optic nerve, extending to near equator as a broad band. Up and out on outer margin of optic nerve is a beautiful star-shaped hemorrhage, one-third the size of normal optic nerve.

December 9.—O. D., swelling of disc has diminished one-half. Arteries are thin. Veins still show some stasis. No hemorrhage. O. S., neuritis less pronounced. The center of the physiologic cup can now be seen. Surrounding optic nerve is a halo of white edematous retina, somewhat striated. The hemorrhage of the macular region has lessened. The veins downward and outward are markedly beaded. Both eyes show improvement.

December 15.—Examinations show about same conditions as on December 9. Distant vision, 20/50.

Jan. 1, 1908.—O. D., optic nerve on a level with surrounding retina. Slight haziness of margin showing some neuritis. Veins clearly defined and above normal in caliber, no blocking at entrance of nerve. Arteries still very thin, showing impeded circulation. Retina has an anemic appearance instead of being a bright red. Chorioidal arteries can be seen. Downward and outward in extreme periphery of fundus is a dark speck, impossible to say if a retina hemorrhage or not. O. S., same general appearance as O. D. Retinal hemorrhages so pronounced two weeks ago are entirely absorbed. General findings show marked improvement.

February 1.—O. D., optic nerve clear and distinct in outline. Blood vessels of normal caliber. No retinitis. O. S., same as O. D. Slight paresis of internal rectus muscles.

March 4.—After the operation the headache disappeared and the vomiting ceased. A swelling about the same of a half of a small orange, soft and fluctuating, appeared at the seat of the opening in the skull. The gait has become much more ataxic, the arms, especially the right arm, are also ataxic, so much so that he feeds himself with difficulty. Babinski's "adiadocoçinesia" is marked in the right arm. Speech is very thick and indistinct. Diplopia is marked and paresis of right third, sixth, seventh, fifth, ninth, tenth and eleventh nerves has developed.

Also some paresis of eighth nerve on the right side. Within the past few weeks the man has had some nausea in the morning and headache has returned, but not nearly so severe as before the operation. Eye sight is excellent for distance.

The question has been put to me several times whether palliative operation might be of benefit when the patient with signs of brain tumor has suddenly fallen into coma. Risien Russell, as already stated, is in favor of trephining when respiration has ceased but the heart continues to beat, even though the chances of saving life may be remote.

Very frequently, in my experience, sudden death has terminated the symptoms of brain tumor, especially

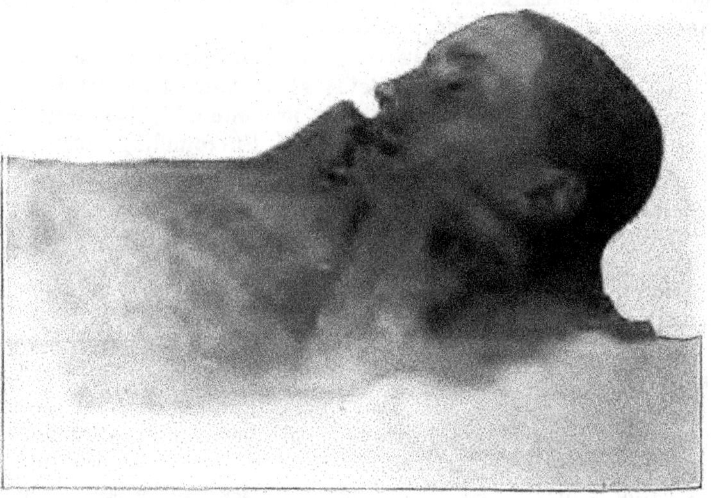

Fig. 1.—Showing the cerebellar position of upper limbs caused by a large tumor at the base of the brain displacing the cerebellum (Fig. 2).

when the tumor is in the posterior cranial fossa. The patient may be no worse than he has been for months, and suddenly he becomes cyanosed, unconscious, possibly has convulsive movements and respiration ceases, but the heart continues to beat. It has seemed extremely doubtful to me whether decompression would be advisable under such circumstances. Death is almost certain, and the physician who performs or recommends a palliative operation when the patient is at the point of death is likely to be regarded by the relatives as having hastened the fatal termination. Such operation, done at a more suitable time, I believe may materially lessen the danger of these sudden and usually fatal attacks.

A patient with brain tumor, who had also been under the care of several of my colleagues, recently died in my service at the Philadelphia General Hospital. A very large tumor was found in the posterior cranial fossa. The occipital lobes had been pushed apart and the cerebellum had been displaced almost to a right angle with the brain stem. Undoubtedly decompression in the posterior cranial fossa, by allowing space for the development of this tumor, would have removed much discomfort (Figs. 1 and 2). A case of sudden death, in which the question of palliative operation in the period of coma was considered, is the following:

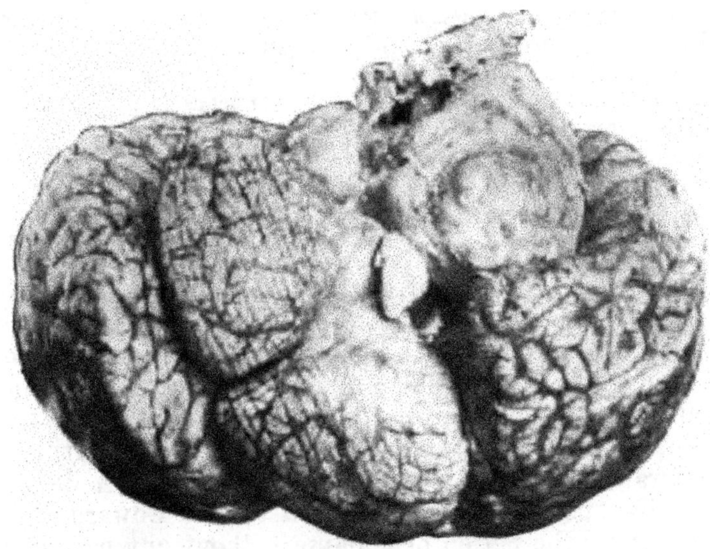

Fig. 2.—The tumor has twisted the cerebellum on its axis and pushed it between the occipital lobes.

Case 6.—*History.*—A man, aged 28 years, was referred to the University Hospital by Dr. J. W. McConnell Jan. 30, 1908. He had been complaining of headache during a year, of vertigo during two months, and of vomiting during one month. He was a brakeman and had been injured frequently. A year before admission he had had attacks of spasmodic movement in the left side of his body. In August, 1907, he had a sudden attack of twitching of the left side of the body, preceded by slight dizziness. He fell and probably was unconscious. He had had syphilis.

Examination.—On admission his gait was unsteady, and the staggering was increased by closing the eyes. The right pupil was larger than the left, and both irides reacted to light and in accommodation. The extraocular muscles were normal. The right nasolabial fold was not so deep as the left. Some ataxia was seen in the finger to nose test, especially on the right side. The right lower limb was stronger than the left. The right patellar reflex was exaggerated, the left slightly so. Ankle clonus was obtained on the right side, but not on the left side. A note made on February 1 is as follows: He has been complaining of severe headache, the face becomes flushed and the pupils dilated. He moans and cries and begs to be put out of his misery, but appears fairly comfortable most of the time.

I saw the patient February 4 about noon. He was suffering intensely from headache, threw himself about in the bed in an agony of pain, and caught hold of the resident when he came near him, begging to be killed and put out of his misery. He was quieted by a hypodermic injection. His suffering was so great that no examination could be made, and, knowing very little of his history, I did not feel justified in requesting an immediate palliative operation. About 3 o'clock in the same afternoon he was found on the floor unconscious, with very difficult breathing. He soon became cyanosed and respiration ceased. The heart action became slow and irregular. Artificial respiration was kept up until about 8:30 p. m., when death occurred. No necropsy was permitted.

I debated whether it would be advisable to have a palliative operation during the collapse, but it did not seem desirable. The chance of benefiting him thereby was very questionable. A similar case of brain tumor of one cerebral hemisphere under the care of Dr. Joseph Sailer was in the University Hospital about a year ago. Cessation of respiration occurred suddenly and artificial respiration was employed for several hours. A decompressive operation was performed by Dr. Edward Martin during the period of collapse without any benefit or any delay to the fatal termination.

Whether pain in itself can cause death or not I think is open to question, and it may be that the intense intracranial pressure with irritation may be the cause of the pain as well as of the sudden death, possibly by paralysis of the important centers of the medulla oblongata. Byrom Bramwell, however, believes that pain alone may kill. Where sudden headache is intense, as described in Case 6, and symptoms of increased intracranial pressure are present, it has seemed to me dangerous to delay decompression, and I regret that in this case it was not done, even though the clinical history was imperfectly known to me. This agonizing headache is sometimes too serious to permit any delay in giving relief by opening the skull.

About four weeks after the experience above related I was asked to see a case in consultation with Dr. Ernest LaPlace, in which symptoms of a focal cerebral lesion were said to have developed gradually within twenty-four hours. The patient, during my examination, had intense headache, and, fearing a fatal termination, I recommended immediate decompression. Trephining with slitting the dura was done and about two ounces of clear fluid escaped, with great temporary relief of the suffering within twelve hours. The opening probably was not sufficiently large.

Decompressive operation is not always beneficial, even when the patient is not in coma, and death may occur within twenty-four hours after a palliative operation, as illustrated by the following case:

Case 7.—*History.*—A. K., male, aged 25 years, was admitted to the University Hospital, March 4, 1907, complaining of blindness, intense headache and vomiting. His mentality was much impaired. He stated that during the winter of 1906-7 he began to have weakness and soreness about the articulation of his jaw. The soreness afterward spread upward in his head. About two months before admission, he became blind in the right eye, and two weeks later he became blind in the left eye. He vomited frequently. He was unable to walk without support, and could not stand with the feet together, but could stand if they were separated. The head was thrown far backward, and any attempt to move it forward caused much pain. The left pupil was considerably larger than the right, and neither iris reacted to light. Corneal and conjunctival sensation and the lachrymal reflex on the right side were lost, as well as the sensation of the mucous membrane on the right side of the nose. The sensations of touch and pain were completely lost in the entire distribution of the right fifth nerve, provided no pressure was made. The mouth deviated to the right, when opened. The patellar reflexes were lost. Babinski's sign was present on the left side.

Dr. de Schweinitz reported: Palpebral fissure about equal in width. Left eye slightly divergent. Left external rectus movement preserved. Movements of internal superior and inferior recti are markedly limited. No wheel movement obtained. Right eye: Loss of movement of external rectus and marked limitation of movements of superior and inferior recti, with almost lost internal rectus movement. There is extensive double optic neuritis with large retinal hemorrhages on the right side.

The case was believed to be one of tumor or syphilis of the base of the brain involving the right Gasserian ganglion.

Treatment.—A decompression operation was done by Dr. Frazier on each side of the head on April 11, 1907, just above the ear. The brain bulged much on the right side. The patient died the following day. An endothelioma was found at the necropsy, implicating the right Gasserian ganglion. Decompression in this case did not prolong life, and it may be, hastened the fatal termination.

In the following cases decompression was of benefit:

CASE 8.—*History.*—Ida K., a woman, aged about 21, consulted me Nov. 3, 1906. She complained of failure of vision during two months. She had aborted four months previously, and headache began about eight days after abortion. It was sometimes frontal, sometimes occipital, and frequent. She had not had nausea, vomiting or convulsions. Menses returned after the abortion and had been regular.

Examination.—The lower part of the right side of the face was weak in showing the teeth; the upper part of the face was not affected. She could not draw up the right side of the mouth separately. The tongue deviated slightly to the right. The grasp of the right hand was weaker than that of the left. The right lower limb seemed a little weaker than the left in resisting passive movements. The patellar reflex seemed to be exaggerated on the right side. The patient later came under the care of Dr. Mills.

An examination of the eyes by Dr. de Schweinitz, Nov. 27, 1906, revealed double choked disc, no external muscle palsy, and very contracted fields.

Treatment.—Dr. Frazier performed a palliative operation Nov. 28, 1906. An osteoplastic flap was made extending one inch behind and three inches in front of the Rolandic fissure. When the dura was exposed, it was found exceedingly tense, and when it was cut, the brain bulged greatly. The veins of the pia were markedly distended. After making a transverse slit in the dura under the middle of the flap, the dura was closed with interrupted silk sutures. A portion of the temporal bone below the flap was then rongeured away for decompression. The skin was closed with interrupted sutures. Hernia cerebri was observed December 6.

The report of Dr. de Schweinitz, December 9, is as follows: Right Eye—Optic neuritis apparently subsiding, + 5 D. (compared with + 7 D. before operation). Both sets of vessels very small. In both maculæ there is some chorioidal disturbance. Left Eye—Optic neuritis + 5 D. Vision (uncorrected), each eye 4/9.

On December 11, the note was made that the patient did not have headache as before the operation and did not vomit. The patient was dismissed from the University Hospital and was admitted to the Philadelphia General Hospital, service of Dr. Mills, Oct. 17, 1907. An examination was made by Dr. Shumway October 22. Pupils respond very sluggishly, are well dilated. Both nerves show advanced optic atrophy following choked disc. The nerve heads are still swollen to a level of 6 diopters (2 mm.) above the retinal level. The macular regions show no changes. The hernia had increased considerably in size.

Death occurred Dec. 7, 1907. A large glioma was found in the left temporal lobe, growing over the left cerebral peduncle (Fig. 3).

The improvement in the condition seems to have been of a duration of months, but as she was not constantly under observation the exact time is uncertain.

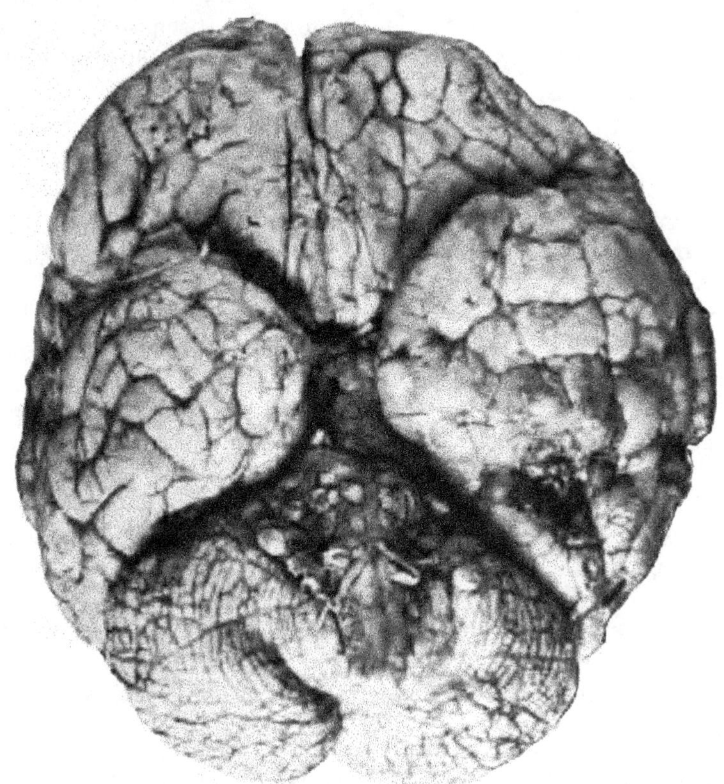

Fig. 3.—A large glioma occupied the greater part of the left temporal lobe and grew as a wedge-shaped process over the left cerebral peduncle (indicated by the line). The left temporal lobe was much enlarged.

CASE 9.—*History.*—A. B., 42 years of age, consulted me June 28, 1906. He had an enlargement of the skull on the left side above and in front of the ear. He complained of weakness on the right side of the body, slight ataxia, some motor aphasia, left-sided headache, some difficulty in reading, and failure of memory.

Examination.—Dr. de Schweinitz found no evidence of optic neuritis, but there was slight over-fulness of the retinal vessels.

Treatment.—Decompression without opening the dura was performed, July 7, 1906. Almost complete disappearance of symptoms followed for about two months, and possibly the improvement would have lasted longer if the dura had been opened. A later operation revealed an endothelioma, which was removed. A full report of this case has been published.[15]

The following case was in the service of Dr. Morris J. Lewis. The operation was not palliative, but was removal of a tumor. It is included because it shows remarkable improvement in the ocular conditions after the operation.

CASE 10.—*History.*—K. H., aged 33, a patient at the Orthopedic Hospital. July 10, 1907, complained of convulsions for past three years. Screams, falls to floor unconscious, bites the tongue. Attack begins in the left arm. She has had about forty attacks in the past ten years and they are becoming more frequent and severe. The eyes were found normal, except for the error of refraction, + 1.5 D. at this visit.

Examination.—Sept. 30, 1907.—Seen by Dr. S. D. Risley at his office; no fundus changes.

October 9.—Seen by Dr. Langdon, and beginning optic neuritis is discovered; discs swollen, 2 D. above fundus level; margins blurred; veins full; no hemorrhages. Fields and vision normal. Brain tumor suspected.

October 19.—Admitted to house. Attacks continuing; vision, fields, muscles and pupils normal; discs swollen; O. D., 3 D. above fundus; O. S., 2.5 D. above fundus. Veins more full and tortuous; numerous transudations of serum, from veins; no hemorrhages.

October 25.—No increase in swelling of discs, numerous hemorrhages in O. D.; none in O. S.

November 4.—Discs swollen, 4.5 D. Several large hemorrhages in O. D. Transudations on O. S. Vision full.

November 15.—Dr. Taylor operated, removing a large tumor (glioma) from upper posterior border of the fissure of Rolando. Patient made an uneventful recovery, with a left hemiplegia.

November 16.—Eyes deviated to right.

November 17.—O. D. disc, 2.5 D. above fundus, and O. S., 1.5 D.

November 22.—O. D., 1.5 D.; O. S., 0.5 D.

---

15. Spiller, W. G.: THE JOURNAL A. M. A., Dec. 21, 1907, p. 2059.

November 24.—Seen by Dr. de Schweinitz and last measurement verified.

December 3.—O. D. disc 1.5 D. above fundus. O. S., no swelling, margins somewhat blurred. No hemorrhages; vision full.

I have attempted to learn the present condition of the patients still alive reported in the previous paper by Dr. Frazier and myself, on whom decompression was performed. This and the results of experimental work will be reported later.

MEMORANDA

THE OPTIC NERVE CHANGES IN MULTIPLE SCLEROSIS.

WITH REMARKS ON THE CAUSATION OF NON-TOXIC RETROBULBAR NEURITIS IN GENERAL.*

WARD A. HOLDEN, M.D.

NEW YORK.

It seems scarcely necessary to dwell on the established facts of the optic nerve changes in multiple sclerosis. These are familiar through the statistical studies of Uhthoff[1] and those who have followed him. We know that ophthalmoscopic changes in the optic discs are found in about half the cases of this disease, that visual disturbances are frequently early symptoms—sometimes preceding any other symptoms by months or years—that the visual disturbances are often of sudden onset, and, if slight, frequently remain long unprogressive, and if excessive usually improve, the course of the optic nerve changes thus differing radically from the slow, steadily progressive atrophy of tabes.

I shall take it for granted, also, that it is the custom to examine the fundus and determine the fields of vision in every case in which multiple sclerosis is suspected. Optic nerve changes, if present, will help to confirm the diagnosis. Thus ophthalmoscopic changes in the discs will exclude hysteria; and since optic nerve changes are rare in early paresis, if not complicated by tabes (I found the discs normal in seventy consecutive cases of early uncomplicated paresis), one can exclude this disease, into which many cases, diagnosed as multiple sclerosis, develop after they come into hospitals for the insane.

---

* This paper has been accepted by the Executive Committee of the Section on Ophthalmology of the American Medical Association, to be presented before the Section at the Chicago Session, June 2-5, 1908. Publication rights reserved by the American Medical Association.

1. Graefe-Saemisch, xi, p. 337.

It will be more to the purpose to base my remarks on a number of illustrative cases, considering them under several headings.

A. THE PATHOLOGIC CHANGES IN THE OPTIC NERVES IN MULTIPLE SCLEROSIS.

The cause of disseminated plaques of sclerosis in the central nervous system is still unknown. It is agreed that the histologic changes consist of localized vascular disturbances, with exudation of round cells, and of degeneration of the medullary sheaths of the nerve fibers, while the axis cylinders and ganglion cells are long preserved. Hypertrophy of the neuroglia usually fills the spaces left by the disappearance of the medullary sheaths.

The degenerative changes may remain limited to the plaque or medullary degeneration may extend upward

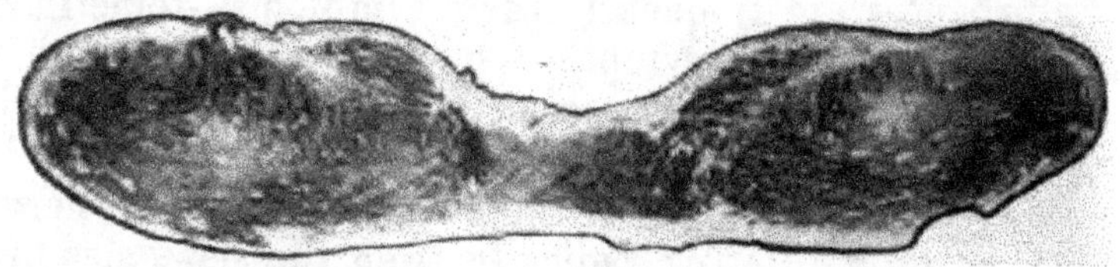

Fig. 1.—Optic nerves in cross section where they emerge from the chiasma. Wolter's medullary stain shows pale areas of degeneration, chiefly in the central bundles of each nerve.

or downward. Restoration of the degenerated medullary sheaths often takes place and the fibers then resume their function.

Typical pathologic changes in the optic nerves and chiasma were found in the following case:

Case 1.—A woman, aged 27, died at the Montefiore Home of infection after cystitis and pyonephritis, which were manifestations of multiple sclerosis.

History.—Seven years before her death she fell and dislocated her right hip. A year later she noticed weakness, numbness, and coldness of her right leg, which lasted for two months. Four months later the same symptoms were experienced in her left leg. These cleared up in two months.

Eye Symptoms.—About this time there was a sudden diminution of vision and it was said that she was "blind in one eye and color blind in the other." Vision improved, and she was comparatively well for a year and a half. Four years before her death her left leg again became weak and numb. Her gait was staggering. There was disturbance of micturition. There were diplopia, nystagmus, poor vision, slow and monotonous speech, deafness, and poor memory for recent events. Three years befor her death temporal pallor of the discs was noted.

Pathology.—At the Pathologic Institute of the New York State Hospitals, serial vertical sections were made under the direction of Dr. Dunlap, through the optic nerves, chiasma, and tracts, and these were stained with Wolter's medullary stain and with hematoxylin-eosin. In a section through the optic nerves at the point of their emergence from the chiasma, there is seen (Fig. 1) a diffuse degeneration, particularly in the

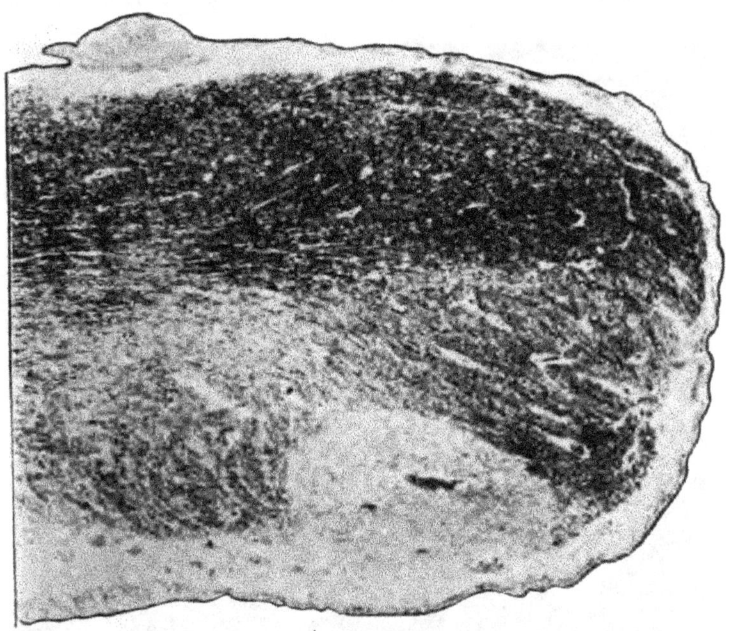

Fig. 2.—A peripheral, sharply-outlined, oval, sclerotic plaque in the chiasma, with a large vessel in its center (below and to the right). Wolter's medullary stain. The fibers which run through the plaque preserve their medullary sheaths in sections anterior to it, but posteriorly a certain degree of ascending degeneration in the optic tract can be made out.

central or papillo-macular bundles of fibers in each nerve, which accounts for the temporal pallor of the optic discs seen in life. This degeneration consists of an absence of a certain number of medullary sheaths in each affected bundle. The degeneration can be followed down the optic nerves toward the eyeballs. Further back in the chiasma there is a sharply outlined oval plaque, in which the medullary sheaths are almost entirely wanting. The affected area appears to be rarified rather than sclerosed, and there is no increase in the number of neuroglia nuclei, and neuroglia fibers form a loosely meshed network (Fig. 2). The degenerations in this case are old, and no inflammatory conditions are found, as was to be expected.

Such being the characteristic pathologic changes in the optic nerves in this disease, it is obvious that they may give rise to a variety of types of visual disturbance.

B. THE TYPES OF FIELDS OF VISION, AND THE CORRESPONDING OPHTHALMOSCOPIC CHANGES IN THE OPTIC DISCS.

The visual disturbances fall chiefly into three groups: (1) Concentric contraction of the field of vision; (2)

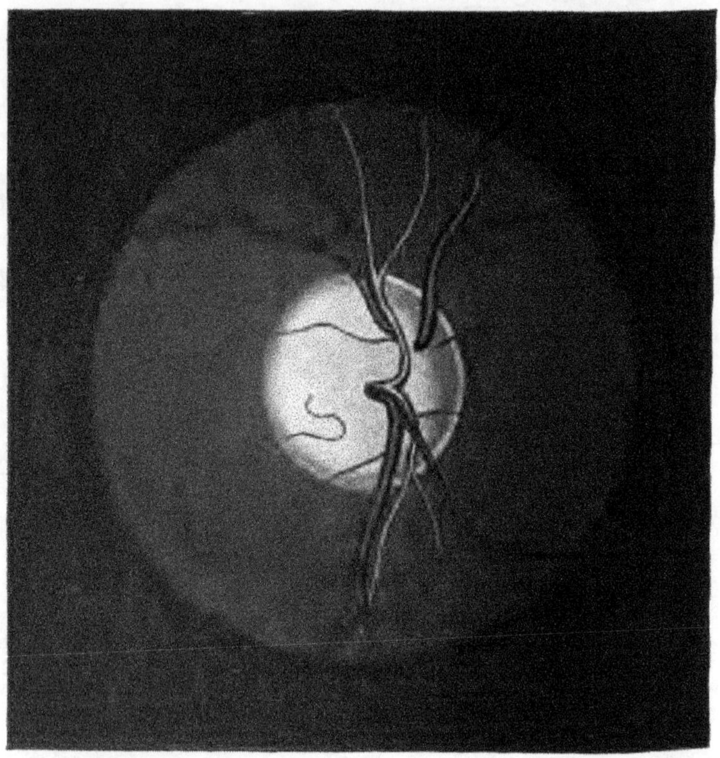

Fig. 3.—Case 2. Concentric contraction of the field for white and red, with well-marked pallor of almost the entire disc.

central scotoma with normal peripheral limits of the field, and (3) a combination of concentric contraction of the field and central scotoma. These types of fields are associated, to a certain extent, with characteristic ophthalmoscopic appearances of degeneration in the optic discs. Discrepancies may occur, however, since in rare instances there may be some degree of papillitis, and, again, a lesion far back in the nerve may cause visual disturbances long before a descending degeneration leads to pallor of the disc, while conversely the clearing up of a lesion in the nerve may lead to improvement in vision while the disc, after once becoming pale, remains so.

Normally, the temporal portion of the disc is paler than the nasal portion, and while in diffuse degenerations of the nerve, with concentric contraction of the field of vision the entire disc may become pathologically pale, this pallor is always more pronounced in the temporal portion of the disc. The axial or papillo-macular

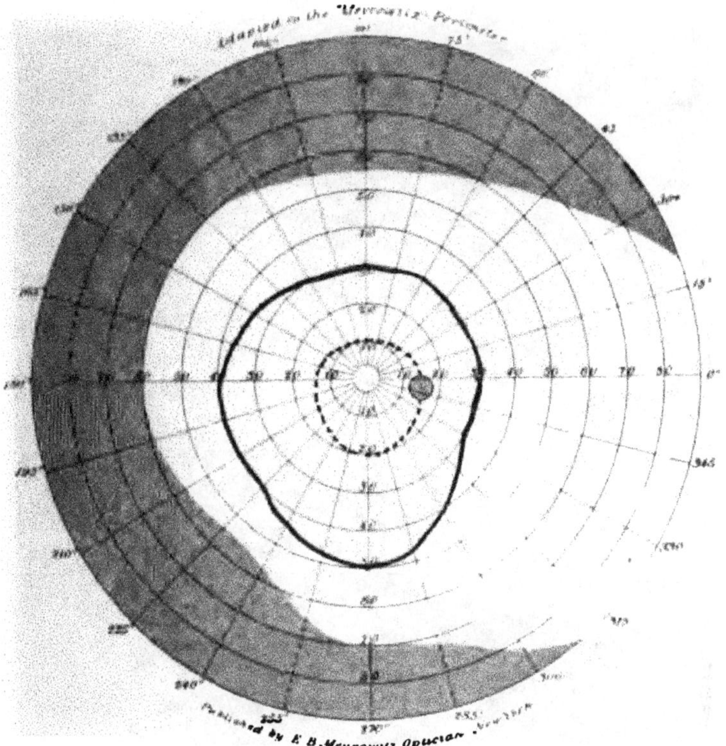

Fig. 4.—Case 2. Diagram of visual field, showing concentric contraction.

bundle of the optic nerve which is distributed to the region of the macula lutea, the center of distinct vision, lies in the center of the optic nerve as it emerges from the chiasma, but when it has descended to the optic disc it occupies the inferior temporal quadrant of the disc. When the papillo-macular bundle alone is involved, in cases with pure central scotoma, the inferior temporal quadrant of the optic disc alone shows a pathologic pallor.

Concentric contraction of the field of vision is well shown in the following case:

CASE 2.—A man, aged 21, four and a half years ago noticed vertigo and a staggering gait. Six months later tremor of the head and hands came on, and there was difficulty in speaking. Now there is marked nystagmus and great difficulty in walking.

Examination.—Three years ago his vision failed during a period of four months and has since been stationary. O. D. = 20/50; O. S. = 20/30. There is concentric contraction of the

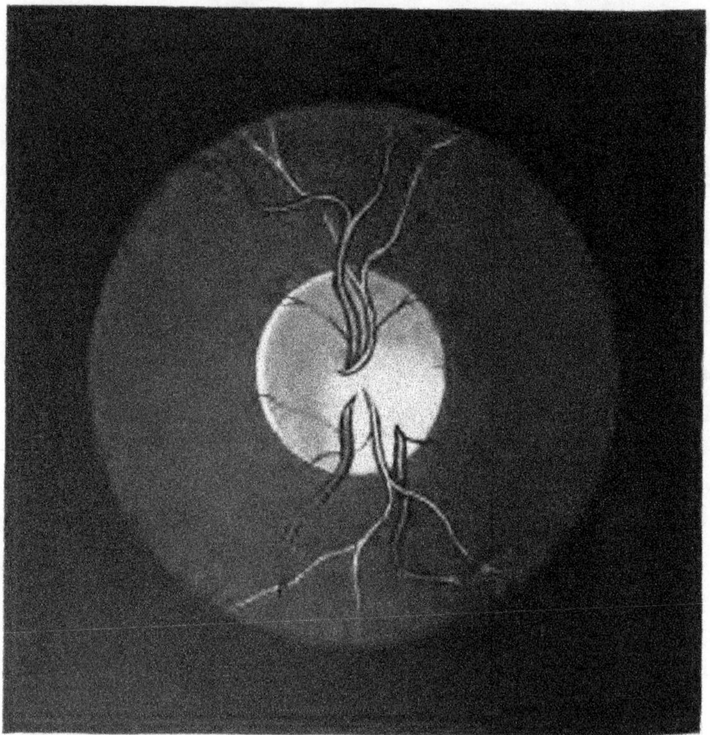

Fig. 5.—Case 3. - A relative central scotoma for red; with pallor of the inferior temporal quadrant of the optic disc, in which lies the papillo-macular bundle.

fields. On the right side, the contracted limits of the field for a 1 cm. square of white on a black ground are shown in Figure 3 by the heavy unbroken line; the contracted limits of the field for a 1 cm. red square on a gray ground are shown by the broken line. The red square can be seen as far away as five feet, and is seen more clearly at the point of fixation than to one side. The disc presents a marked pallor in its entire extent, except in a narrow crescentic zone at its nasal margin.

The outlines of the disc are well defined. The arteries are small, the veins are of normal caliber (Figs. 3 and 4).

The next case exhibits a central scotoma.

CASE 3.—A man, aged 29, noticed five years ago paresthesia of the feet, then weakness and stiffness of the legs, increasing for a year, when he became unable to walk. Two years ago he lost control of his arms. For a time there was diplopia. Now there is constant nystagmus and difficulty in speaking.

Examination.—Five years ago his vision failed gradually for six months, and has since remained stationary. O. D. = 20/50; O. S. = 20/70. For the left eye, the limits of the fields for

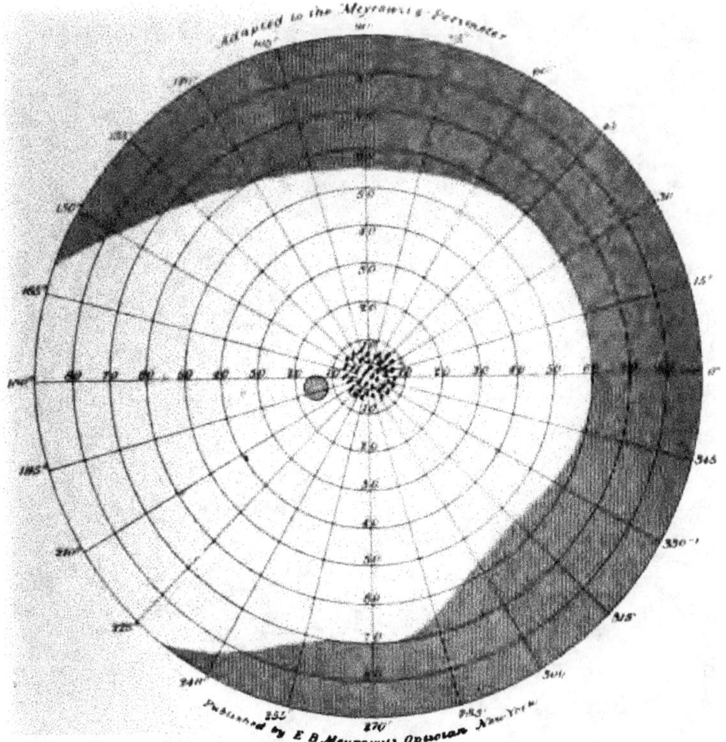

Fig. 6.—Case 3. Visual field. The dotted area represents the relative central scotoma for red.

white, for a 3 mm. black dot and for red are normal, but the red square can not be recognized at a greater distance than eighteen inches, and it is seen at this distance obscurely in a central field 15 degrees in diameter, and more clearly on every side (Figs. 5 and 6).

There is pallor of the left optic disc limited to the inferior temporal quadrant. The outline of the disc is well-defined and the arteries and veins are of normal caliber.

The next case illustrates a combination of concentric contraction of the field and central scotoma.

Case 4.—A woman, aged 27, met with an accident two years and a half ago. Eight months later she had pains in the head, neck, chest, hips and fingers. Her feet felt numb. Now there is constant nystagmus and great difficulty in walking. She has never had diplopia.

Examination.—The vision of the left eye became affected soon after the accident and wnile there have been fluctuations in the sight, no great change has taken place. O. D. = 20/30; O. S. = 20/100. The right optic disc and fields are normal. On the left side there is concentric contraction of the field for white (Fig. 8). In the central portion of the field red is not

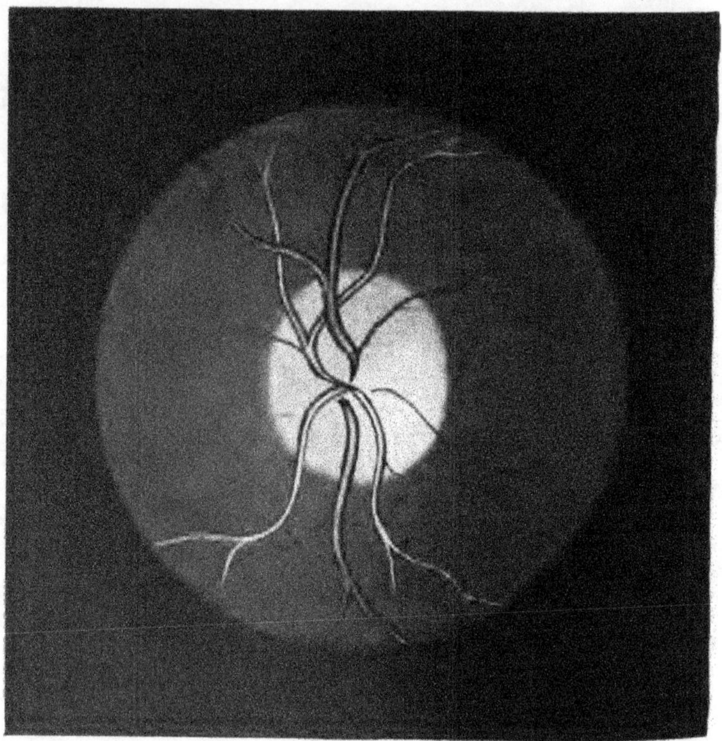

Fig. 7.—Case 4. Concentric contraction of the field for white and for red and also an absolute central scotoma for red. Slight signs of inflammation in the disc and a slight general pallor with more pronounced pallor in the inferior temporal quadrant.

recognized in the area indicated in the chart by the dots. The disc is slightly pale in its entire extent and the *inferior* temporal quadrant is still paler. The outline of the disc is blurred and the veins are dilated.

These three hospital cases examined recently give one a fair idea of the changes in the visual fields and in the optic discs likely to be found in multiple sclerosis.

C. RETROBULBAR NEURITIS THAT IS PROBABLY AN EARLY SYMPTOM OF MULTIPLE SCLEROSIS.

In the cases described above the optic nerve changes clearly were due to multiple sclerosis. But when visual disturbances, suggestive of multiple sclerosis, are not accompanied by other symptoms of the disease there may be much doubt as to their nature. Furthermore, visual disturbances may precede all other symptoms of this disease for years, or, possibly, since this is sometimes

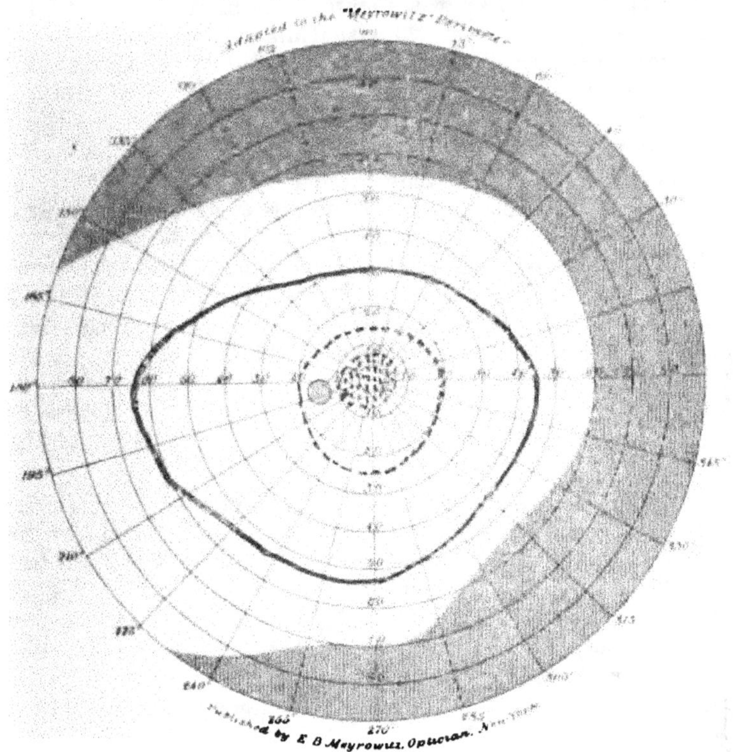

Fig. 8.—Case 4. Concentric contraction of field for white is shown by the heavy unbroken line, and of the field for red, by the broken line. The central dotted area represents the absolute central scotoma for red.

a monosymptomatic disease, the optic nerve disturbances may be the only symptoms.

A case of retrobulbar neuritis suggestive of multiple sclerosis, but unaccompanied by any other pronounced symptoms of the disease, is the following:

CASE 5.—A year and a half ago, I saw a man of 23, who said that the sight of his left eye had become blurred nine months before, and that the sight of the right eye had become blurred three months later.

Examination.—His vision failed rapidly, at first, then remained stationary, and in the few weeks before I saw him, he had noticed some improvement in the vision of the eye first affected. He could count fingers with either eye at a distance of four feet with excentric fixation. The limits of the field for white for each eye were normal. Red could be seen faintly in the periphery of the field of the right eye, but not at all in the field of the left eye. There was an absolute, circular, central scotoma for white, about 25 degrees in diameter, in the field of each eye.

The right optic disc was slightly pale in its temporal half. In the left eye, in which the visual disturbance was of longer duration, there was a slight general pallor of the entire optic disc, more marked in its temporal half. The outlines of the discs were well-defined, and the veins were slightly dilated. His vision was better in reduced illumination.

Other Symptoms.—An only brother, aged 30, had never had any visual disturbance, hence family retrobulbar neuritis could be excluded. The patient was not under weight, his general health was good, and he complained of no nervous symptoms. Tobacco, alcohol, lead, diabetes, and syphilis could be excluded as causative factors. There were no nasal symptoms. There was a slight tremor of the face and also of the hands, but the latter was not pronounced enough to affect his writing. There was at times a slight nystagmus in extreme lateral directions of the gaze. The knee-jerks were active, but not decidedly exaggerated.

Course of Disease.—Examinations by a number of physicians revealed no cause for the retrobulbar neuritis, and various forms of treatment having been of no avail, it was decided to abandon treatment altogether, and the patient went abroad to travel. A few months later, his sight improved so that he was able to read, and he then resumed his occupation. No other symptoms of multiple sclerosis have appeared up to the present time, nearly two and a half years since his vision became impaired.

In this case the optic nerve disturbances, both in character and in course, are characteristic of multiple sclerosis, but up to this time, two and a half years after their onset, no corroborating symptoms have developed. Nevertheless, this case seems to me to be one of multiple sclerosis.

D. THE CAUSES OF RETROBULBAR NEURITIS OTHER THAN MULTIPLE SCLEROSIS.

Frank, in Oppenheim's clinic, found that optic-nerve symptoms appeared before other symptoms in 15 per cent. of the cases of multiple sclerosis. Bruns and

Stölting found this to be the case in 30 per cent. Marx[2] recently sent for all the patients with retrobulbar neuritis and tobacco-alcohol amblyopia who had been seen in recent years in the Strasburg University eye clinic. Cases of toxic retrobulbar neuritis caused by tobacco, alcohol, lead and the toxemias of pregnancy are diagnosed easily and are placed in a category by themselves. Cases due to syphilis, diabetes and trauma also are diagnosed readily.

Among sixteen patients with non-toxic retrobulbar neuritis, whom Marx examined at an interval of from three months to seven years after the first observation, six patients were found undoubtedly to have multiple sclerosis, or 38 per cent. In the remaining ten cases he found the most important etiologic factor to be exposure to cold and wet, followed by coryza.

What was the probable cause of the retrobulbar neuritis in these ten cases? It has long been recognized that since the wall of the sphenoidal sinus is, in part, also the wall of the optic foramen, sphenoidal suppuration may lead to blindness. In this country, more than twelve years ago, Dr. C. R. Holmes operated successfully in such a case by opening the ethmoidal and the sphenoidal sinuses and restored the vision of a blind eye. He stated[3] that sphenoidal disease might be the cause of many obscure cases of retrobulbar neuritis.

Onodi,[4] working for ten years on the relations between the optic nerve and the accessory cavities of the nose, long ago found that frequently the posterior ethmoidal cells are separated from the optic nerve in the optic foramen by the thinnest possible bony wall, and, furthermore, that the distribution of the blood vessels favored an extension of inflammations from the mucous membrane of the ethmoidal cells to the periosteum of the optic foramen. Thus ethmoidal disease may give rise to an affection of the canalicular portion of the optic nerve, which manifests itself in a central scotoma or perhaps in complete blindness. At first there may be no changes in the disc, or merely inflammatory signs, but later pallor from degeneration of the nerve fibers appears.

---

2. Beitr. z. Progn. d. Neur. retrobulbaris u. d. Intoxications amblyopia, Arch. f. Augenh., 1907, lix, 1, p. 28.

3. Arch. Ophth., 1896.

4. Der Sehnerv und die Nebenhöhlen der Nase, Hölder, Vienna and Leipsic, 1907.

Dr. W. C. Posey, two years ago, described vascular changes in the optic disc and surrounding retina in cases of ethmoiditis. And Dr. Arnold Knapp has recently reported a case of retrobulbar neuritis with central scotoma in which, by removing a portion of the middle turbinate and draining the ethmoidal cells, the vision was restored to normal. He believes that the common cases of retrobulbar neuritis following influenza are of ethmoidal origin. An illustrative case is the following:

Case 6.—Three months ago I saw a woman, aged 30, who, two years before, had noticed a sudden diminution of vision in the left eye, which passed off in the course of a few weeks. When I first saw her there had been a rather sudden complete loss of sight in the left eye two weeks before, and this eye had no perception of light. The pupillary reaction to light also was lost. Medicinal treatment had not improved her condition. The optic disc was swollen, and the retinal veins were dilated and tortuous.

Examination and Treatment.—In the right eye, acuteness of vision and the field of vision were normal, hence the lesion on the left side lay anterior to the chiasma. And since nothing could be discovered in the orbit to account for the complete blindness, a diagnosis of disturbance in the canalicular portion of the nerve was made. Examination of the nose revealed an abnormal middle turbinate on each side. A portion of the middle turbinate on the left side was removed by a rhinologist, so that drainage of the ethmoidal cells was established, and vision in the periphery of the field at once returned. The large central scotoma gradually became narrower, and three weeks after the operation vision in the left eye was 20/20, with a normal field.

Course of Disease.—A few days later vision in the right eye sank to 20/70, with a central scotoma and normal peripheral limits of the fields. The middle turbinate on this side showed more evidence of disease than the other had shown, and removal of a portion of it was followed by restoration of normal vision in the right eye in a few days.

As stated above, Marx reported sixteen cases of nontoxic retrobulbar neuritis, and six of these patients were found later to have multiple sclerosis. Most of the remaining patients gave each a history of coryza preceding the diminution of vision. Is one not justified, therefore, in assuming that some of these ten cases of retrobulbar neuritis were of ethmoidal or sphenoidal origin?

Non-toxic retrobulbar neuritis has long been a mysterious disease. but it would seem now that a little more study might rob it of much of its mystery and teach us that although syphilis, diabetes, neoplasms, injuries and the like may be causes, non-toxic retrobulbar optic neuritis, in the majority of cases, if it does not mean disease of the accessory sinuses of the nose, means multiple sclerosis.

RECAPITULATION.

Disturbances of vision are found in about half of the cases of multiple sclerosis. Usually the dimness of vision is noticed early in the course of the disease, and it may come on long before any other symptoms have attracted attention.

More than half of the patients with multiple sclerosis who complain of failing sight have central scotoma in the field of vision, and the ophthalmologic diagnosis of their condition is retrobulbar neuritis. Toxic cases of retrobulbar neuritis, due to poisoning with tobacco, alcohol, lead, and the toxins arising in pregnancy are readily recognized and diagnosed as toxic. The causation of non-toxic retrobulbar neuritis, however, has often been obscure. We have learned recently that many of these cases are due to sphenoidal and particularly to ethmoidal disease, which involves the optic nerve in the optic foramen.

In my opinion, we shall soon come to the belief that a non-toxic retrobulbar neuritis, if not due to a sinusitis or directly to syphilis, diabetes, a neoplasm, or trauma is, as a rule, a manifestation of multiple sclerosis, although no other symptoms of the disease may be present.

MEMORANDA

MIGRAINE, AN OCCUPATION NEUROSIS.*

GEORGE LINCOLN WALTON, M.D.

BOSTON.

It is not claimed that this paper will present a complete explanation of migraine; it is hoped, however, that it will start a suggestive line of thought bearing on a pathogeny which can be at the best only hypothetical.

The form of migraine to which I shall confine myself is the every-day type, the variety which I have found occurring in complete form in 17 per cent. of healthy young adults, and in incomplete form in many more. It reaches its greatest intensity in early life and generally disappears after middle life. It is often preceded by scotomata, by temporary aphasia and numbness, loss of memory, signs of mental incapacity and confusion, and even possibly, as Gowers suggests, by the peculiar feeling that the present is a reproduction of the past, the feeling thus described by Coleridge:

Oft o'er my brain does that strong fancy roll
  Which makes the present (while the flash doth last)
Seem a mere semblance of some unknown past,
  Mixed with such feelings as perplex the soul
Self questioned in her sleep.

Any of these symptoms may appear without the pain in the head. Loss of consciousness never occurs, a fact which sharply distinguishes migraine from epilepsy, though there have been attempts to make them analogous. The frontal and temporal regions are most often involved, the occipital next often, the vertex practically never alone.

At the time of greatest intensity the pain is sometimes accompanied by nausea and vomiting, especially in early

* This paper has been accepted by the Executive Committee of the Section on Ophthalmology of the American Medical Association, to be presented before the Section at the Chicago Session, June 2-5, 1908. Publication rights reserved by the American Medical Association.

life, whence the term "sick headache." The time varies in duration from several hours to a day or more. It does not often materially interfere with sleep, though it frequently appears on awakening in the morning. It does not necessarily accompany extreme use of the eyes, though it is apt to appear after such use, as on the morning following a theater party.

The so-called ophthalmic form of migraine is so rare in comparison with this form, and so distinct in its symptoms, that it seems hardly fair to discuss both types together. The suggestion of Plavec,[1] that the ordinary form is the precursor of the ophthalmic form, seems to have little basis, and his proposed pathology (periodic swelling of the hypophysis), as concerns the ordinary migraine, is purely speculative.

A case reported some years ago by Dr. Cheney and myself has a practical bearing on this question. A man of middle age had suffered many years from what was supposed to be the common type of migraine, though it was accompanied by the unusual symptom of persistent homonomous hemianopsia. The headaches became more severe, various paralyses appeared, mental deterioration ensued, and death followed. The autopsy revealed pituitary tumor.

While this case bears favorably on Plavec's location for ophthalmic migraine, it is far from aiding us in the pathogeny of ordinary migraine. Nor does it suggest that ordinary migraine was the precursor of the more serious trouble. The migrainous headaches in this case should rather be regarded as symptomatic of the local lesion, no more allied to or resulting from ordinary migraine than epileptoid seizures from cerebral tumor are allied to, or result from, idiopathic epilepsy, though they may be mistaken for it at the outset.

Whatever theory is advanced for the pathogeny of ordinary migraine, the use of the eyes can hardly be left out.[2] The arguments connecting the use of the eyes and migraine are easily preponderant. In the first place

1. Deutsche Ztschr. f. Nervenheilk., 1907, xxxii.

2. This statement does not apply to the views of those who find in migraine the precursor of vascular disease and cerebral softening. My conception of migraine is widely at variance with theories which include such outcome. When we weigh the isolated cases supporting this proposition against the hordes of cases running an innocuous course, it seems reasonable to assume that these few cases represent either coincidence of migraine and organic disease or symptomatic headaches which resemble migraine.

too many cases of migraine have been relieved, in part or entirely, by correction of refractive error, particularly of astigmatism, to be explained by coincidence. In the second place, attacks have been frequently aborted by the mere straightening of glasses, as I have many times verified in my own case. In the third place, migraine has lessened and disappeared in innumerable cases after accommodative paralysis has appeared. Finally, study of the blind shows that the greater the blindness the less the migraine. My own examination of a long series convinced me that migrainous headaches are only half as frequent among the blind as among individuals of corresponding age and under like conditions.

It may be objected that migrainous headaches are not quite unknown among the blind. But it must be remembered that it is a common practice for the blind, as for others, to adjust their accommodation to the distance of their work as judged, even in the absence of sight, by the position of the hands.

Assuming, then, that disturbance of the accommodative centers plays a part in migraine, it need not be expected that the blind shall be quite exempt.

Another peculiarity of eyestrain which has an important bearing on my proposition is the almost continuous frown of the astigmatic. This frown involves principally the corrugator supercilii and the anterior part of the occipitofrontalis, which muscles occupy the regions in which the pain most frequently appears.

If one voluntarily contract the brows for fifteen minutes he will experience a disagreeable sensation which suggests migraine in mild form. This leads to the question whether we must assume the pain of migraine to be entirely intracranial, a doubt emphasized by the recent observations of Cushing[3] showing the non-sensitiveness of the dura, the part to which perhaps more than any other the pain of migraine has been credited. It may assist us to recall a somewhat analogous pain which sometimes appears in the back of the neck and "base of the brain" after long-continued eyework in which the head is held firmly in one position. I have been not infrequently consulted for this pain by persons who have undertaken an uncommon line of work, requiring this posture, the commonest illustration being that of the person who has recently undertaken the position of

3. The Journal A. M. A., March 14, 1908.

secretary. This pain so often appears after the completion of the day's work, rather than during the work, that its source is apt to be overlooked. The pain is apt first to appear during the night or in the early morning, and is sometimes decidedly paroxysmal. The only relief is found in discontinuance, or lessening the constancy, of the work (unless, happily, the mere correction of refraction serves the turn). This form of headache is surely muscular rather than intracranial; its analogy to migraine is shown by the fact that it is sometimes preceded by twinkling scotoma.

This occipital form of headache offers a fair illustration of acute occupation neurosis.

The proposition I have to submit is the following:

Migraine is an occupation neurosis, and involves (1) the visual centers; (2) the centers of accommodation (centers of divergence and convergence in the frontal region); (3) the intrinsic and extrinsic muscles of the globe, and (4) the muscles outside the orbit which are called into play in the effort required for accurate vision, principally the corrugator supercilii and occipito-frontalis, but also the muscles inserted in the occipital region, which serve to steady the head.

In order that we may approach the question fairly, it is important that we start with a clear idea of the symptomatology of occupation neurosis in general; its exact pathogeny is hardly susceptible of analysis.

This is a subject not generally understood. "Writers' cramp" has called attention to one symptom (cramp) which is really neither the most prominent nor the most common. Even writer's cramp has its "neuralgic" form, and in other occupation neuroses pain is not only by far the most prominent, but often the only symptom, the other symptoms, weakness, paresthesia and cramp, following with varying frequency and in varying degrees.

An occupation neurosis is a condition resulting from overuse of certain parts. The most constant symptom is pain, generally referred to the overused muscles, but sometimes extending to other parts. Among the less constant symptoms are muscular spasm and paresthesia. The symptoms may be constant or paroxysmal, and are not always synchronous with the muscular overuse which causes them, but sometimes follows after an interval. The disturbance involves the muscles and the sensory and motor cerebral centers which constitute the over-used mechanism.

The following case illustrates a common form of occupation neurosis involving the arm:

Patient.—A woman, aged 30, suffered from pain in the thumb and first finger extending up the forearm, accompanied at night by a numb prickly feeling. She practiced much on the piano, carried a heavy music roll, and often sewed a whole evening without stopping. In short, there was almost constant use, in one form or another, of the hand. There was moderate tenderness of the forearm. There was no objective anesthesia or loss of power. The diagnosis of occupation neurosis was made.

Treatment.—No improvement appeared from simple rest, but when a splint was applied and the arm placed in a sling, thus producing absolute rest, improvement soon appeared, and complete recovery followed. She can now use the hand perfectly, but has learned to keep its use within reasonable limits.

That the pain of occupation neurosis is not always limited to the muscles is shown by the following case, which reminds us also that the excessive use causing this form of neurosis need not be limited to the occupation in the sense of vocation.

A young married woman complained of pain on the inner side of the left thumb. The symptom had lasted about five years, was increasing steadily, and at times the paroxysms were very severe. At first it only came on at night, later it appeared during the day. Sometimes the index finger would become involved, and at times the pain would extend up the arm. The *x*-ray revealed nothing. Close questioning revealed no special use of the thumb beyond piano practice and sewing, in neither of which was this part of the thumb particularly involved. I felt, however, so confident of the diagnosis that I advised rest in splint and sling. It finally occurred to the patient that she was accustomed to read for hours holding the book in the left hand with pressure on the inner surface of the thumb, and illustrating the position in my office promptly produced the pain.

The following case presents a connecting link between such cases and migraine:

Patient.—A successful laryngologist from another state had worked for twenty-five years without vacation. He complained of paroxysms of pain in the left side of the neck and behind the ear, sometimes accompanied by tenderness. The pain would come on when his head was placed in the position of operating, become rapidly unbearable if the posture was maintained, and persist after its discontinuance. It would sometimes come on at an interval after operating. Attempts to read sometimes produced the pain. He had astigmatism with correction by a competent oculist. The condition had naturally given rise to much solicitude, and obvious relief of mind followed the diagnosis of "occupation neurosis." The day following the consultation he spent in and about Boston, and for thirty-six hours was entirely free from pain, an experience which he had not had for some time. On the second day he was feeling so much better that he was tempted to return to his work, notwithstanding my advice for a prolonged abstinence from employment. He was desirous of visiting the Massachusetts General Hospital, and I there introduced him to the throat department, in which he was especially interested. Here he spent about an hour, watching operations, and examining throats. On sitting down to lunch afterward a violent paroxysm of pain appeared and lasted for some time. It recurred during the evening on taking up a paper and putting his head in the position of reading. The evening attack lasted several hours, during which the pain was intense and accompanied by tenderness. The only recourse in this case was absolute cessation from work for many months. He is therefore now taking an extended vacation and reports continued improvement.

This case, like many others which have come under my observation, shows that the pain of occupation neurosis may follow the occupation after an interval, just as that of "theater migraine" may first appear on awakening the morning after attending the theater.

The paroxysmal pain illustrated by such cases of occupation neurosis strongly suggests that of migraine. Nor are the minor symptoms of occupation neurosis wanting in migraine. The analogue of the paresthesia is the scotoma, which represents similarly, disturbance of sensory centers. Analogous to the cramp is the ciliary spasm, to say nothing of the facial spasm which sometimes appears in the lids and spreads to other parts, representing perhaps an effort on the part of the overworked centers to close the eye and relieve the tension. I have seen the most long-standing and obstinate cases of this spasm relieved by the correction of refractive error.

The suggestion that migraine is an occupation neurosis does no violence to the opinion of those who regard all migraine as the result of refractive error, and at the same time may prove more acceptable than the reflex theory to those who insist on the hereditary and constitutional basis of migraine. One need only be reminded that all occupation neuroses are more prevalent among the neurotic and the sensitively organized, in whose families appear the varied signs of feeble resistance. It is surely among this class that we look for migraine —but we have not explained migraine by simply conceding its hereditary tendency.

Furthermore, the theory of occupation neurosis would account for cases of migraine in which the patients have slight error of refraction, but marked psychopathic heredity, and at the same time explain its prevalence among those who have marked error of refraction, since the eyes are here used with an overwhelming handicap, the relief of which may well cause the disappearance of the neurosis.

According to the occupation neurosis theory migraine may even appear without error of refraction, in other words it may result from over-use of the eyes, or, in cases of extreme susceptibility, from moderate use of the eyes, just as writer's cramp may be produced, doubtless, in the absence of a faulty method of writing. The fact is recognized, however, that a faulty method favors writer's cramp, and, similarly, error of refraction is doubtless more potent than any other one factor in the production of migraine.

It is no objection to this theory that some individuals use the eyes continuously without migraine, while others acquire this trouble with comparatively little use of the eyes. The same is true of all occupation neuroses. One individual can practice with immunity on a musical instrument from early morning till late at night; in another individual symptoms of occupation neurosis appear with a few hours' exercise.

It may be objected that no account is taken of the vasomotor phenomena of migraine, a factor on which Eulenberg long ago based his entire theory of the pathology of the condition. But the vasomotor changes, in my view, at least, are so far from constant that they are not to be taken into consideration in the search for causal factors, but are rather to be reckoned, when present, as among the comparatively unimportant accompaniments. This is the view long held by Gowers.

The vasomotor symptoms are not only secondary rather than primary, but, in fact, they are not always present. All suppositions based on dilatation or contraction of blood vessels as a primary cause of migraine lead to theoretical considerations which obscure rather than clarify our ideas of migraine. And, further, all such theories are based on a fallacy, namely, that contraction and dilatation of blood vessels necessarily cause pain. To confute this proposition we need only remind ourselves of the extreme dilatation of blood vessels in the blush of shame or the turgidity of anger, on the one hand, and on the other hand, with the pallor of fear and faintness. Even the extreme degree of vascular spasm which results from cold produces numbness rather than pain. It is true that after exposure to cold with resulting vascular spasm, if warmth is too quickly applied, a vascular dilatation follows which is accompanied by extreme pain, but when we consider the extreme degree of vascular dilatation that produces no pain, it is questionable whether the pain is to be attributed simply to dilatation.

The vomiting is difficult of explanation by the theory offered, but it is not less difficult by any other theory. In point of fact, this symptom is probably not one of the essential features but rather an indirect result appearing generally only in the young and at the height of the paroxysm, representing rather a protective effort on the part of Nature, through producing general and special relaxation, just as fainting may appear at the height of pain, resulting from whatever cause. The fact that relief does often follow the vomiting fortifies this supposition.

CONCLUSION.

Migraine is an occupation neurosis resulting, in individuals of neurotic inheritance, from overuse, or use under the handicap of refractive error, of the parts concerned in vision.

It involves, like other occupation neuroses, disturbance of (1) sensory cerebral centers (those of vision in the occipital region); (2) motor cerebral centers (centers of divergence and convergence in the frontal lobe); and, (3) certain muscles (particularly the intrinsic and extrinsic muscles of the globe, the corrugator supercilii and the occipitofrontalis, and also the muscles which steady the head).

The pain of migraine is not necessarily intracranial, but is localized, in part at least, in the region of the muscles concerned, directly or indirectly, in vision.

AN INFREQUENT TYPE OF OPTIC NERVE ATROPHY.*

HOWARD F. HANSELL, M.D.
PHILADELPHIA.

I am aware that my contribution to the subject of optic nerve atrophy can have but a limited application, and whatever practicability it possesses is clinical and therapeutic only. While the subject is fairly well understood, our knowledge pertains more to etiology and pathology than to therapeutics. Almost without exception inflammation and atrophy are secondary to some other affection, which, either directly by pressure or extension of disease from neighboring parts, or indirectly, following general disturbances of the nervous system, toxemia, alterations in the constituents of the blood or other remote causes impedes circulation and prevents nutrition to the nerve. Rarely does the inflammation arise in, and confine itself to, the optic nerve and its intraocular expansion. The treatment of the optic nerve affections, therefore, is the treatment of the underlying disease. Speaking generally, the ophthalmoscopic findings decide whether the atrophy is a sequel to inflammation, hence more or less acute, or whether it has followed connective tissue increase and destruction of the nerve fiber—the old-fashioned "ascending and descending" atrophy. My purpose in this paper is to confine myself exclusively to atrophy of the optic nerve as a disease in itself and not apparently associated with and dependent on other affections of the nervous system or of other organs of the body.

* This paper has been accepted by the Executive Committee of the Section on Ophthalmology of the American Medical Association, to be presented before the Section at the Chicago Session, June 2-5, 1908.

ANATOMIC RELATIONS.

The optic nerve may be divided arbitrarily for the purpose of clinical study into two sections: that between the chiasm and the optic foramen and that between the optic foramen and the eyeball. The former measures in the adult of average size from 7 to 11 mm. (1/4 in. to 7/16 in.), and the latter from 23 to 30 mm. (7/8 in. to 1 1/4 in.), the entire nerve, from chiasm to globe averaging 35 mm. (1 3/8 in.) in length. The intracranial portion of the nerve lies in the optic canal in the body of the sphenoid bone, and is said to be enveloped only by the pial sheath, since the other two sheaths after passing through the optic foramen become united with the two outer membranes of the brain. The optic canal contains only one other structure, the ophthalmic artery, given off from the internal carotid in close juxtaposition. Between the chiasm and optic foramen the optic nerve runs under the medial root of the olfactory nerve and is separated from it by the anterior cerebral artery. On the medial side it borders on the division between the hemispheres and on the lateral side it lies near the anterior perforated space.

It is important to remember, as a factor of no inconsiderable interest in the clinical study of optic atrophy, that no other cranial nerve lies in close enough proximity to become implicated by paralysis or inflammation by a morbid process that is confined to the optic nerve or its sheath, the third, fourth, the ophthalmic division of the fifth and the sixth nerves entering the orbit through the sphenoidal fissure. Its relation, however, to the sphenoidal sinuses and to the posterior ethmoidal sinuses is significant and throws light on the etiology of optic nerve affections. Professor Onodi, in his recent monograph (1907) on this subject, presents a series of photographs from original dissections which thoroughly explains this relation. He shows clearly how disease of the sinuses, directly by necrosis of the bony walls and extension of the disease through the openings thus made and involvement of the sheath of the nerve and indirectly by pressure from collections of pus or from a growth within the cavities, may affect the optic nerve. The walls of the sinuses are in some individuals exceedingly thin and yield readily to the tension of the contained material. The right sphenoidal sinus seems to be more often the cause of compression of the nerve and chiasm because of its slightly more intimate relation with them.

RELATION OF ACCESSORY SINUS DISEASE.

From this brief résumé of the anatomic relations of the intracranial portion of the optic nerve, it may be inferred that disease of the sphenoid and ethmoid sinuses may be ranked among the prominent causes of inflammation and atrophy. Sufficient stress, I believe, has not been laid either on the frequency or importance of this cause. Posey,[1] Arnold Knapp[2] and others have recently drawn attention to this causative connection and have insisted on the existence of accessory sinus disease despite the negative reports of laryngologists to whom their cases were referred for examination. It is doubtless impossible in the early stages of sinus disease for even the most expert examiners to detect its presence, but in the later stages the electric transilluminator is of great service. I wish here to repeat Posey's admonition that the ophthalmologist shall not be contented with the findings of one examination in cases which point to sinus disease as the cause of the optic nerve affection. In this connection Chance's case is of interest. He reports a case of presumed exostosis of the orbit which proved to be a bulging outward of the outer walls of the ethmoid cells due to an enormous collection of pus contained in the ethmoid and sphenoid sinuses and extending as far forward as the frontal sinus. There were no obstructions in the nasal or faucial passages, no discharge and no indication whatever that the sinuses were diseased. The optic discs were pale and the retinal veins were engorged.

As Bartels[3] has shown in his study of the pathology of blindness in orbital abscess, the optic nerve in purulent disease of the accessory sinuses may be affected by pressure, by extension of inflammation and by necrosis of the sheath and the fiber following impaired nutrition due to thrombosis of the small arteries and veins. First, then, in seeking for a cause the accessory sinuses should be examined thoroughly and repeatedly.

1. The Journal A. M. A., Feb. 23, 1907, 676.
2. Arch. Ophth., January, 1908.
3. Arch. Ophth., January, 1908.

RELATION OF TERTIARY SYPHILIS.

Excluding local causes, no other etiologic factor can be compared in frequency with tertiary syphilis of the structures surrounding the intracranial portion of the optic nerve. The lesions may involve the dura mater, the pia mater, the bones at the base of the skull, the blood vessels and the nerves themselves, and consist of chronic inflammation with exudation, gummatous infiltration, gumma and disease of the vessels. Uhthoff[4] believes that in most instances of intracranial optic neuritis the nerve was affected secondary to surrounding syphilitic lesions. "In Uhthoff's own observations (17 cases), as well as in 150 autopsies of cerebral syphilis reported by others and reviewed bv him, the lesions of the optic nerve were but part of the lesions found at the base of the brain."

Gradle,[5] from whose paper I extract the above quotation, has reported 4 cases, and all of them are believed by him to be syphilitic. In my own 2 cases, to which I shall refer briefly later, one was due to acute disease of the accessory sinuses and the other to syphilis. In view of the prevalence of syphilis in the etiology, I think it would be proper to presume syphilis to be responsible, although there may be no tangible evidence of that disease. To depend on the patient's testimony or on the presence of other lesions pointing to syphilis, would be misleading. It must be remembered that intracranial optic neuritis belongs to the very latest manifestations and the patients may have been in ignorance of their earlier infection or purposely withhold a knowledge of it from the examiner.

According to Gradle, the symptoms are sufficiently marked to make the diagnosis reasonably certain. "Sudden diminution of sight without central scotoma and with nearly normal field, tendency toward recovery, but possibly ending in incomplete atrophy with absence of all other symptoms except initial headache, is the clinical picture of intracranial optic neuritis." He says the transient failure of sight in 3 of his cases can best be explained by the assumption of diffuse optic neuritis involving only the intracranial portion of the optic nerve and the clinical characteristics of this assumed lesion

4. von Graefe's Arch. f. Ophth., xxxix. 1.

5. Arch. Ophth., March, 1907.

are consistent with our knowledge of the topography of the fibers in the intracranial trunk.

When, however, the cause is not syphilis, but disease of the accessory sinuses, the symptoms may vary from those described by Gradle. In Arnold Knapp's case the sight of the right eye had become suddenly affected. V. = 20/70; field: periphery normal, central relative scotoma of 5 degrees; left eye was normal. After relieving the posterior ethmoid cells of a large amount of pus, vision gradually returned and in seven weeks was normal. "A central scotoma always seems to be present if the case is examined early enough and the optic nerve lesion falls into the group of retrobulbar neuritis."

CASE 1.—*History.*—X., a lad of 17, suddenly became partially blind after exposure. He had been driving all day in stormy weather and had become thoroughly chilled. After eating a hearty supper he lay down on the kitchen floor near a hot stove and slept all night. In the morning vision was reduced in each eye to the perception of large objects.

Examination.—The retinal arteries were greatly reduced in size and the papillæ pale. The veins were of normal caliber. He had a large central negative scotoma reducing the seeing field to a small area at the periphery. The cause was laid to intracranial optic neuritis from disease of the sphenoidal sinus, and this opinion was later verified.

Subsequent History.—Treatment was of no avail. The optic nerves became atrophic and a large patch of retinochorioidal atrophy developed corresponding to the scotoma, due probably, as Birch-Hirschfeld[6] has pointed out, to toxic action on the optic nerve fibers.

The ophthalmoscopic appearances of the disc vary from the signs of acute neuritis and retinal edema in the acute cases, to a fine almost imperceptible deeply seated paleness, and this variation seems to be independent of the cause. In Gradle's first case the discs were normal; in the second, the same, in the third, the same at first, but two years later "an unquestionable though very slight atrophy of the left optic nerve while the right papilla was suspiciously pale;" the fourth was healthy. In Knapp's case there was "pronounced neuroretinitis, with a radiating figure of white lines and dots about the macula."

In my first case the atrophy was well marked, and in the second there was apparently good retinal and nerve circulation, but really a slight but positive loss of vas-

6. von Graefe's Arch. f. Ophth., lxv, 3.

cularity in the nerve head. It seems that the diagnosis of affections of the intracranial portion of the optic nerve can not positively be determined by the ophthalmoscope, because its signs do not materially differ from those of atrophy from affections of other parts of the nerve. Yet a "suspicious paleness," remaining unchanged through months and attended with comparatively great loss of vision, points to the situation of the lesion in the intracranial portion. The pupillary symptoms are not significant. The size of the pupils and any difference between them may be accounted for, in uncomplicated cases, by the loss of vision and the difference in vision between the two eyes. Moreover, dilated or unequal pupils may be misleading because they may indicate a lesion farther back in the brain than the chiasm or an extensive disturbance of the nervous system. Pupillary inequalities are present in many different affections, both functional and organic, and are more significant of the gravity of the disease than of the locality of the lesion.

The same statement may be made concerning ocular muscle paralysis. Its presence indicates simply that the lesion is not limited strictly to the intracranial portion of the nerve, but has originated either some distance away or has extended from the canalis opticus backward from the chiasm, involving the fifth, fourth, third and sixth nerves, respectively, or forward into the sphenoidal fissure. Its absence would point to the limitation of the lesion between the anterior border of the chiasm and the foramen opticum. Headache is a common symptom. It is violent and almost continuous in sinus disease and paroxysmal in syphilis. It is not characteristic and does not differ essentially from the headache of refractive errors and many other cerebral and general affections.

CASE 2.—*History.*—Mrs. J., aged 35, was infected by her husband with syphilis eight years ago. She received the usual treatment at the hands of an able and careful physician under whose care she remained for a number of years.

She considered herself well and for four years appeared to be so excepting for an occasional breakdown due to a valvular heart lesion. In the spring of 1906 she consulted me on account of headache and failing vision of the right eye.

Examination.—R. V. = 20/50, L. V. = 20/30. Low hyperopia. Both optic discs were slightly pale with little noticeable difference between them, although the right was possibly a trifle paler, no limitation of either field for white, but concentric contraction for all colors. Urinary analysis showed a trace of albumin, no sugar, no casts.

Treatment.—She was given inunctions of mercury, large doses of potassium iodid, hot baths and sweats, repeated every few weeks. In six months V. had fallen to R. 20/70, L. 20/50; the optic discs were unchanged in color, but the vessels of the retina showed signs of a mild degree of pressure, presumably exerted on the nerve. The veins were dilated and slightly tortuous, the arteries narrowed. The paleness of the discs was peculiar. At first glance the papillæ seemed to be entirely normal and of healthy color, but thorough inspection showed a deep-seated loss of color. At this time the right eye began to diverge, from paresis of the third nerve, fusion of the images requiring a prism of 40 degrees. Central vision was the same, but the fields were limited for white as well as for colors. Vision slowly declined in the right until the spring of 1907, when it equaled only 20/250. In June she stated she had attacks of severe pain, lasting from 12 to 18 hours starting in both eyes and passing back to the occiput and cervical regions. V. R. = 5/200, L. = 20/50. January, 1908, she reported three attacks of pain in right temple with swelling of the soft tissues, attended with transient diminution of vision. At this time there was in the right eye a small central scotoma for red and green. Under treatment vision and fields were improved (R. = 20/100), the scotoma disappeared, but the diplopia remained unchanged. The pupils were equal and responsive throughout, and the patient never seriously suffered in her general health. During the two years of observation of this patient the ophthalmoscopic findings remained without appreciable variation. Even when the vision had sunk to 5/200 and the field for white was limited to a circle of 15 degrees around the fixation point, the deep-lying paleness of the disc had not increased, and again when vision recovered to 20/200 the color was unchanged.

I believe the process in this patient to be a neuritis of varying intensity affecting the intracranial portion of the optic nerve, syphilitic in origin, basing the opinion on the absence of pupillary phenomena and of symptoms of general disturbance of the nervous system, the peculiar deep-seated paleness of the papillæ, the concentric limitation of the fields, the temporary scotoma and the unprogressiveness of the affection.

MEMORANDA

DIFFERENTIAL DIAGNOSIS OF AFFECTIONS OF THE OPTIC NERVE.*

HARRY FRIEDENWALD, M.D.

BALTIMORE.

The subject for consideration is the differential diagnosis of pathologic conditions of the optic nerve between chiasm and retina.

Pathologic investigation has differentiated various forms of inflammatory affection, of traumatic injury, of vascular disease, of hemorrhages and neoplasms within and around the nerve and different kinds of atrophy of the nerve fibers either primary or consequent on the previously mentioned affections. Clinical observation has shown that these conditions differ in the appearance of the nerve head and in their effect on central and peripheral vision, and that variations are not only found between different affections, but even between different cases of the same or similar affections according to location and extent of lesion. The differential diagnosis, therefore, depends in one case on the ophthalmoscopic picture, in another on characteristic changes in the field of vision; but in most cases we must rely for differential diagnosis on careful study of both the appearance of the nerve head and the function of the nerve as tested for acuity of central, peripheral and color vision, on their changes during the progress of the disease; and the facts thus elicited must be considered in connection with the previous history and habits of the patient and with such other ocular, constitutional, organic and especially nervous diseases as may be discovered.

---

* This paper has been accepted by the Executive Committee of the Section on Ophthalmology of the American Medical Association, to be presented before the Section at the Chicago Session, June 2-5, 1908. Publication rights reserved by the American Medical Association.

For the purpose of our inquiry we shall divide the subject into:

(A) **Those cases in which there is ophthalmoscopic evidence of inflammation in the optic disc.**

(B) **Those cases in which the nerve head presents the picture of atrophy.**

(C) **Those cases in which the disc is normal or approximately normal in appearance.**

A. AFFECTIONS IN WHICH THERE IS OPHTHALMOSCOPIC EVIDENCE OF INFLAMMATION IN THE OPTIC DISC.

The recognition of inflammation of the optic disc is sometimes rendered difficult by the great variations which normal optic discs present, and particularly by the markedly hyperemic condition which has been described as pseudo-neuritis. In these cases there may be marked tortuosity of the vessels, but the nerve remains transparent, the vessel walls are normal, there is never great swelling, and we usually find marked errors of refraction, commonly hypermetropic. Continued observation may be necessary for definite diagnosis.

The presence of fine, congenital patches of connective tissue or of hyaline bodies (Drusen) should never lead to errors in diagnosis, the absence of congestion and tortuosity and in the latter condition the characteristic reflexes enable us to recognize these conditions without difficulty.

The inflammatory affections of the optic disc are commonly divided into the descending optic neuritis or neuro-retinitis and choked disc. For clinical reasons it is of great importance to distinguish them, though their differentiation is by no means always an easy matter. The typical choked disc with the narrow arteries, the full and tortuous veins and the great prominence of the optic disc usually occurs as a binocular affection, and when binocular is the expression of increased intracranial pressure, most frequently produced by tumor, symptoms of which are rarely absent. The tumor may be benign or malignant, syphilitic or tuberculous. There is at first little or no visual disturbance, the central vision is unimpaired, the outlines of the field of vision are not reduced and the enlargement of the blind spot is easily overlooked. But there is occasional or frequent obscuration of vision, when, for a moment, everything becomes black before the patient, a symptom rarely found in other conditions than those of increased intracranial pressure. It is only at a late stage when the neuritis gives way to atrophy that there is rapid and marked failure of vision.

The combination of intense neuritis with such slight disturbance of the function of vision is as important as it is characteristic when we bear in mind that ninety per cent. of tumors of the brain, at some time, produce optic neuritis. Cerebral tumor, especially when in the middle fossa, may likewise produce unilateral choked disc or even choked disc of one eye and simple neuritis or optic atrophy of the other. Unilateral choked disc is most frequently due to orbital causes or to a meningeal syphilis passing down and causing lesions of the sheath.

The causes of choked disc aside from brain tumor are too well known to be dwelt on at this time. (Cerebral abscess, meningitis, hydrocephalus, nephritis, anemia, etc.) To one only do I wish to call special attention; namely, to serous meningitis. It is probable that some of the cases in which the diagnosis of brain tumor was made and in which recovery took place should be put in this category.

Case 1.—In December, 1905, I saw a little girl, aged 4, who had been ill for three weeks with high temperature and pain in the ears. Convulsions had occurred. The drums were congested and were punctured without obtaining any exudate. On ophthalmoscopic examination, marked optic neuritis was found and the patient was referred to Dr. Harvey Cushing, who made a decompression operation, followed by complete disappearance of the neuritis. I have seen the child at intervals and find that she has remained perfectly well.

Case 2.—A case still more definite is that of Mary P., colored, aged 32, first seen on Feb. 20, 1906, for acute suppurative otitis media and mastoiditis on the left side. The patient did not consent to an operation until March 3. The operation was performed by Dr. S. Rosenheim and myself. There was pus under some pressure in the mastoid cells and the bone was soft. The lateral sinus was exposed for about one-half an inch; part of it was found covered by granulation tissue. The tip of the mastoid was one large cell filled with pus and granulation tissue on the posterior part of which the sinus was likewise exposed. After packing the latter cavity and withdrawing the packing there was a profuse hemorrhage from the lateral sinus, though no violence had been used. It was controlled by packing with iodoform gauze. Her temperature before the time of the operation was about 99 F., pulse 80 to 98. On the following days the temperature was irregular, reaching 103.6 F. on the fourth day after the operation, while at the same time her pulse dropped on the second day after the operation to 64, and remained below 70 for several days, except when the temperature was very high and the pulse rose to 100.

On the fifth day (temperature between 98.8 F. and 100.5 F.) abducens paralysis set in, and I found mild optic neuritis. From this period on the temperature remained normal, though the pulse continued slow during the entire first week, but the neuritis increased and rapidly became a typical choked disc with hemorrhages in both eyes, more marked in the left. This condition lasted for some time, when the patient ceased coming, the wound having healed.

Seven months after the operation I found very little swelling of the discs, the veins slightly tortuous, but not very full, the arteries somewhat narrow, the color of the discs pink, and margins obscured; the condition of the left eye being more marked than that of the right eye. V. R. E., 16/30; V. L. E., 10/100. While optic neuritis is known to occur in a small number of cases of lateral sinus thrombosis, there was no evidence in this case of thrombosis, and the diagnosis of serous meningitis following injury of the softened wall of the sinus was most probable.

Spontaneous recovery from choked disc with cerebral symptoms, unless due to hemorrhage which is absorbed, or to syphilitic lesions which disappear under treatment, or in very young children whose suture lines break and thus allow expansion, is very rare.

Case 3.—Mrs. G., aged 33, married and mother of two healthy children, whom I saw in 1891, had marked papillitis in the right eye with cerebral symptoms. She recovered after several months. There was no evidence whatever of syphilis. In 1896 she had a recurrence with vertigo and vomiting which again yielded to treatment (iodid of potash). I examined this patient last year and found some retinal pigment atrophy around the disc and normal central and peripheral vision. No evidence of atrophy of the discs, no swelling and no sign of previous neuritis.

Passing on to the other variety of optic neuritis, the so-called descending neuritis, we find but very moderate swelling if at all, no fulness or tortuosity of the veins, but an exudate clouding the disc and blurring the margin and perivascular lines bordering the blood vessels. In these cases, vision rapidly drops and frequently is entirely extinguished. The cause of double descending neuritis is usually some form of meningitis. Meningitis at the base is more prone to produce the optic neuritis and especially tubercular and syphilitic basilar meningitis spreading along the sheath as a perineuritis and thus involving nerve and even retina. Epidemic cerebrospinal meningitis, according to Uhthoff, produces optic neuritis in about 16 per cent. of the cases. It may result from nephritis. When unilateral it is usually due to orbital inflammation or extension from the nasal sinuses.

The differential diagnosis of descending neuritis showing the combination of the great visual disturbance with the characteristic inflammation of the disc presents no difficulty. Both forms of neuritis, the descending as well as the choked disc commonly end in white atrophy, in post-neuritic atrophy.

B. AFFECTIONS IN WHICH THE NERVE HEAD PRESENTS THE PICTURE OF ATROPHY.

Optic atrophy is a term applied clinically to such atrophic conditions as show distinct pallor of the optic disc. They may be due to primary atrophy, as found in locomotor ataxia or secondary to injuries, to the pressure of tumors or of sclerotic blood vessels, to embolism or thrombosis of the central retinal vessels, to retinal or chorioidal atrophy, or to any form of neuritis, choked disc, descending or retrobulbar. The picture presented by the optic disc varies greatly. There may be the grayish pallor, with or without marked narrowing of the larger vessels, but with disappearance of the finer blood vessels and with sharply marked border as is usually seen in spinal atrophy. Or there may be the intensely white disc with irregular margins and perivascular lines usually seen as post neuritic atrophy. But it has been clearly shown that the variations are so great that we can not always determine from the appearance of the disc what form of atrophy it presents. And as in the case of pseudo-neuritis, so here we must also be careful not to regard every pale disc as atrophic, for pallor of the disc is at times very marked in high grades of anemia.

The visual function bears no relation to the appearance of the disc; we may find high grades of apparent atrophy with good vision, and vice versa.

Primary atrophy is with rare exception spinal atrophy. It begins at the bulbar end of the nerve, and therefore the pallor of the disc and the visual disturbance occur simultaneously. Uhthoff has defined three forms in which the field of vision is variously affected and which differ in their course and their prognosis. In the first there is diminution or loss of vision throughout the entire field, central vision is lessened and peripheral vision is restricted, though not uniformly, both for form, but especially for colors. In these cases, vision for green and then for red is lost, later for yellow and blue, thus producing a very great widening of the color blind area of the field. The progress is rapid, is hastened by mercury and the prognosis is absolutely bad.

In the second class sharply cut sector-like defects occur, but the parts preserved are normal in respect to color and form vision. The function of the parts retained may remain stationary, though it is usually lost after a time, one sector succumbing after another. This class, according to Wilbrand and Saenger, presents great similarity to that of syphilitic retrobulbar perineuritis with secondary atrophy of the disc.

The third class shows concentric contraction of the field with good central vision and good color vision in the portion preserved. Similar fields are found resulting from syphilitic affection of the intracranial portion of the optic nerve.

Wilbrand and Saenger have found that the course of the second and of the third class is very favorably influenced by the use of mercury, and they recommend its use here as emphatically as they warn against it in cases of the first class. They suggest as explanation that the differences may lie in mistaking syphilitic pseudotabes for true tabes, or the possibility of a combination of cerebral syphilis with true tabes which would likewise explain the occasional occurrence of "post-neuritic atrophy" in locomotor ataxia.

Uhthoff has shown that true primary optic atrophy never occurs in cerebral syphilis, that it is always secondary. It is, therefore, assumed that it likewise does not occur in spinal syphilis, and that the optic atrophy found in syphilitic pseudo-tabes is secondary and therefore yields to specific treatment. The difficulty of a differential diagnosis between the true tabetic primary atrophy and the secondary is very great. The latter is apt to be slow in developing, while primary atrophy, as has been stated, is observed simultaneously with the first visual disturbances. Monocular affections are likely to be syphilitic; variations in visual function more frequently occur in the syphilitic forms; the latter are apt to be complicated with other syphilitic cerebral nerve palsies; pupillary disturbances may occur in both conditions, but the Argyll-Robertson reaction points to locomotor ataxia; hemiopic defects indicate syphilis and the presence of a central scotoma practically excludes primary atrophy. The last named sign, as may be mentioned in passing, likewise helps to differentiate the secondary atrophy of alcoholic pseudo-tabes from the primary atrophy of true tabes.

Wilbrand and Saenger deny emphatically that syphilitic atrophy is ever primary and regard the latter as spinal in every case. They are in accord with Uhthoff's statement that any adult suffering with binocular primary progressive atrophy must be looked on, not only as suffering from serious ocular disease, but also from grave disease of the central nervous system.

Primary atrophy may, as is well known, precede the appearance of the other spinal symptoms by many years, and it is only the termination which may finally determine the definite diagnosis.

Case 4.—Mr. A., whom I first saw in December, 1895, for left optic nerve affection which had come on suddenly with drooping of the lid, with visions of flashes of light and a large defect in the field of vision, central vision being but slightly affected and the right eye not at all impaired. There was a definite history of luetic infection, but without secondary skin eruptions, mucous patches and other later syphilitic manifestations. Vigorous treatment with iodid of potash and mercury by inunction not only had no effect in arresting the progress of the trouble in the left eye, but did not prevent the same affection arising in the right eye six months later.

The discs at first appeared normal, and showed no atrophy and became pale only after a long period. The sight of the left eye was lost very rapidly, that of the right has shown only slow progress, so that its field is now very small and irregular, but central vision is still almost perfect. In this case, the sudden onset of symptoms, the absence of any early appearance of pallor and the slight ptosis helped to establish the diagnosis as a syphilitic lesion of the optic nerve and even though the treatment did not have the desired effect, the preservation of good central vision in one eye for twelve years and the non-development of any signs of spinal or cerebral disease confirms the diagnosis.

Another case presenting very different appearances is the following:

CASE 5.—A lady, first examined in July, 1890, when her eyegrounds were found normal and with weak convex cylinders her vision was perfect. She was married; her husband had definite syphilis (mucous patches, etc.). In October,. 1899, she again presented herself. She had borne four children and had had one miscarriage. Her younger children were very puny at birth but thrived on small doses of calomel. Subsequently, both had hemiplegic attacks, which were favorably influenced by mercury. An older child had two attacks of paralytic chorea. But though under constant care of her physician, the patient herself never presented a single sign of syphilis. Oct. 1, 1899, she complained of failing vision and the ophthalmoscopic examination showed white discs with V. R. E., 6/12, almost, and V. L. E., 6/24, partly. There were large symmetrical defects in the upper inner quadrants of both fields. Absence of the patellar reflex and slight inequality and loss of light reaction of the pupils were soon noted.

The usual treatment was given, iodid of potash, in very large doses, mercury by inunction for a prolonged period, pilocarpin, nitroglycerin, and later for many years, large doses of strychnia sulphate. The sight of her left eye was soon lost, but the progress of the disease was stayed in the right eye. In 1902 she had lost all color perception for green and red. In 1903, the pupils were noted as equal in size and reacted to light. The patient had had attacks of vertigo and intense headache and a lesion of the mitral valve had recently been discovered.

I last examined the patient in July, 1906, when her vision had dropped to 6/22 almost, and having seen the patient recently, I learned that her vision has not changed perceptibly and that she is still taking large doses of strychnia. The diagnosis made in this case was spinal atrophy, but though eight years have passed, no signs of ataxia have developed.[1]

Among the secondary atrophies aside from the syphilitic those caused by neoplasms must be mentioned. These are usually monocular; the tumors produce ocular motor disturbances and displacements of the eyeball,

1. This case is an interesting example of Colles' law of apparent immunity of a mother who has borne a syphilitic child. The case shows that though immune to the primary and secondary manifestations, she is not immune to the late nervous sequelæ. Since this paper was written, within the month of April, 1908, signs of tabes have set in very acutely and intensely: Ataxia, loss of the patellar reflexes, lightning pains, and disturbance of the function of the bladder.

or if at the chiasm produce the characteristic hemiopic defects in the fields by which they can be recognized. The secondary atrophies due to pressure of the sclerosed carotid or ophthalmic arteries should be thought of in slowly developing secondary atrophy in the aged. Atrophies following embolism or thrombosis of the central retinal artery need no special consideration at this time. The history of their onset, their unilateral character and the excessively altered vessels help to establish the diagnosis.

The atrophies following descending neuritis or choked disc are sufficiently characterized by well marked signs of the neuritis, by the perivascular lines and the connective tissue developed from the inflammatory exudate to permit of ready diagnosis, usually borne out by the previous history. The atrophy occurring in deep glaucomatous excavation of the disc presents so pathognomonic a picture that it can not be mistaken.

Secondary atrophy depending on retinal and chorioidal degeneration bear the diagnosis in their yellowish, muddy appearance; in the thread-like blood vessels and especially in the evident retinal or chorioidal lesions.

Traumatic secondary atrophies, when unaccompanied by traumatic changes in the retina or the chorioid are usually recognized by other scars and by the clinical history. One class deserves special mention. I refer to the monocular atrophies resulting from blows on the head, most commonly on the upper margin of the orbit. The blindness and secondary atrophy in these cases is due tc injury of the optic nerve in the optic foramen through which the fracture passes. The blindness is usually permanent and distinct atrophy of the nerve head can be made out within four or five weeks after the injury.

C. AFFECTIONS OF THE OPTIC NERVE WITH NORMAL OR APPROXIMATELY NORMAL DISCS.

The affections comprised within this group are the various forms of retrobulbar optic neuritis. It occurs in acute and chronic forms. The most common and best known form is the toxic, produced by tobacco and alcohol, and is characterized by a long but narrow paracentral scotoma, reaching from the blind spot of Marriotte to the point of fixation and later embracing it. Its development is very slow. The vision within the area of the scotoma is partially or completely lost. The course of the affection is usually very slow and great improvement and even complete recovery is possible. As stated above, the disc shows little change. There is usually pallor of the temporal sector. The lesion is a neuritis of the papillo-macular fibers of the orbital portion of the optic nerve, a bunch of fibers which possesses peculiar vulnerability to certain poisons. Autointoxication in diabetes may affect it in a manner similar to that just described.

In acute toxic affections resulting from quinin, salicylic acid, methyl alcohol and other substances the blood vessels of the nerve and retina show marked contraction, and there is blindness or a high degree of amblyopia. often followed by early atrophy. The effect of lead poisoning on the optic nerve is to produce a papillitis, together with marked vascular changes.

Numerous infectious diseases may produce retrobulbar neuritis in one or both eyes, with central scotoma or peripheral defects in the field of vision. Central scotoma is more commonly met with and is usually much larger than in the tobacco-alcohol form. Syphilis, rheumatism and influenza may be mentioned as the more important underlying affections. Syphilis, it is thus seen, may produce any one of the forms of optic nerve disease that we have described (except primary atrophy). As an illustration of syphilitic retrobulbar neuritis the following case may be mentioned:

Case 6.—Mr. A., aged about 45, was seen in November, 1905, with the history of recent syphilis which had not received regular treatment. His right eye, which had always been his better eye (almost emmetropic) had V. 6/30; his left eye (with myopic correction) was normal. There were fine dust-like opacities in the vitreous and on the cornea, but the ophthalmoscopic image was clear. No evidences of chorioiditis.

The right disc showed slight edema. The extent of the field of vision was normal, but there was a large absolute scotoma in the form of a vertical oval below the point of fixation extending as a relative scotoma over this point. Vigorous mercurial treatment, together with iodids and sweats, was ordered and persisted in with the result of obtaining very slow improvement of vision beginning after ten months and not reaching approximately normal vision until more than one year had passed. Since that time, the patient has normal eye-grounds and has had no further trouble.

Acute retrobulbar neuritis in one or both eyes with high degree of amblyopia due to large central scotoma, sometimes with rapid and complete loss of all light perception, is seen in women at the menopause and in young women suffering with sudden disturbances of the menstrual function. Vision is usually regained in great measure, though permanent defects in the field of vision and white optic discs are commonly left. Cases similar to these are sometimes, though indefinitely, classed as rheumatic.

An interesting group of cases of retrobulbar neuritis are those known as hereditary amblyopia, in which there is loss or great impairment of central vision usually without involvement of peripheral vision. The disease commonly attacks male members of a family in early adult life.

Besides the cases thus far mentioned, there are many others, characterized by large central scotoma, which, for want of satisfactory explanation, are commonly diagnosed as idiopathic retrobulbar neuritis. In recent years it has been shown that a number of these cases, apparently more than generally supposed, are to be attributed to inflammation extending from the sphenoidal sinus and the posterior ethmoidal cells. Birch-Hirschfeld has recently shown that this neuritis is apt to present the clinical picture of retrobulbar neuritis with central scotoma. It is further commonly characterized by being monocular and by its sudden appearance and its tendency to rapid extension of the scotoma so as to involve large parts of the field.

Another important contribution to the etiology of a large number of cases of retrobulbar neuritis has been made in the study of the bearing of multiple sclerosis to the ocular affection. It has long been known that retrobulbar optic neuritis, at times showing inflammation or atrophy of the nerve head, frequently occurs in cases of multiple sclerosis and is of great aid as a diagnostic sign; that it is often characterized by great variability in the visual defect and by the possibility of complete recovery after great loss of vision; and that central scotoma is of frequent occurrence. Fleischer has lately followed and studied the cases of retrobulbar optic neuritis observed during the last twenty-five years in Tübingen. His results show that a large number of the cases of retrobulbar neuritis subsequently developed multiple sclerosis. The interval varied from a few weeks to four, five, eight, ten, twelve and fourteen years. If these observations are confirmed it will bear seriously on the nature and prognosis of many of the so-called idiopathic and other forms of retrobulbar neuritis.

Cases are observed in which the typical central scotoma of retrobulbar neuritis is associated with well-marked inflammation of the optic disc. They belong etiologically to the same classes as those described and must be interpreted as retrobulbar neuritis with involvement of the bulbar end of the nerve.

The differential diagnosis of these affections from each other depends chiefly on the previous history and general examination of the patient. The character of the visual disturbance differentiates them from affections due to lesions behind the chiasm, the careful determination of the form and color defects of the field of vision being the main guide. The most difficult diagnosis often lies between these conditions and those of hysterical amblyopia and of simulated blindness. The difference in the fields of vision in hysterical amblyopia and retrobulbar neuritis usually serves to distinguish these affections. And for the detection of simulation the ingenuity of the examiner is often taxed to the utmost.

RELATION OF SO-CALLED OPHTHALMIC MIGRAINE TO EPILEPSY.*

ALVIN A. HUBBELL, M.D.

BUFFALO, N. Y.

I venture to offer a word on the subject of the relation of so-called "ophthalmic" migraine to epilepsy—a subject on which discussion is by no means closed.

The "ophthalmic" migraine of Charcot I do not regard as essentially an ophthalmologic subject, but the accompanying, and often quite alarming visual and other sensory disturbances, many of which are naturally referred to the eyes, lead the afflicted to consult an ophthalmologist. This, together with its frequency of occurrence, gives the ophthalmologist a large opportunity to see and study cases of this kind—an opportunity which is unequaled by any other class of practitioners.

From the time of Airy's graphic description,[1] in 1868, and of Liveing,[2] in 1873, to that of Gowers[3] of the present day, the symptoms of this affection have been presented to the profession over and over again, and are, or should be, familiar to all. Therefore, I shall at once invite attention to the relation of this disease, expressed by visual scintillations and scotomata, motor and sensory disturbances, aphasia, etc., to epilepsy.

That a difference of opinion still exists in regard to the relationship of these two diseases is shown by the following quotations from two excellent authorities. Dr. William P. Spratling[4] says: "I believe it (mi-

---

* This paper has been accepted by the Executive Committee of the Section on Ophthalmology of the American Medical Association, to be presented before the Section at the Chicago Session, June 2-5, 1908. Publication rights reserved by the American Medical Association.

1. Philosoph. Trans. Royal Soc., Lond.
2. Megrim or Sick Headache, London, 1873.
3. Subjective Sensations of Sight and Sound, etc., London, 1904.
4. Epilepsy and Its Treatment, 1904, p. 180.

graine) is associated with the disease (epilepsy), especially in women, who more frequently show a periodicity in convulsive phenomena than men. Unquestionably some of the lighter forms of epilepsy pass for periodic sick headaches. It is a rule for psychic seizures to be followed by an intense, protracted pain in the head, that may persist for several days." On the other hand, Dr. James Hendrie Lloyd[5] says in regard to the possibility of the transition from migraine to epilepsy: "This claim is made by some authors, but the present writer has never seen or heard of an authentic case, and does not believe in the doctrine."

Most authorities endorse the conclusions of Liveing and some of his predecessors, which are voiced by Spratling. Believing that migraine and epilepsy are two distinct forms of neurosis, I desire to do what I can toward disabusing the profession of the idea that a kinship exists between them, or that a genuine transformation of one into the other ever takes place.

By way of illustration, one of the more recent efforts to establish such kinship has been made by Dr. Spiller of Philadelphia, who has described in detail two cases.[6]

CASE 1.—A man, 51 years of age, who, since 44, had had attacks occurring twice a year at first, but now quite frequently. During the first four years there was numbness of the tongue on the right side, and inability to speak, the attacks lasting a minute or two. At 48 he began to have similar attacks of numbness in his right upper limb, and after a short time in his right lower limb. The paresthesia was always confined to the right side of the body, and was associated with impaired function of speech and weakness of the hand. There was also a feeling of tension in the limbs at times, and the right eye would feel drawn upward, to the right, and backward when the numbness passed to the right side of the head. When seen in the attacks, however, the eyes were not drawn upward. In the lighter attacks there was no loss of consciousness, but in the "major" attacks there was loss of consciousness and he would fall. These attacks were preceded for twenty minutes by an unusually "well" feeling, followed by drowsiness, and as they came on he would utter a sound like "uh-uh-uh."

He sometimes remained unconscious in severe attacks for half to three-quarters of an hour. The attack was followed by bewilderment for a short time. There was a slight tremor of the hands, but no jerkings or twitchings. He had not

5. Posey and Spiller's "The Eye and the Nervous System," 1906, p. 710.

6. Am. Jour. Med. Sci., January, 1900.

suffered from headache, was seldom dizzy and never had hemianopsia, scintillating scotoma, or other visual disturbances.

This case Dr. Spiller considers one of epilepsy in which the absence of convulsions is a noteworthy feature.

CASE 2.—A well-developed woman, 21 years of age, when $4\frac{1}{2}$ years of age, fell and struck her head, leaving a red spot on the right side. She was at first confused, and in a few minutes became unconscious. After a short time she began to scream and could not be quieted for several hours. For several days afterward her mind was exceeedingly active. Some months after the fall she had an attack in which the right arm fell powerless to the side of the body, and the whole right side seemed paretic for about half an hour, and she complained of headache.

These attacks recurred for several years, sometimes being on the right side and sometimes on the left, but never on both sides. As she grew older she explained that in the attacks there was numbness and paresis of the limbs, paraphasia, and intense headache on the side opposite to the affected limbs. The numbness began in the fingers and passed upward. She was unable to speak correctly when the numbness reached the tongue. The visual disturbances were doubtful. In one attack during the past year there was dimness of vision. No convulsions ever occurred. The headache, when frontal, was attended by a sense of sweet odor, when none existed.

On Oct. 4, 1899, she was suddenly attacked by severe headache, a few minutes after which she became quiet, and her father, a physician, thought she was unconscious. She soon began to complain of pain again, and a very small amount of chloroform was administered. After the attack was over she had a very imperfect recollection of what happened. This was doubtfully interpreted as an epileptic seizure.

In these two cases Dr. Spiller believes that he finds a connecting link between epilepsy in the first and migraine in the second by means of the transitory paresis, paresthesia, and disturbance of speech found in both.

Sir William Gowers, Féré, Charcot, Diller, Möbius, and others, refer to their experiences corroborating the theory that the two diseaes are related to each other. Gowers,[7] in speaking of the pathology of migraine, and especially of its relation to other diseases, says: "The most important and one of the most frequent of these associations is the relation of migraine to epilepsy. The connection of the diseases is of especial interest because the sensory disturbance of the two has so many common

7. Diseases of the Nervous System, Am. Ed., 1888, p. 1182.

features." He then refers to cases of epileptics in whom migraine was present in themselves or in their ancestors or descendants. He says he has met with a number of cases in which there was both epilepsy and migraine. In some, epilepsy developed after many years of migraine or seemed to grow out of it. In one, the migraine which had existed for years almost disappeared when the fits occurred, and vice versa. In some there were similar sensory symptoms preceding the epilepsy to those in migraine.

In all that Dr. Spiller or others have said it has not been proved that these supposed "connecting-link" symptoms belong essentially to true epilepsy, or that they are necessarily forerunners or development-symptoms of it. Undoubtedly among those affected by transitory paresis and paresthesia there are thousands who never have epilepsy to one who has. They are, however, common in those affected by migraine. Again, undoubtedly, there are thousands who are subject to migraine, even the typical "ophthalmic" form, who are not epileptic, to one who is. My own observations serve to prove this assertion.

The effort has been made to establish a relationship not only between migraine and epilepsy, but also between migraine and other disorders. Gowers[7] says that gout bears a causal relation, and adds that "an alternation is often observed with some other forms of neurosal disorders or at least a transition from one to another. Migraine occasionally ceases, and is replaced by simple neuralgia." Liveing[2] has collected many instances of such transition of migraine to gastralgia, laryngeal spasm, anginal seizures, and paroxysmal insanity. In one case, acute mania came on.

In my opinion, more proof than these and similar citations is required to establish a kinship or transition (transformation, according to Liveing), of migraine to other diseases. In the first place the pathology and pathogeny of migraine is very obscure. Second, certain symptoms may or may not attend it, such as aphasia, paresis, paresthesia, etc. Some of these are complained of by persons who are neither migrainous nor epileptic. Third, altered states of the nervous system and of metabolism in various ways may induce or aggravate migraine, or, on the contrary, so act as to alleviate it, or perhaps even to stop it entirely, at least for a time. In my own case, an ocean voyage does away with attacks of migraine entirely, during the time, and often for many months afterward; but it can scacrely be assumed that there is a direct transition or relation between migraine and seasickness. A change, however, is undoubtedly effected, etiologically, by which the migraine is abated.

DIFFERENTIAL DIAGNOSIS.

The argument that there is a similarity of symptoms of migraine to those of epilepsy does not seem to me to be well sustained. A paroxysm of epilepsy is sudden in its onset, begins almost without warning, and at once reaches a climax. Its duration is short and the patient soon becomes normal again. That of migraine begins with slight symptoms which gradually increase in severity and reach their climax after a half hour or one hour. Even the visual disturbances which sometimes usher in an attack are at first slight and gradually become more pronounced for ten or fifteen minutes, when they reach their height, and then slowly disappear in the course of another ten or fifteen minutes. In epilepsy there are convulsions, in migraine there are none. In epilepsy there is unconsciousness, in migraine there is not. In epilepsy there are varied sensory and mental disturbances which do not belong to migraine, and vice versa. Epilepsy often leads to insanity; migraine does not. Epilepsy has the character at first of an "explosion," while migraine is at first more like a "nervous inhibition." The sequence of an attack is different in both diseases.

I may add that my personal experience and observation also serve to establish a separate, individual entity, functional, or otherwise, for the two diseases. Having been myself affected from childhood with typical migraine, ushered in by "fortification" and "spectral" visual scotoma and having been somewhat disturbed by the idea of its kinship to epilepsy, a disease to which death would almost be preferable, which Liveing and other high authorities had promulgated, I have been led to take deep interest in the subject. I have had migraine in all its variations as to intensity, frequency, accompanying motor and sensory disturbances, length of interval between attacks, etc., but have never had a single symptom of epilepsy. In my mother's family and my own, there have been, besides myself, twelve who have been subject to migraine, but not one has had epilepsy in any form.

My practice has given me a large opportunity to extend my inquiries far beyond my family limitations, with results that are not only enlightening, but, as it seems to me, comforting to one afflicted with "ophthalmic" migraine, and who has an intense abhorrence of becoming an epileptic.

Since 1888 I have been consulted by a very large number of migrainous patients. I have not collected the full number, but it must have exceeded two thousand. But to keep the number within the bounds of absolute certainty, I will place it at fifteen hundred, or an average of seventy-five a year. I have questioned these patients in regard to symptoms of epilepsy, and not one of the fifteen hundred had had epilepsy in any form or degree, nor had it existed in any ancestors or descendants, so far as could be ascertained.

It is not impossible that migraine and epilepsy may exist in the same individual. In fact, I know a few epileptics who are also subject to migraine, but the attacks are entirely separate and independent. Neither will I question the changed manifestations of one disease in the presence of the other, but I do not think that this proves a kinship or transformation. If migraine is related, either etiologically or pathologically, to epilepsy, it does seem that during its existence for a period of years, varying from one to fifty, a certain proportion of fifteen hundred would have become epileptics or shown some symptoms of epilepsy. But no such result has taken place.

I have no doubt that some epileptics may be migrainous, and that occasionally out of so many who have migraine there may be, now and then, one who is also epileptic or who may develop epilepsy. But this does not prove a pathologic kinship. It might as well be assumed that there is a relationship between dyspepsia and epilepsy because certain epileptics have dyspepsia, or certain dyspeptics have epilepsy.

I might enlarge on this subject, perhaps with profit, but Sir William Gowers, apparently with a decided change of views, has most clearly, as it seems to me, epitomized in his late volume[8] conclusions that nearly approach my own. I will make a single quotation: "The traces of a definite relation of migraine to epilepsy are slight. In extremely rare instances one affection may develop, while the other goes on, and as we have seen, the same premonitory disturbance may even be attached to each. But such cases are so rare as rather to emphasize the rule to which they form exceptions. When the exceptions are carefully examined they show that any relation to epilepsy is indirect."

---

8. The Borderland of Epilepsy, London, 1907, p. 77.

MEMORANDA

HISTORY OF IRIDOTOMY.

KNIFE-NEEDLE VS. SCISSORS—DESCRIPTION OF AUTHOR'S V-SHAPED METHOD.*

S. LEWIS ZIEGLER, A.M., M.D., S.C.D.

Attending Surgeon, Wills Eye Hospital; Ophthalmic Surgeon, St. Joseph's Hospital.

PHILADELPHIA.

To Cheselden has been conceded the honor of being the father and originator of iridotomy. Nearly two centuries have elapsed since he first published the report of his procedure in the Philosophical Transactions for 1728. Ever since that time, his signal success has been acknowledged by all except those who either failed to equal his dexterity, or who were prejudiced by their ambition to originate a new method.

A careful review of the medical literature of the century and a half following Cheselden's announcement can not fail to impress the reader with the great interest attached to operations for the formation of an artificial pupil, which subject was considered second only in importance to that of cataract itself. Not only were a large number of monographs devoted wholly to this subject, but every work on general surgical topics set aside one or more chapters for the discussion of artificial pupil. This is in great contrast to the limited space which modern works on ophthalmology grudgingly yield to this still important subject.

It is difficult for us to appreciate the conditions which brought about so large a percentage of cases of pupillary occlusion. Crude surgical procedures, poor operative technic and the utter lack of asepsis often resulted in iridocyclitis or iridochorioiditis. The couching of the

---

*** This paper has been accepted by the Executive Committee of the Section on Ophthalmology of the American Medical Association, to be presented before the Section at the Chicago Session, June 2-5, 1908. Publication rights reserved by the American Medical Association.**

lens, the free discission of both hard and soft cataracts, the frequent introduction of the knife-needle through the dangerous ciliary zone, and the bungling efforts at extraction all increased the tendency to inflammatory reaction, while inadequate therapeutics and lack of antiphlogistic measures frequently permitted the deposit of plastic exudate in the pupillary area, thus resulting in membranous occlusion of the pupil.

OPERATIONS FOR ARTIFICIAL PUPIL.

For the sake of historical completeness, and in order to better emphasize the special domain of iridotomy, I will mention briefly the various methods that have been employed in making an artificial pupil. These are:

(1) *Division* of the thickened iris-membrane by an incision made either through the sclerotic or through the cornea. This is true *iridotomy.*

(2) *Excision* of a portion of the iris through a previously made corneal opening. This is now known as *iridectomy.*

(3) *Separation* of the iris from its ciliary attachment. This was generally known as *iridodialysis,* but sometimes called *iridorrhexis.*

(4) Simple *incision* of the pupillary margin, and of the free iris tissue. This has been designated *sphincterotomy* by some, and *coretomy* or *iritomy* by others. Either one of the latter terms is to be preferred, because it is more clearly descriptive.

(5) *Detachment* of the synechiæ at the pupillary margin, either anterior or posterior, thus allowing the pupil to retract. This was known as *corelysis.*

(6) *Strangulation* of the prolapsed iris in the corneal incision was called *iridencleisis.* The prolapse was sometimes tied with a ligature.

(7) *Trephining* of the iris-membrane, by passing a small trephine or punch through a corneal incision.

(8) *Section* and removal of a portion of the sclerotic and chorioid by knife or trephine, with replacement of the conjunctiva over this opening, the conjunctiva thus acting as a substitute for the cornea in transmitting light. This was called *sclerectomy.*

(9) *Transplantation* of the cornea for total leucoma. This was usually preceded by partial or complete trephining of this membrane.

In addition to these nine distinct methods certain combinations of these have been described and successfully practiced:

(10) *Division* and *excision* have frequently been performed together.

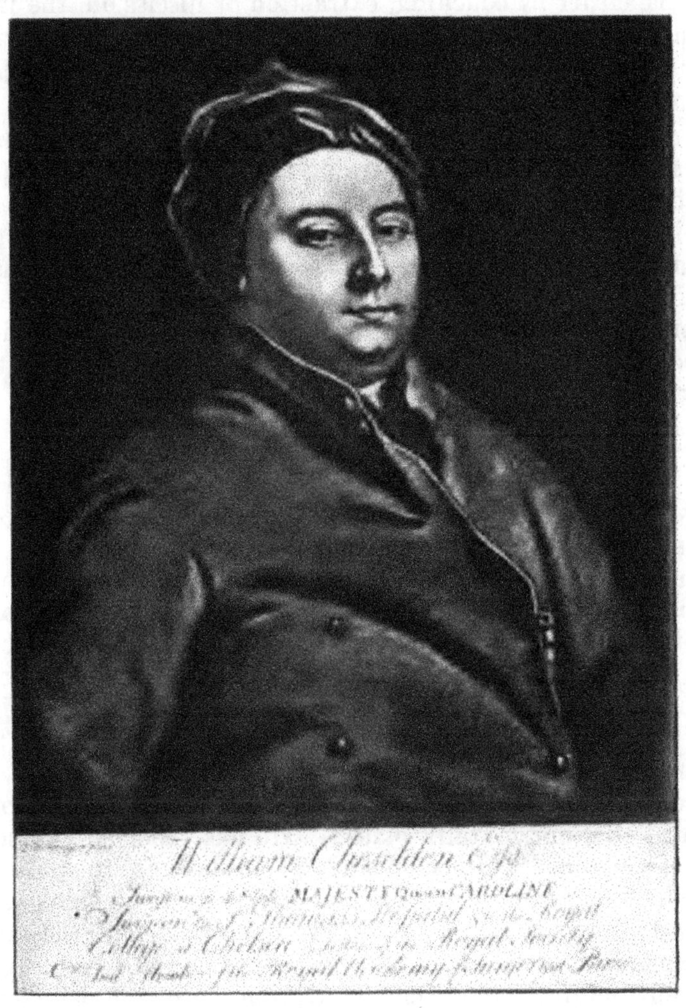

Portrait of William Cheselden, 1688-1752. Painted by Richardson.

(11) *Separation* and *excision* have likewise had some vogue.

(12) *Separation* and *strangulation* have occasionally been practiced.

(13) *Detachment* of the synechiæ and *excision* have also been performed.

HISTORICAL REVIEW OF IRIDOTOMY.

In this brief review of iridotomy,[1] we shall confine our attention to the methods that have been advanced for the formation of an artificial pupil in cases of membranous occlusion of the pupil following removal of the lens, either by couching, extraction or discission, the iris-membrane in these cases being chiefly composed of inflamed iris tissue, glued down by a retro-iridian exudate to the thickened lens capsule.

The early history of iridotomy shows that the advocates of this operation were divided into two schools, (1) those recommending the use of the *knife-needle* for incising the iris-membrane, and (2) those adopting the method of introducing *scissors* through a previously made corneal section and freely incising the iris-membrane, or excising a portion of the same. We will first consider the school which advocated incision by the knife-needle.

I. KNIFE-NEEDLE METHOD.

Cheselden,[2] a renowned surgeon, and oculist to Her Majesty, Queen Caroline of England, first announced, in 1728, his success in making an artificial pupil by means of his knife-needle. He made his puncture back of the corneoscleral junction on the temporal side, passing the knife across the posterior chamber, and making a counter-puncture in the iris-membrane near the nasal margin. He then cut through the iris from behind forward as he withdrew the knife, the incision being carried through two-thirds of its extent. The pupillary opening thus made was a long oval slit, horizontally placed. He has reported two successful cases[3] (Figs. 1 and 2), occurring in patients who had previously undergone couching of the lens. His instrument, strange to say, was practically of the same general shape as the Hays knife-needle, but was larger, and judging from the description more clumsily constructed, as there was danger of leakage of the aqueous and sometimes of the vitreous when it was used. Its form resembled a combination of a bistoury and a sickle-

1. Wagner, Karl Wilhelm Ulrich: Inaugural Thesis, Göttingen. 1818. He invented the designation iridotomia, which he formed from the original Greek, ἶρις ἴριδος the iris and τομή cut.

2. Cheselden, William: Philosophical Transactions, 1728, xxxv. p. 451.

3. Ibid. abridged, vii. pl. v. Figures 2. 3 and 5.

shaped knife, having a sharp edge on one side, a rounded back, and an acute point. We possess two good illustrations of this knife-needle, one by Cheselden himself (Fig. 3), and the other by his pupil, Sharpe[4] (Fig. 4).

For more than a century the method of Cheselden seems to have been the storm center of controversy. Some doubted his veracity, others essayed his operation but failed, while a few had a moderate degree of success. Many attributed to him statements which do not appear

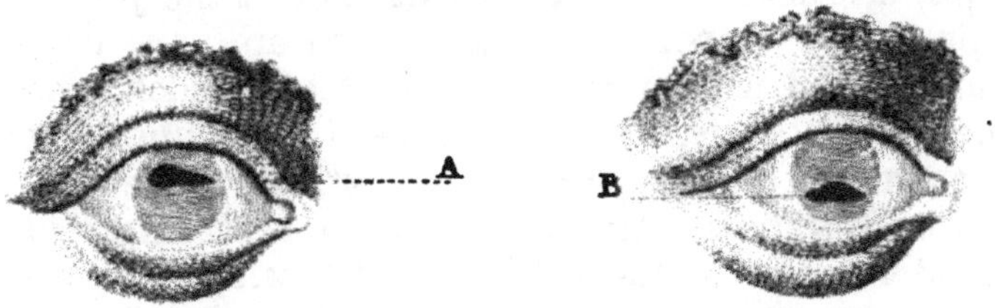

Fig. 1. Fig. 2.

Fig. 1.—Original case of iridotomy. Iris incised above (Cheselden). Fig. 2.—Second case of iridotomy. Iris incised below (Cheselden).

in his published report. He says clearly that in each of his cases couching had previously been performed, and yet some have insisted that the lens was present, and must have been wounded. He also states that his incision was made from behind forward, and yet his followers, Sharpe[4] and Adams,[5] both describe the incision

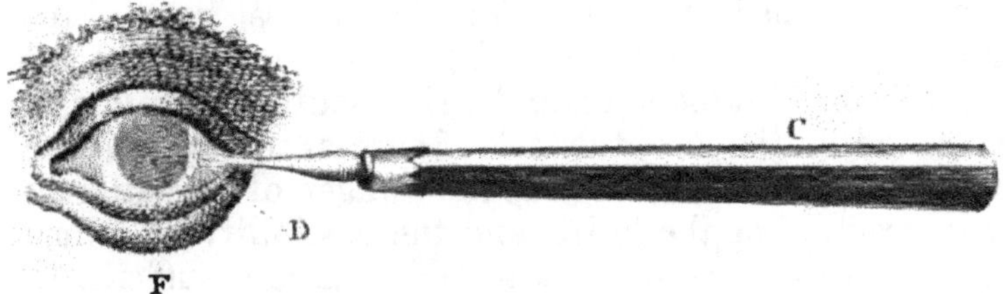

Fig. 3.—Original knife-needle in situ, behind the iris (Cheselden).

as being made from before backward. As Sharpe was his pupil, and presumably had seen him operate, Guthrie[6] suggests the possibility of his having made his incision both ways, the technic being practically the same.

---

4. Sharpe, Samuel: A Treatise on the Operations of Surgery, London, 1739, p. 169.

5. Adams, Sir William: Practical Observations on Ectropium, Artificial Pupil and Cataract, London, 1812, p. 37 et seq.

6. Guthrie, G. J.: Operative Surgery of the Eye, London, 1830, p. 428.

Morand,[7] in his "Eulogy of Cheselden," claims to have personally seen him operate "on an eye in which the iris was closed by an accident," and gives a more detailed description which closely follows the original method. He states that Cheselden presented him with one of his knife-needles as a souvenir of the occasion. Although Morand does not record the exact date of his visit to London, he does state that it occurred during the year 1729. Huguier,[8] in his exhaustive thesis on artificial pupil, also places the date of this visit in the year 1729. This fact is important, as some writers have declared that Morand neither made the visit to London nor saw Cheselden operate, but only quoted the original account given in the Philosophical Transactions. The publication of Morand's high encomiums in 1757 attracted renewed interest to the subject of Cheselden's operation among men of scientific and medical attainments.

Sharpe,[4] in 1739, performed this operation in the same manner as Cheselden, except that after he had entered the knife-needle through the sclerotic he passed it through the iris and across the anterior chamber, and then incised the iris-membrane from before backward. Although he was Cheselden's pupil, and dedicated his small volume on surgery to him, he probably did his master more harm than good, as all the objections to Cheselden's method seemed to be based on the deprecatory remarks of Sharpe. He says, "I once performed it with tolerable success, and a few months after, the very orifice I had made contracted and brought on blindness again." He mentions the danger of wounding the lens, the lack of success in paralytic iris with affection of the retina, the danger of iridodialysis from traction of the knife, and the possibility of failure because the incision would not enlarge sufficiently. Thirty years later (1769) he published the ninth edition of his book without recording a single additional case, but added the thought that, since extraction of the crystalline lens showed the cornea was not so vulnerable as had been believed, he would "imagine" that a larger knife might be introduced perpendicularly through the cornea and iris and a similar incision made. In his first eight editions he pictures Ches-

---

7. Histoire et Mémoires de l'Académie Royale de Chirurgie. Paris, 1757, iii, p. 115.

8. Huguier, Pierre Charles: Des Opérations de Pupille Artificielle, Paris, 1841.

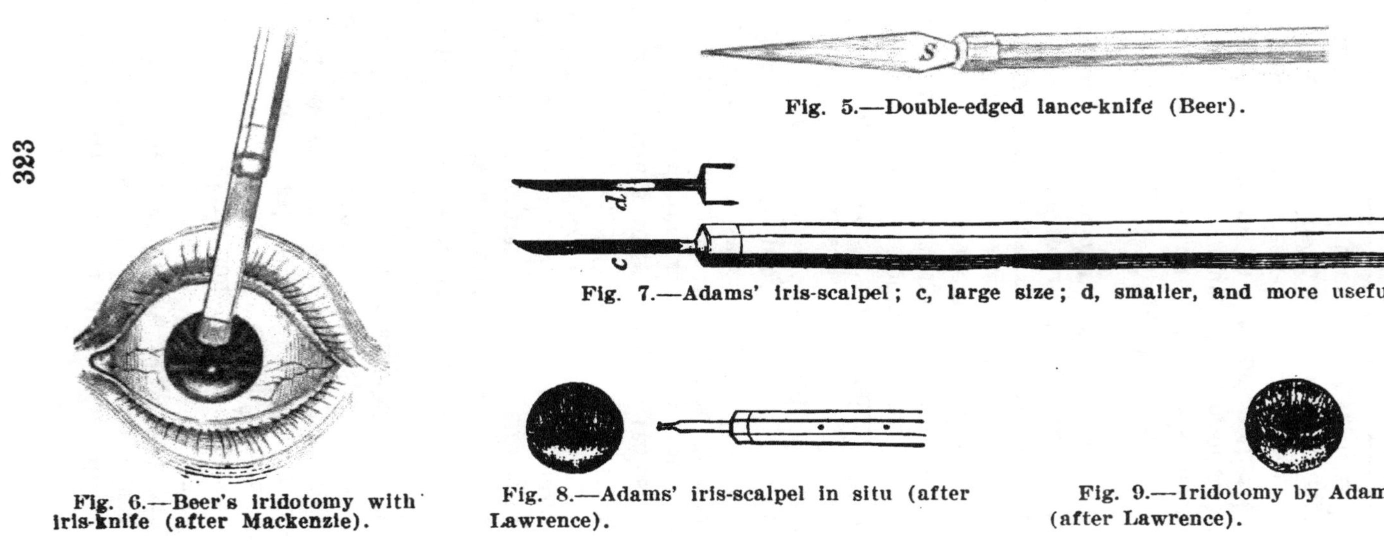

Fig. 4.—Cheselden's knife-needle (after Sharpe.).

Fig. 5.—Double-edged lance-knife (Beer).

Fig. 6.—Beer's iridotomy with iris-knife (after Mackenzie).

Fig. 7.—Adams' iris-scalpel; c, large size; d, smaller, and more useful size.

Fig. 8.—Adams' iris-scalpel in situ (after Lawrence).

Fig. 9.—Iridotomy by Adams' method (after Lawrence).

elden's iris-knife (Fig. 3), but in his ninth edition he substitutes a broad lance-knife with two edges, which closely resembled the one Wenzee (Fig. 15) had just introduced (1767), and which Sharpe suggests "can also be used for the extraction of the cataract." He evidently did not have a very clear idea of the subject, and only succeeded in casting doubt and discredit on the method of Cheselden, which, judging by his own statement, he had tried only once.

Heuermann,[9] in 1756, had already antedated these thoughts of Sharpe by practising a similar method. He passed a double edged lance-knife through the cornea instead of through the sclera, and then made a sweeping incision through the iris-membrane without enlarging the corneal wound. He was probably the first to puncture the cornea with the iris-knife.

Janin,[10] about 1766, performed Cheselden's operation several times with but little success owing to reclosure of the wound by plastic exudate. He adopted Sharpe's modification, but later on changed the incision from a horizontal to a vertical one with better results. He, however, afterward abandoned this procedure and became the originator of the other school, composed of those who preferred to use the scissors.

Guérin,[11] in 1769, made a free corneal incision with a large cataract knife, and then introduced a small iris-knife, with which he made a crucial incision from before backward in the center of the iris-membrane. Although Guthrie[6] distinctly states that Guérin afterwards removed the four angles of the cross with a pair of scissors in order to prevent reclosure of the incision, no direct confirmation of this statement can be found in his writings.

Beer,[12] in 1792, first published his method, which he designated as "an improvement on Cheselden's method." Although the technic is somewhat different, the procedure is practically the same as that originated by Heuermann in 1756. Beer selected certain cases in which a prolapsed iris had followed the lower incision for cataract, causing adherent leucoma with a tensely

9. Heuermann, Georg: Abhandlung der Vornemsten Chirurgischen Operationen, Copenhagen and Leipzig, 1756, ii. p. 493.

10. Janin, Jean: Mémoires et Observations sur l'Oeil, Lyon, 1772, p. 191.

11. Guérin, M.: Maladies des Yeux, Lyon 1769, p. 235.

12. Beer, Georg Joseph: Lehre der Augenkrankheiten, ii, Wien, 1792, p. 12.

drawn iris-membrane. He plunged his double-edged lance-knife (Fig. 5) through the cornea and stretched out iris, from above downward and a little obliquely (Fig. 6), so as to incise the center of the tense iris fibers crosswise, at right angles to the line of traction; cutting horizontally when the traction was vertical, and vertically when this was horizontal. In his monograph on artificial pupil,[13] 1805, he substitutes for the lance-knife his new broad iris-knife, which is practically the same as that later shown by Walton (vide Fig. 12), as,

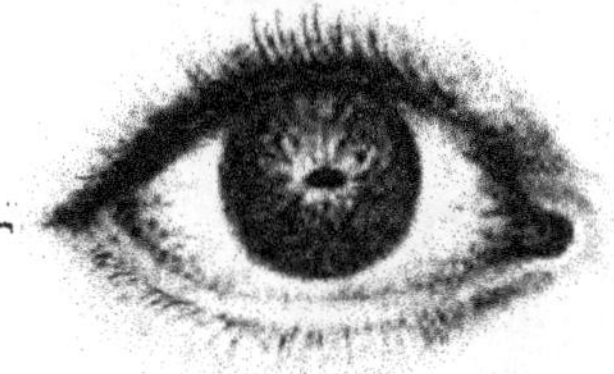

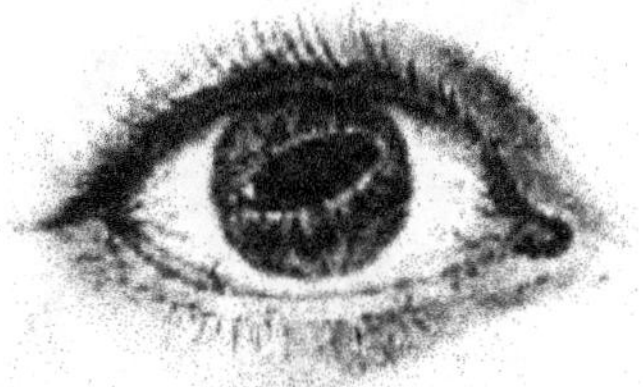

Fig. 10. Fig. 11.

Fig. 10.—Occlusion of pupil (Adams). Fig. 11.—The resulting pupil after iridotomy (Adams).

indeed, Walton's procedure (vide Fig. 13) was almost identical with that of Beer. For other conditions he usually employed Wenzel's operation until by chance he encountered a puzzling case which led him to perform the operation we now know as iridectomy (1797) and which thereafter became his favorite procedure for artificial pupil.

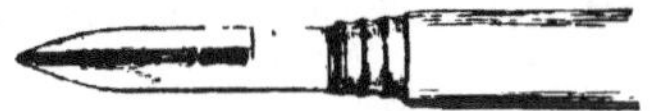

Fig. 12.—Iris-knife (Walton, after Beer).

Adams,[14] in 1812, revived the operation of Cheselden with certain modifications. While his puncture was made in the same location, his technic was different. He entered the sclera with a small iris-scalpel[5] of his own special design (Fig. 7), which, like Sharpe, he passed through the iris-membrane into the anterior chamber, carrying it across to the nasal side (Fig. 8). From entrance to exit he always kept the edge of the knife turned back toward the iris, so as to cut from before

---

13. Beer, Georg Joseph: Ansicht der Kunstlichen Pupillen-Bildung. Wien, 1805, p. 105.

14. Adams, Sir William: A Treatise on Artificial Pupil, London, 1819, p. 34, et seq.

backwards. He was thus able by the most delicate pressure of his instrument, to make a long horizontal incision, without causing iridodialysis (Fig. 9). If the first incision appeared to be too short, he did not withdraw the knife entirely, but again carried it forward and partially withdrew it, always cutting in the same plane. To quote his own words, "by repeating the efforts to divide the iris (taking care in so doing to make as slight a degree of pressure as possible upon the instrument, instead of withdrawing it out of the eye at once, as recommended by Cheselden), a division of that membrane

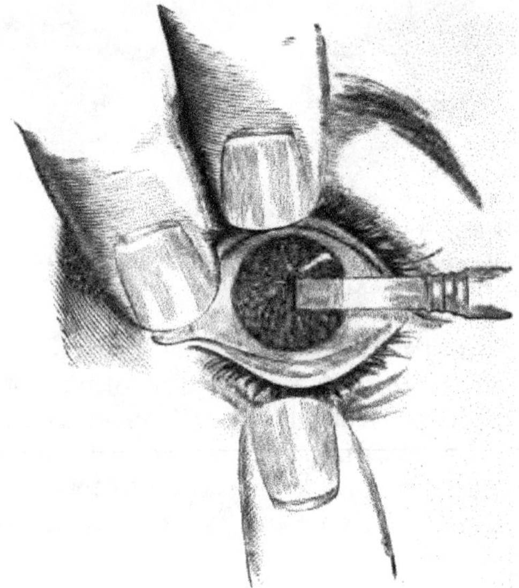

Fig. 13.—Iris-knife in position to make central pupil (Walton, after Beer).

may, in almost all cases be effected, of a requisite size to establish a permanent artificial pupil" (Figs. 10 and 11).

Here were three elements of success, a sharp knife, a gentle sawing movement, and the most delicate pressure of the instrument. His method was a decided advance, and he reported success in nearly one hundred cases. Others, less skilful, however, failed of success, and the severe criticisms of Scarpa,[15] though evidently unjust and tinged by personal animosity,[16] cast a shadow of doubt on the method.

15. Scarpa, Antonius: Trattato Della Principali Malattie Degli Occhi, Ed. quinta, Pavia, 1816, translated by Biggs, London, 1818. p. 373.

16. Edin. Med. and Surg. Jour., No. 58.

From that time on for nearly half a century this form of iridotomy was practically abandoned, the pendulum swinging toward the use of scissors, which Maunoir had popularized and Scarpa had indorsed. Walton,[17] however, about 1852, proposed a method closely resembling that of Heuermann (Fig. 12) and almost identical with that of Beer (vide Fig. 6). His iris-knife (Fig. 12) was practically the same as the broad iris-knife of Beer. He incised the cornea near the limbus, and passed the knife across the anterior chamber to the middle of the iris-membrane which he punctured with a sweeping vertical incision (Fig. 13). If the tissue still retained its elasticity there appeared a long pupillary aperture, elliptical and vertical (Figs. 14 and 15). This incision, however, like all those made through a single set of the iris fibers, was only successful when there was sufficient

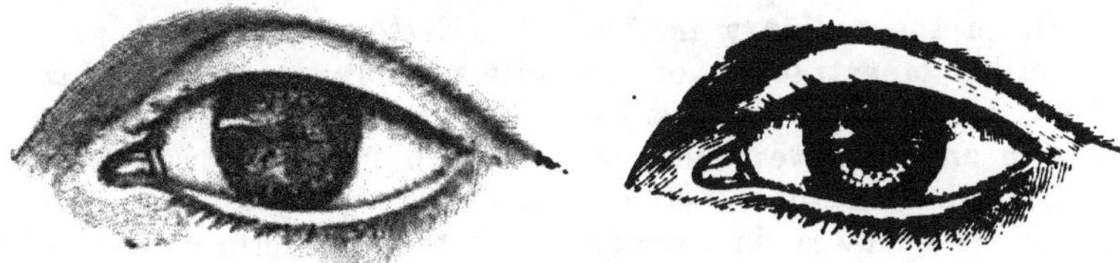

Fig. 14. Fig. 15.

Fig. 14.—Occlusion of pupil (Walton). Fig. 15.—New pupil after incision with iris-knife (Walton).

resiliency remaining in the iris tissue to draw the slit open, and thus keep the edges from uniting. While this method never became very popular, there were some who later practiced it by substituting a very narrow Graefe knife for the iris-knife of Heuermann, Beer and Walton. In fact, this latter procedure still has considerable vogue, both for iridotomy and capsulotomy.

During the following seventeen years no notable advance was made, the scissors method still retaining its hold on the profession, until in 1869. von Graefe, after long reflection, became convinced of the dangers of that method, and communicated to one of his pupils, M. Meyer, his method of simple iridotomy performed with the knife-needle. Meyer[18] quotes his views as follows:

17. Walton, H. Haynes: The Surgical Diseases of the Eye, London, 1861, p. 604.

18. Meyer, Edouard: Traité Pratique des Maladies des Yeux, Paris, 1880, translated by Freeland Fergus, Philadelphia, 1887, p. 396.

"For such cases von Graefe has suggested another method of operation, the principle and execution of which are contained in the following note written for us by that illustrious savant in 1869:

"When, in consequence of a cataract operation, the lens is absent, and when there is highly developed retro-iritic exudation, with disorganization of the iris tissue, flattening of the cornea and the other sequelæ of a destructive iridocyclitis, I substitute simple iridotomy for iridectomy, which is the operation hitherto performed, generally without success. The operation consists in inserting a double-edged knife, resembling in shape a very sharp pointed lance-knife, through the cornea and newly formed tissues till it pierces the vitreous body, and immediately withdrawing it; and, while withdrawing it, enlarging the wound in the membranes without increasing the size of the corneal wound. Experience shows that such plastic membranes attached to the atrophied iris and to the capsule of the lens have a tendency to contract sufficient to maintain, to a certain extent, the opening which has been made.

"If, in the ordinary method of iridectomy, combined with laceration or extraction of the false membranes, we find that the artificial pupil usually becomes closed, we must attribute this to an excessive vulnerability, which immediately sets up proliferation in those tissues which have been touched, and which are endowed, in consequence of their structure, with an irritability altogether peculiar. We know that even the transitory reduction of the intraocular pressure, which follows the evacuation of the aqueous humor, is sufficient to give rise to hemorrhage in the anterior chamber, which interferes with the perfect success of the intended operation; but most of our failures in the ordinary methods are due to the irritation caused by the forceps and the traction on the surrounding structures. Simple iridotomy is free from such inconveniences; it is, so to speak, a sub-corneal act, and enjoys the immunity which belongs to subcutaneous operations.

"I have also reduced the corneal wound to a minimum, by using small falciform knives. These are passed through the false membranes, which are then cut from behind forward."

Von Graefe thus proposed two methods, (1) by cutting from before backward with a double-edged lance-knife, according to the method of Heuermann, and (2) by cutting from behind forward with a sickle-shaped knife, after the original suggestion of Cheselden. Later in the same year, as he lay on his last bed of illness, he became so absorbed in the study of this subject that he sent a telegram to the Heidelberg Congress[19] (September, 1869), in which he advocated the method by the sickle-

19. Klinische Monatsblätter für Augenheilkunde, 1869, p. 431.

shaped knife-needle as the best procedure. His last message to his colleagues showed, therefore, that through mature conviction he strongly favored the use of the knife-needle, and the making of a sub-corneal incision in the iris-membrane without evacuating the aqueous humor. His untimely death, however, prevented him from further perfecting this procedure and presenting it to the profession.

Galezowski,[20] in 1875, published a somewhat similar method in which he used his falciform knife, *aiguille-a-serpette* (Fig. 14), which he introduced through the cornea and iris-membrane, making either a horizontal or a vertical incision, with a "go-and-come" (sawing) movement, after the suggestion of Adams. If this single cut was not sufficient, he made a linear incision of the cornea with a Graefe knife, drew out the iris and cut it off with scissors. By a process of evolution, however,

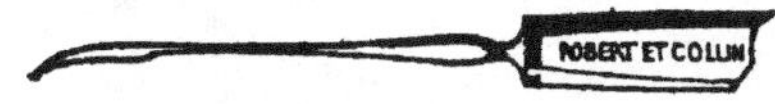

Fig. 16.—Sickle-shaped knife, Aiguille-à-serpette (Galezowski).

he perfected the former procedure and eliminated the scissors. This latter method was published in the third edition of his book in 1888. He punctured the cornea and iris-membrane with the sickle-shaped knife, making first a horizontal incision by the sawing movement of Adams, and finishing with a second cut in the vertical direction, thus forming a T-shaped incision. In actual practice, however, he almost always prolonged this second cut, thus making a crucial incision after the manner of Guérin.[11]

The writer,[21] in 1888, was led to devise an operation with a modified Hays knife-needle, in which through a corneal puncture he made a converging incision in the iris-membrane which resembled an inverted V. The resulting pupil opened up and formed either a triangular or an oval-shaped pupil depending on the degree of stiffness or resiliency of the iris-membrane. This method will be described in detail later on.

20. Galezowski, Xavier: Maladies des Yeux, 2d. ed., Paris, 1875, p. 401, and 3rd. ed., Paris, 1888, p. 384.

21. A brief description of the author's method was first published in de Schweinitz on Diseases of the Eye, Philadelphia, 2nd. ed., 1896, p. 607.

II. SCISSORS METHOD.

We will now return to the consideration of the second school in which scissors were introduced through a previously made corneal section and a free incision was made in the iris-membrane, or a portion of the membrane excised.

Janin,[10] in 1768, having abandoned the procedure of Cheselden, proposed a new method. He incised the cornea below as for cataract extraction, and raised the corneal lip with a spatula while he introduced a pair of curved scissors, the lower blade of which was pointed. He plunged this sharp blade through the iris-membrane, and with a single vertical cut made a crescentic pupil which gaped sufficiently for visual purposes. As this is the first known description of iridotomy by the scissors method it is probable that Janin was the originator of this procedure.

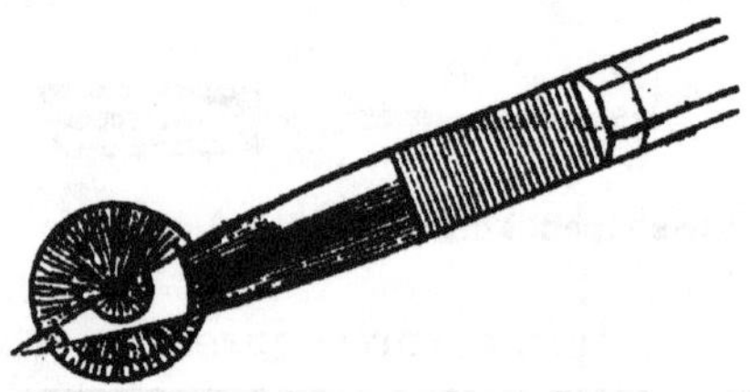

Fig. 17.—Wenzel's cataract knife, and method of incision (after Mackenzie).

Wenzel,[22] in 1786, employed a different method. With a lance-shaped cataract knife he entered the cornea, dipped through the iris-membrane, returned to the anterior chamber, and continuing to cut made a counterpuncture on the opposite side of the cornea, following which he completed his cataract incision. This gave a semilunar flap of iris tissue which could easily be excised by scissors passed through the large corneal opening (Fig. 17).

Maunoir,[23] in 1802, took up the method of Janin, with the object of improving it. He made an incision near the corneal margin, through which he introduced a pair of long, thin, angular scissors of his own design (Fig. 18), one blade of which was sharp-pointed like a lancet, and the other button-pointed like a probe. The

22. Wenzel, Baron de: Traité de la Cataracte, Paris, 1786, translated by James Ware, London, 1805, ii, p. 256.

23. Maunoir, Jean Pierre: Mémoires sur l'Organisation de l'Iris, et l'Opération de la Pupille Artificielle, Paris, 1812.

iris-membrane was then punctured by the sharp blade at about the natural location of the pupil, and an incision executed toward the ciliary margin of the iris. Finding that this single incision did not always succeed,[24] he subsequently improved this method by making a second incision from the pupillary area toward the iris margin, in the line of the radiating iris fibers, thus making a divergent V (Fig. 19). This triangular flap was then allowed to shrink back, or if too stiff, was drawn out and excised. The resultant pupil assumed the shape either of a triangle, a parallelogram (Fig. 19), or a crescent (Fig. 20). He always made his incision parallel with the radiating fibers of the iris and across the circular fibers.

Scarpa,[15] in 1818, having abandoned his own method of iridodialysis as wholly unsatisfactory, adopted Mau-

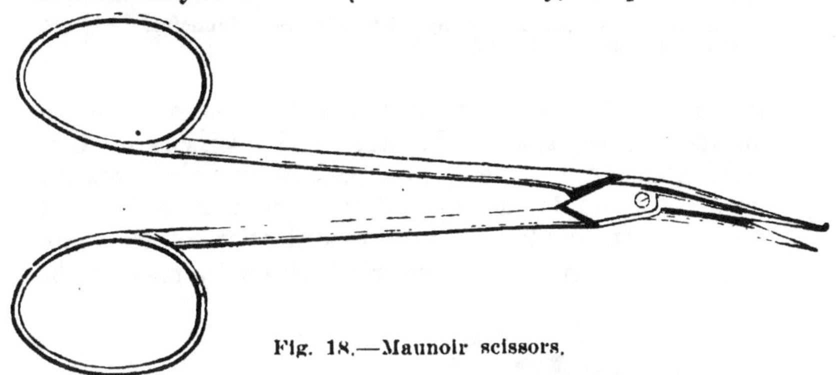

Fig. 18.—Maunoir scissors.

noir's procedure with enthusiasm, chiefly because he had by a friendly correspondence[24] personally encouraged Maunoir with advice and suggestion during its development. He indorsed Maunoir's plan of a double incision when he stated his conviction that "experience has proved that in order to obtain, with the most absolute certainty, a *permanent* artificial pupil, it is necessary to make *two* incisions in the iris so as to form a triangular flap in the membrane, in the form of a letter V, the apex being precisely in the center of the iris and the base near the great margin." Some have claimed that Scarpa himself originated the V-shaped incision, but he gives Maunoir full credit for its successful accomplishment, although he does suggest some additional indications for its practical application.

His opposition to the knife-needle incision of Chesel-

24. Medico-Chir. Trans., London, 1816, vii, p. 301, and ix, p. 382.

den arose from the fact that the pupil either did not open, or if it did open would not remain permanent, chiefly because of the single iris incision. His antagonism to the more successful procedure of Adams was the result of a caustic personal controversy[16] with that skilful surgeon, who ably parried his charges.[14] His great influence with the profession of that day, however, served to check the sentiment in favor of Adams' procedure, and when the weight of his indorsement was cast

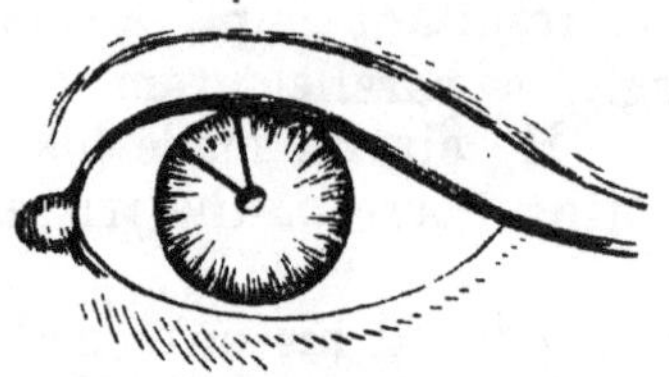

Fig. 19.

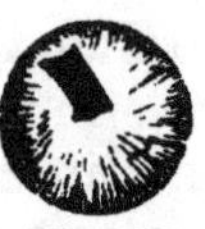

Fig. 20.

Fig. 19.—V-shaped iridotomy with scissors (Maunoir). Fig. 20. —Parallelogram pupil (Maunoir).

in favor of Maunoir's operation the scales were decisively turned toward the side of the scissors method.

Mackenzie,[25] in 1840, practiced Maunoir's operation with considerable success, but in certain cases found it necessary to employ a slight modification of this procedure. He reversed Maunoir's incision by making the

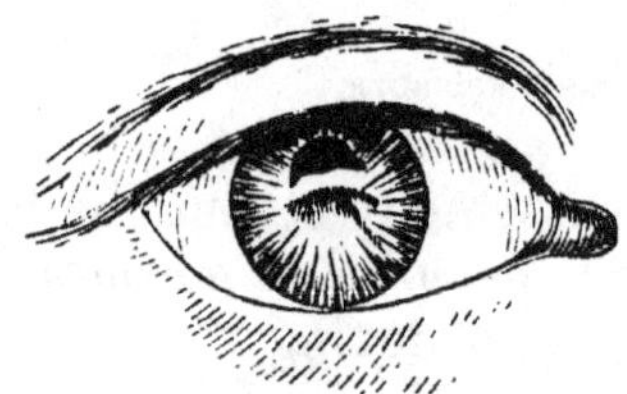

Fig. 21.

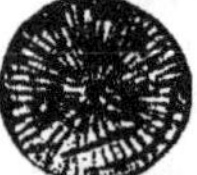

Fig. 22.

Fig. 21.—Crescent pupil (Maunoir). Fig. 22.—Mackenzie's incision in cornea and iris-membrane (Mackenzie).

same divergent V across the radiating fibers of the iris instead of parallel with them (Fig. 22), thus securing a triangular pupil (Fig. 23), which Lawrence[26] thought might succeed in some cases where Maunoir's method would not be available.

---

25. Mackenzie, William: Diseases of the Eye, 3rd. ed., London, 1840, p. 746, American edition, edited by Hewson, Philadelphia, 1855, p. 815.

26. Lawrence, Sir William: Diseases of the Eye, edited by Hays, Philadelphia, 1854, p. 478.

Bowman,[27] in 1872, proposed a method which, though surgically difficult to execute, was quite ingenious, and may have been the initial suggestion that stimulated DeWecker to write his monograph in the following year. I will quote his description as follows: "We make a double opening simultaneously on opposite sides of the cornea. It is more convenient, of course, to make these two openings in a horizontal than in a vertical direction. I then run a pair of scissors in two diverging lines (V) from each incision, thus enclosing between the incisions a large square or rhomboidal portion of the iridial region

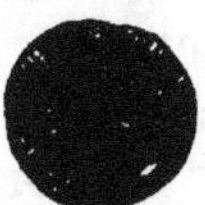

Fig. 23.—Resulting pupil from Mackenzie's incision (Mackenzie).

including the pupil, and all the structures there. You then withdraw the portion thus cut out. There is no drag on the ciliary region; whatever is withdrawn has been cut away from its connections beforehand." This method is simply an elaboration of the one proposed by Maunoir, in which, instead of forming one divergent V, Bowman has made a duplicate incision on the opposite side, and by joining the bases of these two resultant triangles has caused them to take the shape of a rhomboid, thus <>.

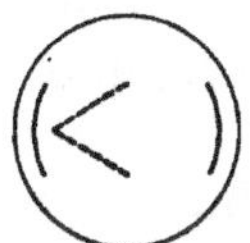

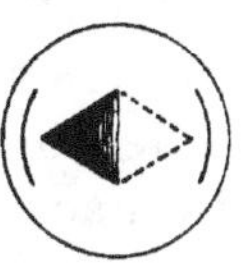

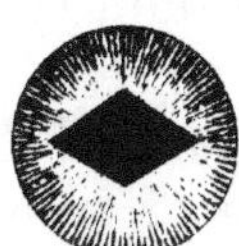

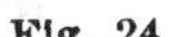

Fig. 24. Fig. 25. Fig. 26.

Fig. 24.—Plan of Bowman's first iris incision. Divergent V. Fig. 25.—First incision completed. Plan of second, showing double V. Fig. 26.—Rhomboidal pupil, resulting from Bowman's iridotomy.

DeWecker,[28] in 1873, published his admirable monograph on iridotomy, in which he proposed the operation which bears his name, and which has long stood as the best recognized method of this procedure. He advocated two different ways of performing this: 1, simple iridotomy, and 2, double iridotomy.

---

27. Transactions, Fourth Int. Ophth. Cong., London, 1872, p. 170.

28. De Wecker, Louis: Annales d'Oculistique, Sept., 1873, p. 123, et seq.

1. *Simple Iridotomy.*—This is practically the same operation as Critchett's sphincterotomy and Bowman's visual iridotomy, although differently executed. It has been supplanted in our day by iridectomy, and does not, therefore, come within the purview of this discussion.

2. *Double Iridotomy.*—He rightly claimed this was both antiphlogistic and optical in its purpose. He employed two distinct methods, which he designated as (*a*) iritoectomie, and (*b*) iridodialysis. The instruments he used were a small stop-keratome (Fig. 27) and a pair of specially devised fine iris scissors (pinces-ciseaux) (Fig. 28), one blade being sharp pointed and the other blunt. These scissors were a great mechanical advance over all previous instruments of this kind, and undoubtedly proved to be a most important element in the success of his procedure.

(*a*) *Iritoectomie.*—He entered the stop-keratome through the cornea, made an exact 4 millimeter incision, and then partly withdrew it while letting the aqueous slowly escape. As soon as the iris-membrane floated up against the knife, he pressed forward, making a 2 millimeter incision in the iris. Slowly withdrawing the knife, he introduced the sharp point of the scissors through the iris buttonhole and cut obliquely from either extremity of the incision toward the apex of a triangle, thus making a convergent V (Fig. 29). He then grasped the resulting triangular flap with the forceps and removed it, leaving an open central pupil.

(*b*) *Iridodialysis.*—His second method was a counterpart of Maunoir's earlier operation, with the addition of iridodialysis. He made the corneal and iris incision with the stop-knife, as in the previous method. Slipping in his scissors he cut from the center of the iris-membrane toward the periphery, and duplicated this incision at an oblique angle to the first, thus making a divergent V (Fig. 30). This formed a triangular flap which he grasped with forceps and tore from its ciliary attachment by iridodialysis.

DeWecker's procedure was planned by a skilled operator, and required great dexterity in its execution. When successful, however, the result was most brilliant. Nevertheless, it was impossible to eliminate the danger of hemorrhage and loss of fluid vitreous in iritoectomie, while in iridodialysis there was the added danger of a torn ciliary surface and traction on the ciliary body. His strict injunction to have a trained assistant hold up the speculum blades in order to avoid the loss of fluid vitreous, showed how much he feared this disastrous contretemps. The success of his method of incision is well shown in the illustration of his two cases (Figs. 31 and 32).

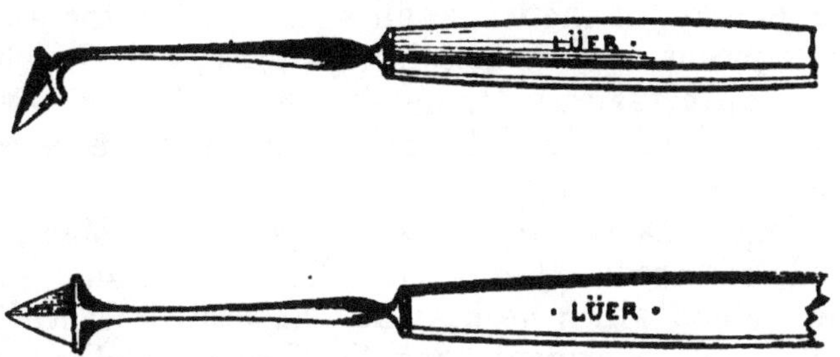

Fig. 27.—Stop-keratomes, straight and angular (DeWecker).

I have already suggested the possibility of Bowman's paper before the London Congress of 1872, having given origin to DeWecker's monograph in 1873. This seems quite reasonable when we consider that Bowman proposed two methods of iridotomy, one his double V operation with a rhomboidal pupil (previously quoted). and the other a visual iridotomy or sphincterotomy, by cut-

Fig. 28.—Forceps-scissors (pinces-ciseaux) (DeWecker).

ting through the pupillary margin with a blunt corneal knife. These two methods are exact prototypes of DeWecker's proposals. Furthermore, DeWecker was present at the London Congress where he heard Bowman's paper, and took part in its discussion. In fact, thirteen years later DeWecker acknowledged[29] that after

29. De Wecker et Landolt: Traité Complet d'Ophthalmologie, Paris, 1886, ii, p. 393.

considering the objections to Bowman's method of iridotomy "I addressed myself at that time to the search for an instrument which allows the avoidance of all traction on the iris, and which can be handled through a narrow opening, while exerting its cutting action in a plane parallel to the surface of the cornea, against which the diaphragm of the iris applies itself, after the escape of the aqueous humor. The forceps-scissors having been discovered, it was easy for me to cause to be revived the procedure of Janin, and to make it decisively take rank in modern ocular surgery."

DeWecker makes only a casual reference to Maunoir's method, but credits Janin with the original suggestion of the method which he has thus elaborated. Nevertheless, it is quite evident that DeWecker's method was simply a modification of the one outlined by Maunoir seventy years before. Furthermore, he lays down the same rule that Maunoir first offered: "Always cut parallel to the radiating fibers and perpendicularly to the circular fibers of the iris."

RELATIVE ADVANTAGES OF KNIFE-NEEDLE VS. SCISSORS.

In reviewing the questions at issue between these two schools of iridotomy, one can not help noticing the constant oscillation from one method to the other as certain advances were made. The method by the knife-needle seemed to possess the advantage of easy accomplishment and less postoperative disturbance, but with the disadvantage that often the pupillary opening was inadequate and promptly reclosed by plastic exudate. On the other hand, the method by the scissors was more difficult of accomplishment, caused more traumatism to the eye, was often complicated by great loss of fluid vitreous, and was frequently followed by severe inflammatory reaction. If, however, it proved successful, the resulting pupil was permanent and sufficiently large for visual purposes. The inclination of all operators seemed to be toward the use of the knife-needle. and it was only necessity that forced them to adopt the more complicated procedure of the open operation with scissors. Von Graefe seemed to recognize this when he referred to the knife-needle incision as "a sub-corneal act which enjoys the immunity of subcutaneous operations."

The chief advantages of iridotomy by the knife-needle are the ease of incision, the lack of traction on the ciliary body, the freedom from postoperative inflammatory reaction, the avoidance of opening an eyeball which may contain fluid vitreous, the lessening of the tendency to iris hemorrhage from lowered tension, and the avoidance of the nebulous scar which often follows a large corneal incision in old inflammatory eyes. The disadvantages revealed in the method of the knife-needle lay partly in the method and partly in the faulty instruments constructed in that day. Cheselden, Morand,

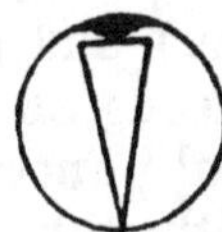

Fig. 29.

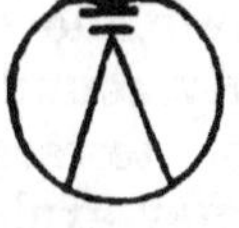

Fig. 30.

Fig. 29.—Iritoectomie. Convergent V (DeWecker). Fig. 30.—Iridodialysis. Divergent V (DeWecker).

Sharpe and Adams all made the mistake of entering the eye back of the corneoscleral junction, which is so near to the danger zone of the eye. Adams, however, made a two-fold improvement in adding to his operation a sawing movement and in advocating the "most delicate pressure of the instrument" in order to make a free incision. Heuermann was apparently the first to make the puncture through the cornea instead of through the sclera.

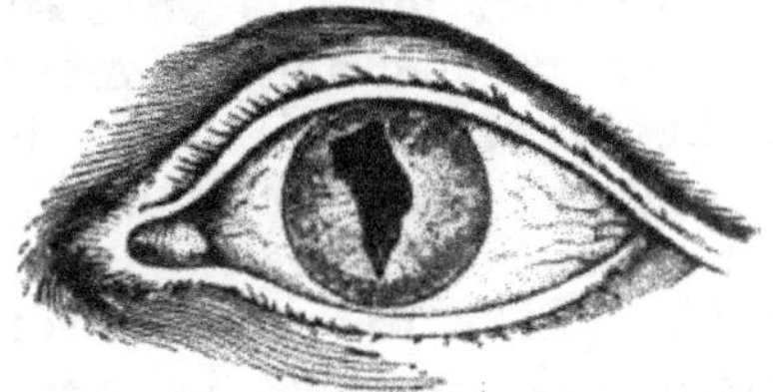

Fig. 31.

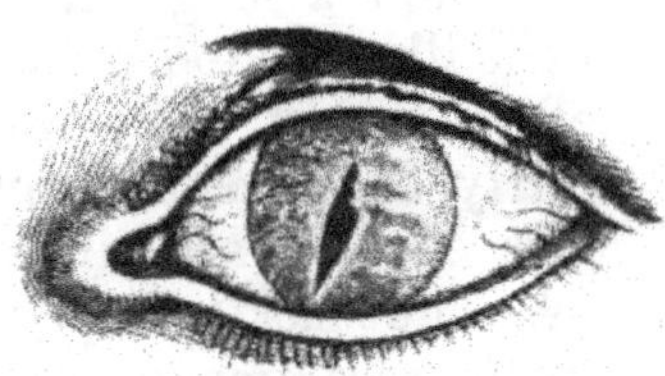

Fig. 32.

Fig. 31.—Pupil by iritoectomie. Two incisions. Convergent V (DeWecker). Fig. 32.—Stenopaic pupil. Single iris incision (De Wecker).

The advocates of the knife-needle method long labored under the disadvantage of making a single iris incision, while those who employed the scissors early discovered that a double incision was necessary to success. Although Janin was the originator of the scissors method, Maunoir was the first to deliberately try a triangular flap, which DeWecker later elaborated and made a permanent success. The many disastrous results of the open operation, however, compelled conservative surgeons, like von Graefe, to revert to a study of Cheselden's method, and to seriously consider the great advantages which a successful iridotomy by the knife-needle method would confer on surgeon and patient alike.

THE CHOICE OF A KNIFE-NEEDLE.

1. Cheselden's knife-needle (Figs. 3 and 4) was a splendidly designed instrument, but a poorly executed one. The blade was too large (11 mm.) and the shank improperly rounded, so that both aqueous and vitreous were liable to escape through the scleral puncture. This leakage may explain many failures, although the single iris incision was undoubtedly the most serious fault of the method.

2. The iris-scalpel of Adams (Fig. 7) was poorly designed but splendidly executed, the long blade completely filling the wound and thus preventing the escape of any fluid. The cutting edge, however, was too long (15 to 20 mm.), and especially so for the execution of the sawing movement advised by Adams.

3. The double-edged lance-knife (Fig. 28) employed by Heuermann, Beer and von Graefe, was useful for the long sweeping incision in the iris-membrane which they advocated, but is not adapted for the method which will be described later. The same shaped knife with a small blade and a long shank is also used for this purpose, but is likewise too broad, too oval pointed and too much bellied to cut well, while the upper edge is liable to scarify Descemet's membrane at the same time that the lower edge is executing the incision in the iris tissue.

4. The sickle-shaped knife (Fig. 16) which von Graefe recommends and Galezowski employs, is excellent for making the puncture, but for the go-and-come movement, which Galezowski advises, is not nearly so good as the straight blade with a slight falciform point. It closely resembles the older falciform knife of Scarpa.

5. The knife-needle of Knapp (Fig. 34), which is so generally used for capsulotomy, is unfortunately not well adapted for iridotomy. The point is too oval, the cutting edge is too much bellied, and the blade is too short (5 mm.). It will not easily puncture a dense iris-membrane, and the long sawing incision can not be well executed, because the short blade either persists in

slipping out of the iris incision or else allows the membrane to ride up on the shank, in either case interfering with the completion of the operation.

6. Sichel's iridotome (Fig. 35) closely resembles Knapp's knife-needle, and although specially designed for this purpose, has the same faults, an oval point and a bellied edge. On the other hand, the blade is too long (11 mm.) to be easily manipulated in the anterior chamber.

7. The Hays knife-needle (Fig. 31), as suggested in the early part of this paper, has the same general shape as Cheselden's instrument, although much smaller. It

Fig. 33.—Double edged lance-knife (modern model).

was devised by Dr. Isaac Hays, an early surgeon of the Wills Hospital, and, although not well known to the profession at large, has been in constant use by the staff of that hospital for more than half a century. I may be pardoned for briefly quoting the original description of the instrument as published by Hays[30] in 1855:

"This instrument from the point to the head, near the handle (a to b, Fig. 36), is six-tenths of an inch, its cutting edge (a to c) is nearly four-tenths of an inch. The back is straight to near the point, where it is truncated so as to make the

Fig. 34.—Knapp's knife-needle.

point stronger, but at the same time leaving it very acute, and the edge of this truncated portion of the back is made to cut. The remainder of the back is simply rounded off. The cutting edge is perfectly straight and is made to cut up to the part where the instrument becomes round, c. This portion requires to be carefully constructed, so that as the instrument enters the eye it shall fill up the incision, and thus prevent the escape of the aqueous humor."

8. The knife-needle, which I invariably use, is a modified pattern of that devised by Hays. The form of this instrument lies midway between the falciform knife and the bistoury, and possesses the advantages of both. It has a very delicate point which punctures easily, and

30. Amer. Jour. of the Med. Sciences, July, 1855,, p. 82.

an excellent cutting edge of sufficient length (7 mm.). If the shank is properly rounded it can be used with a sawing motion, sliding backward and forward through the corneal puncture without injuring the cornea, and without allowing the aqueous to escape. To accomplish this the more easily, the shank has been made 4 mm. longer than the original model. This instrument, therefore, seems to meet all the requirements of a perfect iris-knife, viz., a falciform point which makes the best puncture, a straight edged blade which makes the best incision, and a cutting edge 7 mm. long, which is the best length for properly executing the sawing movement. My model[31] of knife-needle (Fig. 37) resembles Cheselden's knife, as shown by Sharpe (Fig. 4), even more closely than the original pattern of Hays does.

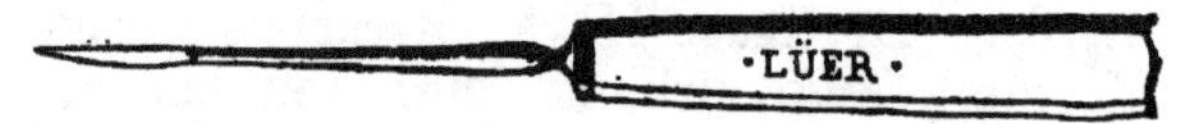

Fig. 35.—Sichel's iridotome.

ESSENTIALS OF SUCCESS IN IRODOTOMY BY THE KNIFE-NEEDLE METHOD.

1. A good knife-needle must be carefully selected. We have already concluded that the modified Hays knife-needle is the best model for this purpose. The knife-needle must, of course, have a well sharpened point and edge.

2. The character of the incision in the iris-membrane is of vital importance. It should be a double incision. Guérin, Maunoir, DeWecker and Galezowski recognized this. Guérin made a crucial incision, Maunoir and DeWecker adopted the triangular flap, while Galezowski advocated the T-shaped cut. Our choice is the V-shaped incision, which is undoubtedly the only one that will cut through all the iritic fibers in such a way as to give us the greatest retraction of the membrane.

3. Absolutely no pressure should be made in cutting with the knife-needle. This must be recognized as the main secret of success, whether you are incising a dense, felt-like iris-membrane, or a thin filmy capsule. If this rule is observed all traction on the ciliary body will be avoided.

31. This knife needle has been carefully made for me by Luer, Paris. and by Ferguson, Philadelphia.

4. The knife-needle should slide backward and forward through the corneal puncture with a gentle sawing movement.

5. The corneal puncture and membrane counterpuncture should be far enough apart to make the corneal puncture a good fulcrum for the delicate leverage necessary in executing the iris incision.

6. The knife-needle should be so manipulated that no aqueous shall be lost, as this accident may prevent the completion of the operation, and may increase the tendency to iris hemorrhage by lowering the ocular tension.

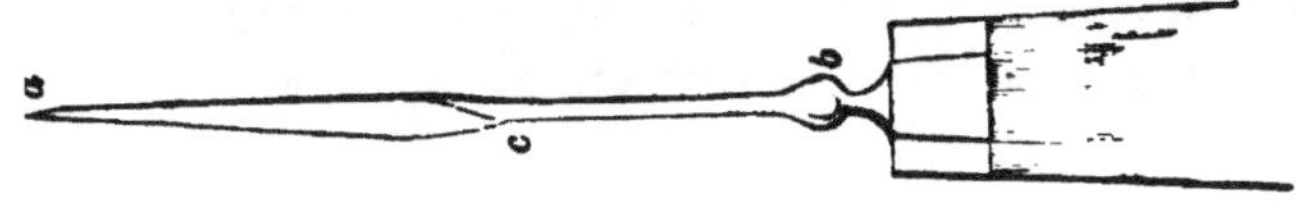

Fig. 36.—Hays' knife-needle, exact size and enlarged (Hays).

7. Every incision should be made a thoroughly clean cut, and all tearing of the tissues should be avoided.

8. The most perfect artificial illumination should be secured, either by an electric photophore or a condensing lens, as both iridotomy and capsulotomy require constant and close inspection of the operative field.

Fig. 37.—Author's model of knife-needle.

AUTHOR'S V-SHAPED IRIDOTOMY:

The method of V-shaped iridotomy, performed by me with my modified Hays knife-needle, may be described as follows:

First Stage.—With the blade turned on the flat, the knife-needle is entered at the corneo-scleral junction, or through the upper part of the cornea (Fig. 38), and passed completely across the anterior chamber to within 3 millimeters[32] of the apparent iris periphery. The knife is then turned edge downward, and carried 3 millimeters to the left of the vertical plane (Fig. 39).

Second Stage.—The point is now allowed to rest on the iris-membrane, and with a dart-like thrust the mem-

32. Compare with millimeter scale beneath each diagram.

brane is pierced. Then without making pressure on the tissue to be cut, the knife is drawn gently up and down with a saw-like motion, until the incision has been carried through the iris tissue from the point of the membrane puncture to just beneath the point of the corneal puncture. This movement is made wholly in a line with the axis of the knife, the shank passing to and fro through the corneal puncture, and the loss of any aqueous being carefully avoided in the manipulation.

Third Stage.—The pressure of the vitreous will now cause the edges of the incision to immediately bulge open into a long oval (Fig. 35) through which the knife-blade is raised upward, until above the iris-membrane, and then swung across the anterior chamber to a cor-

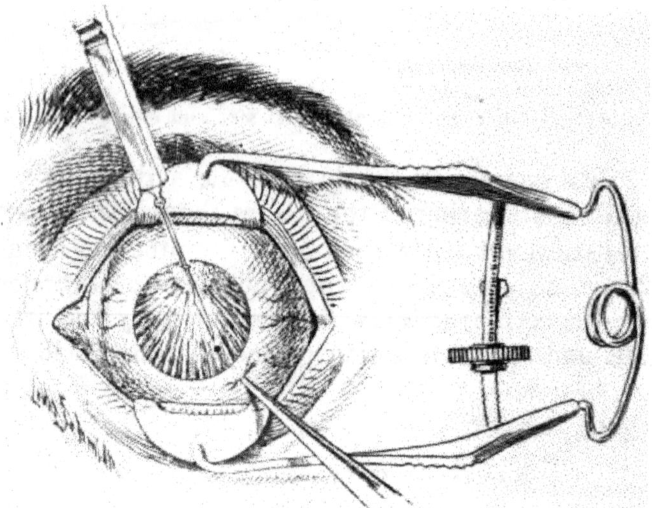

Fig. 38.—Author's V-shaped irodotomy.

responding point on the right of the vertical plane, which, owing to the disturbance in the relation of the parts made by the first cut, is now somewhat displaced and the second puncture must be made at least 1 millimeter farther over, i. e., 4 millimeters to the right of the vertical plane (Fig. 40).

Fourth Stage.—With the knife-point again resting on the membrane, a second puncture is made by the same quick thrust, and the incision rapidly carried forward by the sawing movement to meet the extremity of the first incision, at the apex of the triangle, thus making a *converging* V-shaped cut (Fig. 41). Care must be taken at this point that the pressure of the knife-edge on the tissue shall be most gentle, and that the second incision shall terminate a trifle inside the extremity of the first, in order that the last fiber may be severed and thus allow the apex of the flap to fall down behind the lower part of the iris-membrane. If the flap does not roll back of its own accord it may be pushel downward with the point of the knife. When the operation is completed the knife is again turned on the flat and quickly withdrawn.

CAUSES OF FAILURE.

The most fruitful sources of failure are, first, a poorly sharpened knife-needle; second, a badly planned incision; third, inability to sever the apex of the triangle; fourth, the early loss of aqueous; fifth, too heavy pressure with the knife-edge, and sixth, rocking or rotating the knife backward instead of making the sawing movement. All of these can easily be avoided, if the surgeon will only exercise care and good judgment.

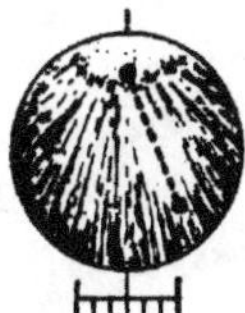
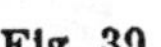
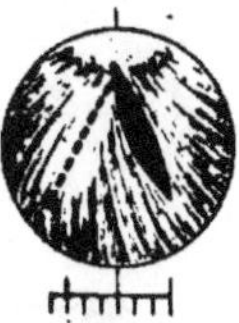
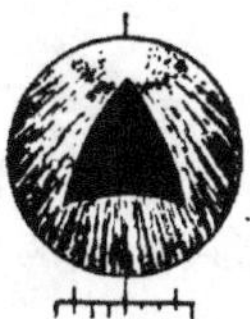

Fig. 39. Fig. 40. Fig. 41.

Fig. 39.—Plan of first incision. Fig. 40.—First incision completed. Plan of second incision. Fig. 41.—Pupil resulting from V-shaped iridotomy.

In an occasional case, the iris-membrane may be so stiff that the apex of the flap will not retract. If the apex can not be pushed down by the tip of the knife turn the blade on the flat, puncture the base of the flap by a quick thrust, and with a sawing motion cut across its fibers so that it will fall back as though hinged; or, if positive that the vitreous is not fluid, introduce a keratome in the cornea below, draw out the triangular tongue, cut it off with the iris scissors, and dress back the base with a silver spatula.

It is possible that the capsule, or iris tissue, may lose its anchorage. In that event we must either reverse the procedure by entering the knife-needle below, and cut from above downward, or else pass a second knife-needle through the loosened edge of the membrane to fix it, and then proceed with the usual method.

Occasionally, the apex of the triangular flap will hold

fast, because the last fiber of tissue has not been severed. If the leverage is too short to incise it from above, withdraw the knife-needle and reintroduce it far enough from the apex to secure the proper leverage, and again incise it gently, until it falls back.

Traction on the ciliary processes, accidental puncture of the ciliary body, or the tearing of the membrane from its ciliary attachment may all set up iridocyclitis or glaucoma, and should therefore be avoided. As tense capsular bands are liable to engender a similar condition they should be incised. If any of these traction bands should remain in the edge of the coloboma, we may enter the knife behind them and gently saw through into the already cleared pupil, before withdrawing the knife.

ILLUSTRATIVE CASES.

I will briefly cite a few examples of the V-shaped operation, two that were my first efforts, and two that were

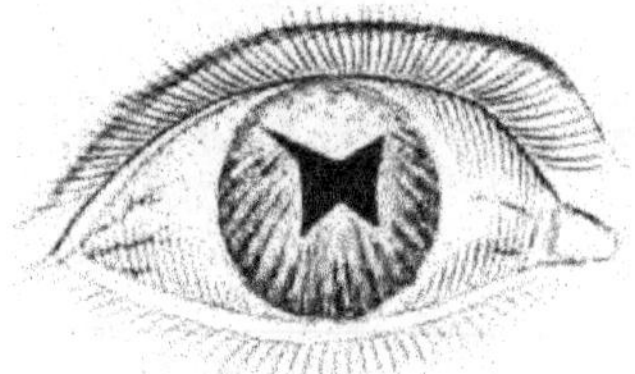

Fig. 42.

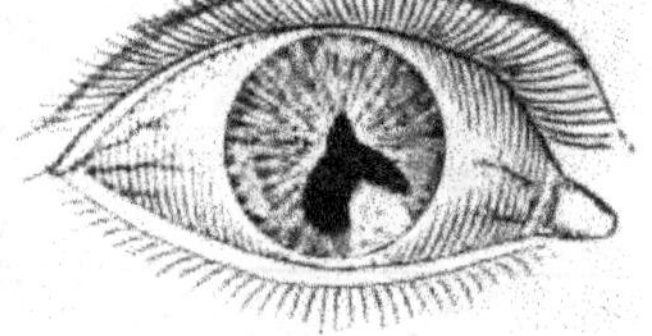

Fig. 43.

Fig. 42.—Iridotomy in a stiff iris-membrane (author's original case).
Fig. 43.—Iridotomy in a soft eyeball, with dense iris-membrane.

recent cases. They were all of the class that are often abandoned as hopeless; hence the visual result is far below the operative success.

CASE 1.—*History.*—F. M., aged 65 years. O. D. complete membranous occlusion of pupil from iridocyclitis, following cataract extraction. The iris and capsule are tensely drawn up toward the ciliary border. Light perception and projection good. Several efforts have been made to incise the membrane, but without success. Admitted to Wills Hospital by the late Dr. Goodman, through whose courtesy I operated.

Operation.—On Jan. 15, 1889, I made two long incisions, almost crucial, and extending beyond the apex of the V, resulting in a W-shaped pupil, on account of the stiff iris membrane (Fig. 42). With S. + 10 D. he saw 20/50.

CASE 2.—*History.*—J. S., aged 30 years. O. S. injured and enucleated. O. D. sympathetic inflammation, chorioidal cataract; three discissions and one iridectomy, down and in.

Membranous occlusion of pupil. I first saw him in 1888 while house surgeon at the Wills Hospital, where iridotomy was skilfully performed nine times by one of the surgeons, the methods being varied and ingenious, but without success, as the incision was invariably closed by plastic exudate. My interest in this series of operations first drew my attention to the subject of iridotomy, and stimulated me to develop the method I have here submitted and which I first tried in Case 1.

One year later this patient came to my clinic at St. Joseph's Hospital. Iris was discolored, capsule thickened and visible through the coloboma, down and in; areas of scleral thinning, with pigmented chorioid showing through. T—3. Light perception good, projection only fair.

Operation.—On June 17, 1889, I made a V-shaped iridotomy along the outlines of the former iridectomy. The membrane freely opened up into a triangular or pear-shaped pupil (Fig. 43), which proved permanent, but was only useful for quantitative vision, about 5/200. No further test could be made because the disorganized vitreous was filled with floating

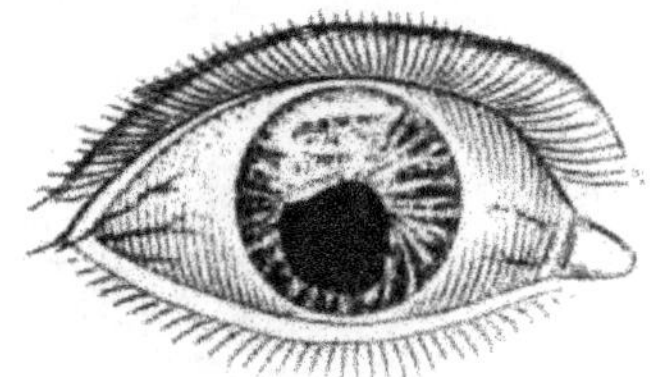

Fig. 44.

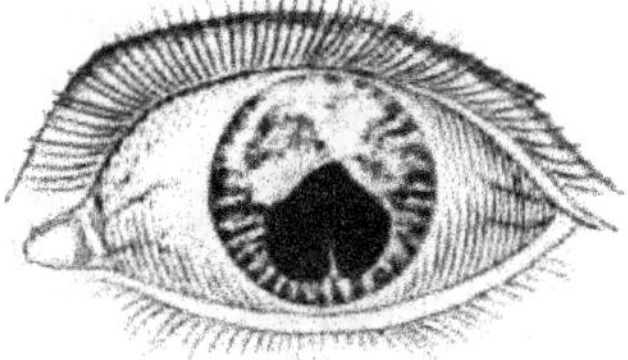

Fig. 45.

Fig. 44.—Iridotomy in a soft eyeball, with thin membrane and iris bombé. Fig. 45.—Iridotomy showing apex of iris flap after incision.

masses. I have seen him within a year, going about and earning his living. From an operative standpoint I have always considered this early effort one of my most successful cases, chiefly because of the great density of the iris-membrane and the lowered tension of the eyeball.

Case 3.—*History.*—Mrs. A. D., aged 45 years. O. D. iridectomy for glaucoma seven years ago. O. S. iridectomy two years ago by another surgeon, at which time there occurred slight incarceration of iris, followed by sympathetic ophthalmitis in O. D. The severe iridochorioiditis resulted in cataract and some shrinkage of globe. The cataracts were extracted from both eyes in 1907, followed by dense opacity of cornea above, iris bombé, shallow anterior chamber, T—2. Here was a soft, distensible, iris tissue with shallow anterior chamber and greatly lowered tension of the eyeball, constituting one of the most difficult conditions to operate on.

Operation.—On May 13, 1907, the eyes being quiet, and light perception and projection fair, V-shaped iridotomy was performed on both eyes. The leucomatous areas in the upper part of cornea necessitated making the pupil below. In O. D. the pupil opened up beautifully (Fig. 39), but in O. S. a tag of iris hung fast (Fig. 45) and was again incised two months later. The artist has illustrated the remaining portion of this tag very well. As soon as the iris tissue was incised it retracted, making the pupils larger than the area of incision. The test for glasses, nearly a year later, March 15, 1908, yielded the following result:

O. D. S + 13 D = C + 4.75 D ax. 105° = 20/40.
O. D. S + 13 D = C + 3 D ax. 65° = 20/40.
Add
O. D. S + 4 D = J. 10.
O. S. S + 4 D = J. 10.

These were ordered in biconvex torics. She had worn glasses for a year, but claims vision is much better with the new ones. This seems like an excellent result when we consider that these eyes had passed through glaucoma, iridochorioiditis and cataract, followed by membranous occlusion of pupil, lowered tension and fluid vitreous. The high hyperopia and astigmatism show the phthisical condition of each globe. There is marked cupping of both nerve heads and the fields are contracted.

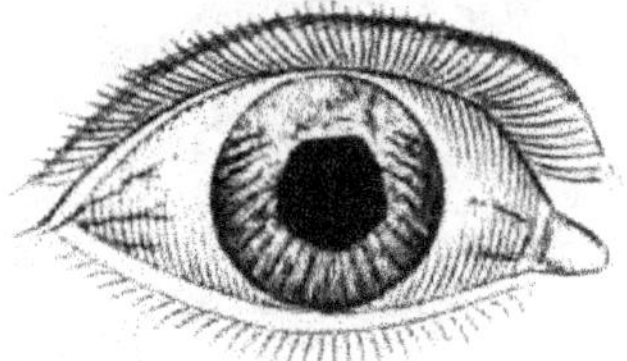

Fig. 46.

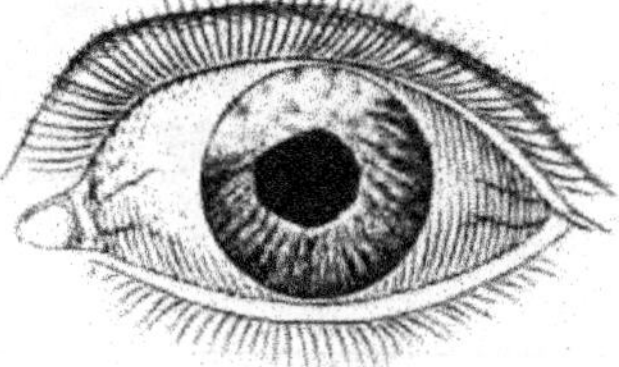

Fig. 47.

Fig. 46.—Irido-capsulotomy, with band of iris, and capsule in coloboma above. Fig. 47.—Iridotomy with round central pupil.

Case 4.—*History.*—Mrs. B. M., aged 64 years. O. S. struck by a stone in childhood, destroying vision. Dense leucoma above, chorioidal cataract, calcareous deposit; exclusion of pupil. T—1. Lpc. good. Lpj. fair. O. D. recurrent attacks of inflammation for seven years, posterior synechiæ and cataract. Counts fingers at 6 inches. Extraction with iridectomy, both eyes, in 1907. Site of incision has become densely leucomatous. O. D. shows capsular area above, iris drawn up. O. S. complete membranous occlusion of pupil.

Operation.—Oct. 7, 1907, V-shaped incision was executed entirely in the iris tissue of O. D., the pupil spreading out into an ovoid shape (Fig. 46), leaving area of capsule and small band of iris above. O. S. was operated on Jan. 13, 1908, by the same method, the resulting pupil being almost round (Fig. 47) owing to the resilient iris tissue.

The test for glasses, March 10, 1908, gave the following result:

O. D. S + 12 D ⌢ C + 1.25 D ax. 135° = 20/50.
O. S. S + 12 D ⌢ C + 1.25 D ax. 135° = 20/70.

Add

O. D. S + 5 D — J. 6.
O. S. S + 5 D = J. 12.

These were ordered in biconvex torics, which she now wears with great comfort. It is worth noting that O. S. still retained good visual acuity, although blinded by an injury nearly fifty years ago.

CAPSULOTOMY BY THE V-SHAPED METHOD.

The application of the V-shaped method to capsulotomy shows an even greater field of usefulness, as this method is par excellence the best way of incising a delicate secondary capsular cataract. This should be done under artificial illumination. The pupil should be dilated, as the area of incision is necessarily smaller than in iridotomy, and unnecessary wounding of the iris

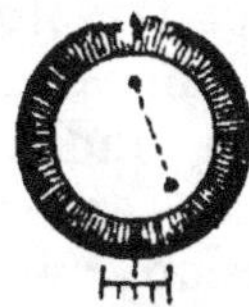

Fig. 48.

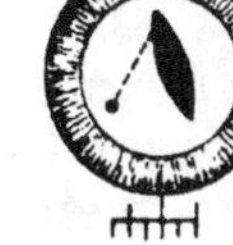

Fig. 49.

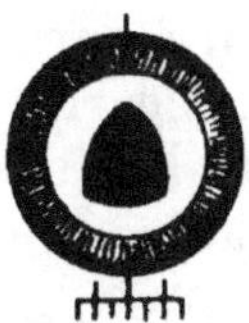

Fig. 50.

Fig. 48.—Author's V-shaped capsulotomy. Plan of first incision. Fig. 49.—First incision completed. Plan of second incision. Fig. 50.—Pupil resulting from V-shaped capsulotomy.

should be avoided. The proposed capsular opening must be so calculated as to fall within the area of the undilated pupil, or partly within the coloboma if an iridectomy has been previously performed.

The knife-needle is entered at the upper corneal margin, passed across the anterior chamber to a point 2 mm. to the left of the vertical plane (Fig. 48), the capsule punctured by a quick thrust, and the saw-like incision carried from below upward, as in iridotomy. The knife is then raised up above the capsule and swung 3 mm. to the right of the vertical plane (Fig. 49), the capsule is again punctured, and a duplicate incision carried up to join the first, at the apex of the converging V (Fig. 50).

Where the pupillary margin is adherent to the underlying capsule, or the pupillary space is too small, it may be necessary to start the incision in the iris tissue, a little below the pupil, and then cut upward until the knife emerges into the pupillary area, thus making an irido-capsulotomy. The soft iris tissue is easily incised if no pressure is made with the knife, and the sawing motion is maintained.

AFTER-TREATMENT.

Postoperative inflammatory reaction is infrequent, but if it should occur the usual antiphlogistic treatment of atropin, calomel, ice-pads and leaching should be actively instituted and continued until the eye is absolutely quiet. The operation itself is frequently an antiphlogistic measure, because it relieves iris-tension and traction on the ciliary body. The usual compress of gauze and cotton, covered with a Liebreich patch, may be applied to the eye for the first twenty-four hours and rest in bed enjoined for that period.

IN CONCLUSION.

We have carefully reviewed the history of iridotomy for nearly two centuries, and noted how the pendulum has swung from knife-needle to scissors, and back again. We have learned that Cheselden, the father of iridotomy, originated the method of incision by the knife-needle, which Heuermann modified, and Adams later revised and improved. We have seen how Janin abandoned this procedure and originated the scissors method, which Maunoir greatly improved and caused to hold sway for more than half a century. We have been deeply impressed by the fact that the mature, judicial mind of von Graefe led him to abandon the scissors and revert to the knife-needle method. We have seen how, soon after his death, the great influence of De Wecker had swerved the thought of the ophthalmic world back to the adoption of the scissors method in a greatly improved form.

Whether I have succeeded in citing sufficient facts and arguments to establish my thesis in favor of the knife-needle, or not, I nevertheless submit to the profession my V-shaped iridotomy and capsulotomy with a confidence born of twenty years' successful experience in its use, and with the hope that it may prove equally efficient in the hands of others who will take pains to study and understand the method, and who may have the patience to put it in practice.

MIOTICS VERSUS IRIDECTOMY IN THE TREATMENT OF SIMPLE CHRONIC GLAUCOMA.

AN ANALYTICAL STUDY OF 65 CASES TREATED BY MIOTICS OVER A SERIES OF YEARS.*

WM. CAMPBELL POSEY, M.D.

PHILADELPHIA.

In 1906 I presented a paper before the Section on Ophthalmology on "The Treatment of Simple Chronic Glaucoma by Miotics",[1] in which attention was called to the very satisfactory results which attend the use of these drugs in this variety of glaucoma, and their more intelligent and persistent administration was urged. It was pointed out that "while the results of operation are known to be less favorable in simple chronic glaucoma than those obtained in other forms of this disease, yet it is almost commonly conceded that even in this type iridectomy gives a better chance for retaining vision than any other form of treatment."

It was questioned, however, whether there is positive evidence that miotics are of less value than iridectomy in the treatment of chronic glaucoma, as no statistical study had ever been made of a series of cases of this variety of glaucoma which had been treated by miotics long enough or in sufficiently great numbers to permit a comparison to be made with series of cases which had been operated upon by iridectomy. I referred, in this connection, to a study which had been made of 167 cases of chronic glaucoma which were taken from the records of the Wills Eye Hospital, by Dr. Wm.

* This paper has been accepted by the Executive Committee of the Section on Ophthalmology of the American Medical Association, to be presented before the Section at the Chicago Session, June 2-5, 1908. Publication rights reserved by the American Medical Association.

1. The Journal A. M. A., 1907, xlviii, 676.

Zentmayer and myself in 1895, and I remarked that while many of these cases had been observed over a very protracted period, the miotics which were employed were doubtless administered indifferently in many instances, so that the full advantage which might have been gained from them was not obtained in any of the cases.

Notwithstanding this failure to obtain a maximum effect from the miotics, the comparison which was made between the medicinal and operative form of treatment, and which was based on a careful analysis of all the cases, was very favorable to the former.

Among the conclusions which were arrived at may be cited the following:[2] "When the drug was well borne it was found that the central visual acuity improved in 62.16 per cent. of the cases, while it remained unaltered in 21.62 per cent. In only 16.21 per cent. did the vision diminish, the drug being powerless to prevent it. Its influence on the extent of the visual field was not so great as on the degree of visual acuity, for an improvement was noted in the former symptom in but 50 per cent. of the cases. The field remained stationary in 18.75 per cent., while in 31.25 per cent., it steadily diminished. Contrasted with these figures are those obtained from a study of the cases on which iridectomy was performed. As a result of this procedure, vision was improved in 60 per cent., and remained the same in 20 per cent. of the cases. In another 20 per cent. the operation failed to prevent the loss in visual acuity. The extent of the visual field was increased in 30 per cent., and remained unchanged in 20 per cent. and diminshed in 10 per cent."

The limitations of these conclusions were, however, recognized, though it was asserted that from observations which I had made over a very considerable number of cases, both in private and dispensary service, since the publication of the report 12 years previously, that I was convinced that were it possible to compare an equal number of cases which had been subjected to iridectomy and to the action of miotics, properly administered over a similar period, the results would be shown to be far greater in favor of the former.

The present communication is offered in proof of this assertion, inasmuch as I have been enabled to collect sufficient and suitable data from cases of simple

---

2. Wills Eye Hosp. Rep., 1895, 1, No. 1.

chronic glaucoma treated by miotics, which were observed in my own practice and from notes generously given me by colleagues, to render a comparison with a similar series of cases treated by iridectomy possible.

I desire at this point to publicly acknowledge my indebtedness to the gentlemen who aided me with their cooperation, as without their notes, such a statistical study would have been impossible, for one observer can scarcely acquire sufficient data from his own practice to draw conclusive results. As a rule, only private cases can be depended on for statistical purposes, for there are but few hospital patients who can be trusted to follow the miotic treatment. Again, chronic simple glaucoma is uncommon, and since as a rule, it affects those who are advanced in years, death often ensues before observations can be extended over many years, even when the subjects of the disease remain constant in their attendance on one surgeon.

TABLE I.

Showing Length of Time Under Observation.

16 years	1 case
15 years	2 cases
13 years	3 cases
12 years	2 cases
11 years	2 cases
10 years	2 cases
9 years	1 case
8 years	5 cases
7 years	4 cases
6 years	6 cases
5 years	7 cases
4 years	8 cases
3 years	6 cases
2 years	9 cases
1 year	7 cases

Sixty-five cases have been analyzed, all, so far as it was possible to ascertain, being pure types of simple chronic glaucoma. It is necessary, however, to refer once more to the difficulty there is in distinguishing between this variety of glaucoma and atrophy of the optic nerve with excavation. All of the cases which are reported, however, manifested increased intraocular tension at some time while they were under observation, and all were observed sufficiently often to enable the diagnosis to be established as convincingly as the present state of our knowledge of the pathology of the two affections renders possible.

All were treated by miotics, in most instances in sufficient dose to keep the pupils very small, the strength of the drug being increased from time to time to secure this, which is so essential in order to obtain the desired effect on the intraocular tension.

All but seven of the cases were observed over a period of two years; 12 had been carefully followed for more than 10 years.

The average period of time each patient was under observation was five years and eight months.

As most advocates of iridectomy in simple chronic glaucoma urge the necessity of early operation, and as it is generally recognized that the treatment and the prognosis of the affection is much influenced by the stage in which the disease comes under observation, I have divided the cases into three classes, according to their degrees of development: (1) Beginning cases; (2) moderately advanced cases; (3) very advanced or desperate cases.

Of the total number, 19 are recorded as beginning cases, 28 as moderately advanced and 7 as far advanced cases. The histories of 8 cases are added in which iridectomy had been done on one or both eyes, but always in conjunction with the employment of a miotic. Finally, the notes of two additional cases are given: Of one case, because, though many of the signs of glaucoma were present, the diagnosis of the true nature of the case is in doubt, and of the other as it demonstrates the slow progress of the disease, even without treatment.

Observations could be made of but 110 eyes, 13 out of the 130 which were presented for examination being blind or nearly so from glaucoma, while in two instances the eye was blind from other causes, i. e., sarcoma of chorioid and phthisis bulbi. Five eyes were normal.

Of the 110 glaucomatous eyes it was found that vision had either improved or held its own during the entire time the case was under observation, over a varying period of years, in 88 eyes, or 80 per cent; that there had been a slow deterioration in both central and peripheral vision in 13 eyes, or 11.8 per cent., while in 9 eyes (8 per cent.) the miotics seemed to exert no influence whatsoever on vision, the eyes going gradually blind, and passing into absolute glaucoma. The form field was maintained as long as the case was under observation in 51 eyes, or 45 per cent. Loss in form field was observed in 59 eyes, or 55 per cent. The average length of time vision was maintained in each case was 5 years and 3 months.

TABLE 2.

Vision and field improved in 3 eyes for a period of 2 years.
Vision and field improved in 1 eye for a period of 5 years.
Vision improved but field contracted in 1 eye during period of 1 year.

TABLE 3.—NORMAL VISION AND NORMAL FIELD MAINTAINED.

Beginning cases.

In 4 eyes for 13 years.
In 2 eyes for 12 years.
In 2 eyes for 11 years.
In 1 eye for 8 years.
In 1 eye for 7 years.
In 2 eyes for 6 years.
In 4 eyes for 5 years.
In 3 eyes for 4 years.
In 2 eyes for 3 years.
In 3 eyes for 2 years.
In 2 eyes for 1 year.

TABLE 4.—NORMAL VISION MAINTAINED, BUT WITH CONTRACTED FIELD.

(a) *Beginning Cases* (11).

In 1 eye for 16 years.
In 1 eye for 10 years.
In 1 eye for 8 years.
In 3 eyes for 6 years.
In 1 eye for 5 years.
In 4 eyes for 4 years.

(b) *Moderately Advanced Cases* (23).

In 1 eye for 15 years.
In 2 eyes for 12 years.
In 3 eyes for 3 years.
In 1 eye for 6 years.
In 3 eyes for 5 years.
In 4 eyes for 4 years.
In 4 eyes for 3 years.
In 4 eyes for 2 years.
In 1 eye for 1 year.

(c) *Far Advanced Cases* (2).

In 1 eye for 15 years.
In 1 eye for 4 years.

TABLE 5.—BOTH CENTRAL VISION AND FIELD REDUCED AT TIME OF COMMENCEMENT OF TREATMENT, BUT BOTH MAINTAINED WHILE CASE WAS UNDER OBSERVATION.

(a) *Moderately Advanced Cases* (13).

In 2 eyes for 8 years.
In 2 eyes for 5 years.
In 3 eyes for 4 years.
In 4 eyes for 4 years.
In 2 eyes for 2 years.

(b) *Far Advanced Cases* (7).

In 1 eye for 3 years.
In 5 eyes for 2 years.
In 1 eye for 18 months.

TABLE 6.—SLOW DETERIORATION IN BOTH CENTRAL AND PERIPHERAL VISION.

(a) *Beginning Cases* (4).

In 2 eyes for 8 years.
In 2 eyes for 4 years.

(b) *Moderately Advanced Cases* (9).

In 2 eyes for 10 years.
In 2 eyes for 8 years.
In 3 eyes for 2 years.
In 1 eye for 1 year.
In 1 eye for 2 months.

TABLE 7.—MIOTICS POWERLESS TO PREVENT LOSS OF VISION, BLINDNESS ENSUING.

1 eye going blind in 6 years (beginning case).
1 eye going blind in 5 years (moderately advanced).
1 eye going blind in 4 years (moderately advanced.)
2 eyes going blind in 3 years (moderately advanced).
2 eyes going blind in 2 years (beginning case).
1 eye going blind in 2 years (moderate).
1 eye going blind in 18 months (moderate).

Iridectomy was performed on 11 of the 68 cases. Two doubtful cases maintained vision 3 years. Four beginning cases maintained vision 14 months (miotics useful in other eye); one, 6 years (miotics useful in other eye); another, 18 months (miotics useful in other eye); iridectomy powerless in one case.

Five moderately advanced cases: Maintained vision 2 years in 1 case after visual acuity had been raised by miotics; 6 months in 1 case after miotics had failed; 10 months in 1 case after miotics had failed; 1 year in 1 case after miotics had failed; 6 months in 1 case after miotics held the disease in check 3 years.

Such are the figures obtained from an analysis of 110 eyes treated by miotics. The interesting question now arises, how do they compare with similar series treated by iridectomy?

Fortunately, there are available for this purpose two groups of cases which are admirably adapted to a comparative study, for Bull, of New York, in 1902, gave the postoperative history of 50 cases of simple chronic glaucoma, before the American Ophthalmological Society, and last year before the same society gave the history of 60 additional cases. All of the cases of both groups had been under observation for varying periods and all occurred in Bull's own practice. This series, therefore, possesses a peculiar value, as the expression of the personal experience of one of America's most eminent surgeons and observers, and may be taken as a fair index of the maximum effect which may be gained by iridectomy.

In Bull's first series (50 cases, 94 eyes iridectomized), there was a maintenance of the existing vision at the time of operation while under observation in 24 eyes, or 25.5 per cent., and a gradual failure in 58 eyes or 61.7 per cent. The average length of time the maintenance of vision was noted in any given case was 2 years and 5 months.

The form fields remained as they were at the time of operation in seven cases (14 per cent.), which were under observation for a period ranging from 15 months to 11 years, but became more contracted in 60 eyes. Absolute glaucoma resulted in 11 eyes. Total loss, 75.5 per cent. Average length of time each case was under observation was 4 years and 11 months.

In Bull's second series (60 cases, 115 eyes iridectomized), the average length of time each case was under observation is not mentioned, the general statement being made of from 5 to 11 years.

Vision—Temporary improvement in central vision in 14 eyes, 12 per cent.; no permanent improvement in central vision in any eye; maintenance of vision for a period of years (the longest being 8 years) in 21 eyes, 18 per cent.; gradual failure in central vision in 94 eyes, about 70 per cent.

Field—No maintenance of field while case was under observation in any case. Steady increase in the concentric narrowing of the field in 92 eyes. In 16 eyes the final result was absolute glaucoma. Total in which field sank, 108 cases, or 90.3 per cent.

Summary.—Apparent arrest of the progress of the disease as to central vision, condition of the field and tension in 21 eyes, or 18.2 per cent.; 16 eyes passed into absolute glaucoma.

When comparison is made of both of these series with that analyzed by me, it will at once appear that miotics exerted a much more beneficial influence than iridectomy. Thus, if central vision is considered, it will be found that in my series, each case of which was observed over an average period of 5 years and 8 months, vision was maintained in 80 per cent. of the cases, to 25 per cent. in Bull's first series and to 18 per cent. in his second; while there was a loss of central vision in 20 per cent. of my cases to 61 and 70 per cent. of Bull's first and second series respectively, each case in his first group being observed over an average period of 2 years and 5 months, while those in the second group were noted as being observed over a period ranging from 5 to 11 years.

Miotics exerted a more favorable influence on the form field also than iridectomy, the field being maintained as long as the case was under observation (each case an average of 5 years and 8 months) in 45 per cent. of my series, while the same was true of but 14 per cent. of Bull's first series (over an average period of 4 years and 10 months for each case), while in the second series there was no maintenance of the field while the case was under observation in any instance. In

Bull's first series, 11 eyes passed into absolute glaucoma, in the second, 16 eyes, while in my series only 9 eyes became totally blind.

There are other groups of cases, also, which may be used for purposes of comparison. Of these by far the most interesting for the purposes of this paper are the observations of Schleich, in Tübingen, which were based on the study of 102 cases which had been iridectomized and of 46 cases treated by miotics. In the series of cases which were submitted to operation, vision became worse immediately after the iridectomy in 30 per cent. of the cases, and of this number 26 per cent. became totally blind in a short time, the remainder growing gradually worse, with the exception of 3 per cent, in which vision after the first loss was maintained. Of the 70 per cent. who did not show an immediate deterioration of vision after the operation, sight remained unchanged for 2 years and even longer in 21 per cent., but there was a gradual loss in 79 per cent. In other words, 7.8 per cent. became blind directly or shortly after the operation; vision gradually failed in 76.5 per cent., being maintained in only 15.7 per cent. for a period of at least 2 years. In the 46 cases treated by miotics, the results were more favorable, as vision was maintained in 39 per cent., progression of the disease being observed in the remaining 61 per cent.

Another valuable communication is by Karrewiz, who reviewed the operations performed for the relief of glaucoma by Koster, in the Ophthalmic Clinic in Leyden during a period of 10 years. The results obtained in other forms of glaucoma are foreign to the scope of this paper and will not be dwelt on, of 20 eyes, however, with chronic glaucoma, which were iridectomized, record is made that vision was improved or remained *in statu quo* in 75 per cent. and diminished in 25 per cent.

Of the 75 per cent. in which loss of vision did not follow the operation, the visual acuity soon diminished in 74 per cent. of the cases, a lasting improvement being observed in but 26 per cent. Tension remained normal in 79 per cent. of the operated cases, increasing after the operation in 11 per cent. from various causes. Notwithstanding the good effect on tension, the vision in 53 per cent. of the cases, in which tension was benefited, deteriorated.

Although giving no figures to support his statement, Koster's experience with miotics in patients refusing operation leads him to conclude that while there are cases which can be held in abeyance by drugs, they are very exceptional, and that under their use glaucoma progresses steadily. He admits their value, however, both before and after operation.

In a discussion on the therapy of glaucoma before the Hungarian Ophthalmological Society, Grosz of Budapest reported that of 237 cases of glaucoma operated on by him, and which were under observation for a long time after the operation, 62 cases were instances of glaucoma simplex and success was attained by operation in 70 per cent. of the cases. In the discussion Béla insisted on the necessity of keeping the eyes under the full control of miotics, and Csopodi reported a case of glaucoma simplex in which good vision had been preserved for 4 years in one eye, the other eye which had been iridectomized being blind from glaucoma.

Strong evidence in favor of the beneficial effect of iridectomy in simple glaucoma is advanced by von Hippel, of Göttingen, who based his statistics on the study of 58 patients with 74 glaucomatous eyes taken from among a total of 70,000 eye cases. Iridectomy was performed 65 times, sclerotomy 6 times and iridectomy with a later sclerotomy 3 times. Of this number only 66 eyes, for various reasons, could be utilized in preparing statistics. von Hippel is of the opinion that the long continued use of miotics in chronic glaucoma is dangerous, inasmuch as it obscures the symptoms and prevents iridectomy being done sufficiently early. He believes that they should not be used before the operation, therefore, but employs them regularly and continuously after operation, as he is convinced that they exert an appreciable effect in preventing the progress of the glaucomatous process. In no case was central vision diminished by the operation, notwithstanding that many of the cases operated on by him had markedly contracted fields and pronounced cupping of the disc. The summary deduced by von Hippel from his statistics is as follows: Forty-one per cent of the cases operated on showed no aggravation of symptoms after 2 years; 20 per cent. showed none after 5 years; 14 per cent. after 10 years, and 9 per cent. after 14 years. He considered that 9 eyes (about 14 per cent) could be considered "as cured for the present," as 6 showed no loss in vision during a period of 1 to 2 years and 3 during a period of less than a year. A slow loss of vision, however, appeared in 17 eyes (about 26 per cent). All of these cases could be included under the class designated by me as "moderately advanced." Thirteen eyes (20 per cent) went blind in spite of iridectomy, though a period of partial vision was attained in half of the cases for a period ranging from 3 to 5 years.

To these statistics should be added the figures mentioned by Uhthoff, in the discussion of Berry's paper before the British Medical Association, in 1904, to the effect that after iridectomy he had found a perceptible improvement of vision in 5 per cent. of the cases. The disease remained stationary in about 45 per cent.; it advanced slowly, in spite of the operation, in approximately 40 per cent, and grew much worse in fully 10 per cent.

In the discussion of Schleich's paper, Königshofer said that as years go by he has grown to doubt the value of iridectomy, and he treats all cases first with miotics, iridectomy being resorted to as a last resort. He has even seen loss in the visual fields gradually improve under miotics. Adamük,[3] referring to Wygodski's contention that it is necessary to operate in cases of glaucoma as soon as possible, and even in the prodromal period, maintains that although originally he had been a strong advocate of iridectomy, since the development of the miotic treatment and particularly with the ability to secure good miotics, he doubts the value of operative interference in these early and prodromal periods. No matter how correctly the iridectomy may be performed, it gives rise to a certain diminution of visual acuity. After the operation the patients are more disposed to atrophy of the optic nerve, not to mention the complications of hemorrhage, explosive and otherwise, which may occur during the operation. Fully admitting the great utility of iridectomy, he does not think that it is applicable to all the cases from the very start, but that first there should be medicinal treatment, and if this is faithfully carried out the necessity for operation will grow less frequent.

It is interesting to note that this distinguished ophthalmologist, who died in September, 1906, shortly after

3. Ophth. Year Book, 1907, p.198.

Table of Comparison of Series of Cases of Chronic Glaucoma Treated by Miotics and by Iridectomy.

	Zentmayer and Posey; 167 Cases.	Schleich.	r; 20 Eyes. (Iri- ›my.) Per cent.	Grosz; 62 Cases. (Iridectomy.)	Uhthoff. (Iridectomy.) Number of Cases not Mentioned. Per cent.	Hippel. 66 Eyes. (Iridectomy.) Per cent.
Central vision Maintained in. .				70 "Favorable result attained." Details of what constituted "a favorable result" not given.	50 (Actual improvement of V. in 5.)	14 ("Cured for the present.")
Gradually lost in					50 (40 gradual; 10 rapidly.)	41, no aggravation of symptoms after 2 years. 20, no aggravation of symptoms after 5 years. 14, no aggravation of symptoms after 10 years. 9, no aggravation of symptoms after 14 years. 26, slow loss in vision. 20, went blind in spite

the publication of the above, had been a sufferer from attacks of glaucoma from the age of 36 years, which were always readily combated by eserin, normal vision being retained by the miotics until his death, which occurred 31 years after the first attack.

In addition to these foreign statistics and expressions of opinion, a number of our own countrymen have given voice to their views regarding the various forms of treatment of chronic glaucoma. Lack of space prevents detailing what these views are, but those who are interested are referred to papers by Bull and Weeks before the American Ophthalmological Society in 1902, and to the discussion of their papers by Gruening, Theobald, Pooley, Chandler, Standish and Ring; to the discussion of my paper[1] by Weeks, Bull, de Schweinitz, Wilder and Callan; to a paper by Risley[4] on "The Surgical Treatment of Chronic Glaucoma," and finally to a paper by Cheney,[5] of Boston, and to the discussion which it evoked by Hansell, Zentmayer, Ziegler, Veasey, de Schweinitz, Risley and myself.

From a careful consideration of the views, both of these latter and of foreign observers, it is apparent that while a better technic has improved the results which are attained by iridectomy in skilful hands, and while there are some who still maintain the greater value of this procedure over any other means of therapy, the miotic form of treatment is gaining in adherents, and that those even who prefer iridectomy, insist on the adminstration of miotics after the operation has been performed, acknowledging their belief in the power of such drugs to control the glaucomatous process. While I do not believe that the series of cases which I have collected offers absolute proof of the superiority of the miotic over the operative form of treatment, its comparison with the percentages obtained by iridectomy makes it appear at least likely that such is the case. The types of the disease are so varied, however, and there are so many factors which are misleading in the compilation of statistics of cases of chronic glaucoma, that it is very desirable that very many other cases and groups of cases both of those treated by iridectomy as well as

4. The Journal A. M. A., 1907, xlix, 291.
5. Ophthalmology, April, 1907.

by miotics, should be followed and carefully studied over long periods of years. I venture to suggest, therefore, that the Section may undertake a compilation of further statistics under its own auspices, the members following their cases of chronic glaucoma as carefully and as long as possible, making frequent and accurate notes of the course of the disease, so that their reports may be available for statistical purposes.

Just as the advocates of iridectomy find beginning cases to be more amenable to treatment than those in more advanced stages of the disease, so cases treated by miotics from the early stages give better percentages in so far as the maintenance of central and peripheral vision is concerned. Thus, of the 19 cases recorded as "beginning," vision deteriorated in but 4 and even then only after a considerable period, a slow deterioration in both central and peripheral vision being noted in one case over a period of 8 years, and in another over a period of 4 years. Absolute glaucoma supervened in but two cases which were under observation from their very incipiency, miotics being powerless to prevent one eye going blind in 6 years and another in 2 years. In view of such favorable statistics from the use of miotics alone, and with the possibility of error in the diagnosis complicating the situation and iridectomy being performed upon merely atrophic nerves, is operation ever justified when both central and peripheral vision are normal, without trial of what miotics can do?

As argument against the propriety of early iridectomy, two cases may be cited, in one of which though the nerves presented all the signs of a commencing glaucomatous excavation, and the sclera were distinctly rigid, typical glaucoma cups never developed, though the case was observed for eleven years. Eserin was continuously employed, though in weak doses, as I never have felt justified in relinquishing its use. Had an iridectomy been performed on what were still normal eyes, though possessing decided glaucomatous tendencies, it is possible that the eyes might have been lost, or sight at least impaired by the procedure, whereas vision is still normal. Vision is still safeguarded in both eyes by a miotic, the continuance of this treatment demanding nothing more of the patient than a few moments' attention to dropping night and morning.

Case 1.—Female, aged 67. When first seen, discs in both eyes noted as being congested and the excavations large temporally, the macular vessels being distinctly kinked as they passed over the edges of the disc. O'Tn. Fields normal.

O. D. + S. 0.75 D. ⊂ + C. 0.50 D. ax. 180° = 5/5

O. S. + S. 0.75 D. ⊂ + C. 0.50 D. ax. 160° = 5/5

Eserin, gr. 1/10, gtt. ii, b. d., prescribed for both eyes.

This patient has reported on an average of once each year. Vision and fields have remained normal in each eye, though the anterior chambers have perhaps become somewhat shallower, the nerves grayer, and the excavations more extended and deeper. Both scleras are rigid and tension is somewhat elevated. The miotic has been but slightly increased, being now employed in the strength of ¼ gr. to fl. oz. i, gtt. ii, b. d.

The second case was under observation for fifteen years, and during the past nine years of this period typical glaucomatous cups, with all the other signs of advancing glaucoma, slowly manifested themselves. Miotic treatment was prescribed, but was not persisted in, so that the patient was practically without treatment. Notwithstanding this, however, central vision is still normal in one eye, and almost so in the other, while the fields of vision are not greatly restricted. The patient is now 79 years of age, and has had the uninterrupted use of his eyes during the entire period of the development of the glaucoma. An iridectomy might have robbed him of his sight or might, at least, have occasioned hemorrhage or other complications which would have seriously interfered with vision.

Case 2.—Male, aged 79. Under observation fifteen years, March, 1893, to March, 1908. When first seen, nerves hyperemic. Central excavations.

O. D. + C. 0.50 D. ax. 90° = 5/5

O. S. + S. 0.75 D. ⊂ + C. 0.50 D. ax. 60° = 5/5

Six years later came for change of glasses; nerves grayer, excavations becoming depressed to T. side. Three years later (1902), large shallow glaucomatous excavation in right eye and forming one in left. T. +. Anterior chamber shallow.

O. D. + S. 1.25 D. ⊂ + C. 1.25 D. ax. 120° = 5/6

O. S. + S. 0.50 D. ⊂ + C. 0.50 D. ax. 180° = 5/7½

(Fields as per Fig. 1.)

Eserin, gr. 1/6, to fl. oz. i, gtt. ii, in each eye, b. d., prescribed.

Not seen until two years later, eserin having been used but irregularly in the interval. Central vision in each eye as in 1902. Fields more contracted, especially in O. S. Eserin continued in ascending doses, but patient failed to report until 1908, when he confessed to not having used the miotic.

O. D. V. + C. 0.50 D. ax. 160° = 5/5 partly

O. S. V. — C. 0.50 D. ax. 60° = 5/9 partly

Tension is decidedly elevated in both eyes. The anterior chambers are shallow and the pupils one-third dilated. Both optic nerves are the seat of glaucomatous excavations, that in the right eye being the larger.

In the 28 "moderately advanced" cases, 9 eyes showed slow loss of vision, while blindness supervened in 6. The best results of all, however, were attained in the "far-advanced" or desperate cases, for of the 7 so designated, all maintained vision in a very remarkable manner, and in several instances over a long period of years, the most remarkable example of this being Case 48, the details of which were reported fully[6] in June, 1906.

As even the most enthusiastic advocates of iridectomy realize the danger of operating on cases in this stage of the disease, all can at least agree that in the treatment of this type of cases miotics should be employed energetically and continuously, the pupils being kept at pinpoint contraction.

A number of the cases were seen from their very incipiency, the glaucomatous cupping of the head of the nerve being preceded in each instance by a low-grade neuritis, similar to that noted by Zentmayer and myself[7] thirteen years ago. Miotics were employed early in all these cases, but notwithstanding their energetic use, the glaucomatous process slowly became more manifested in each case, the excavations extending and deepening, the chambers becoming shallower and the sclera more rigid. While the disease in each instance gave decided evidence of progression, vision, however, and the visual field remained normal, showing that the glaucoma, while not entirely checked by the miotics, was in any event greatly retarded in its progress. Miotics can not, therefore, be regarded in any sense as curative, and must be relied on solely as measures which may hold chronic glaucoma in abeyance.

In conclusion, I desire to emphasize what I have already said elsewhere: First, that miotics should be relied on as the sole means of treatment only in those cases which are free from attacks of so-called "glaucomatous congestion," the presence of such congestive symptoms

---

6. The Journal A. M. A., 1907, xlviii, 676.
7. Wills Eye Hosp. Rep., 1895, i, No. 1.

being in my opinion the chief indication for iridectomy; and second, that to gain the full benefit of miotics it is necessary that they should be administered properly. Beginning in doses small enough to avoid creating spasm of the ciliary muscle, and rapidly increasing the dose until the pupil of the affected eye is strongly contracted, this degree of contraction should be maintained as long as life lasts by gradually increasing the strength of the solution, from time to time, and by instillations of the drug at intervals of every three or four hours. Conjunctival irritation may be avoided by employing only fresh and sterile solutions of the drug. Suitable cleansing washes should be administered, and attention given to the general health and especially to the condition of the blood vessels. Careful and repeated correction of the refraction error should be made and restrictions enjoined on the use of the eyes.

REPORT OF BEGINNING CASES.

CASE 1.—*History.*—Female, aged 75 years. (The age given in all of the cases refers to what it was at the time of last observation.) Under observation nearly sixteen years.

First sought treatment on account of secondary glaucoma in the right eye, following iritis. Iridectomy performed, but without avail, vision soon being reduced to 2/40 eccentrically, and the field being much contracted.

Examination.—Even at time of first consultation, O. S. manifested signs of chronic glaucoma, the anterior chamber being shallow, the sclera rigid, and the excavation on the head of the nerve embracing its outer two-thirds, with undermined edges. O. S. V. + S. 0.50 D. ⊃ + C. 0.25 D. ax. 20° = 5/5. Field normal. Eserin, gr. 1/20 to fl. oz. i, prescribed. This patient has been seen at intervals of at least every six months during sixteen years, the miotics being gradually increased in strength until pilocarpin, gr. 4 to fl. oz. i, gtt. ii, t. i. d., is now employed to keep the pupil contracted *ad maximum.* The anterior chamber has become very shallow and there is now a typical glaucoma cup embracing all but a small part, the nasal third of the nerve. (Fields as per Fig. 2.)

O. S. V. + S. 0.37 D. ⊃ + C. 0.75 D. ax. 155° = 5/5.

Despite the long-continued use of miotics, there has never been any appreciable irritation of the conjunctiva caused by it.

Remarks.—Glaucomatous process held in check while under observation for almost sixteen years, central vision being still normal and the field but slightly contracted.

CASE 2.—*History.*—Female, aged 52 years. Under observation thirteen years. At time of first observation O. D. + S.

0.75 D. = 5/5; O. S. + S. 1 D. = 5/5. Both discs were dull gray to the nasal side, especially in the left eye. Seen at intervals of every two or three years.

Examination.—Ten years after first observation nerves noted as paler and forming pathologic excavations observed in each eye. Tension elevated. Eserin, gr. 1/10, gtt. ii, b. d., prescribed. Fields of vision and vision normal. Now large shallow excavations in each eye, sclera rigid. Marked pulsations or retinal vessels on compression of the eyeball.

O. D. V. + S. 0.25 D. ⊂ + C. 0.50 D. ax. 20° = 5/5

O. S. V. + S. 0.25 D. ⊂ + C. 1.25 D. ax. 160 = 5/5

Fields of vision normal, using eserin, gr. ¼, gtt. ii, b. d.

Remarks.—Development of glaucoma cups while under observation, though vision and fields continue normal.

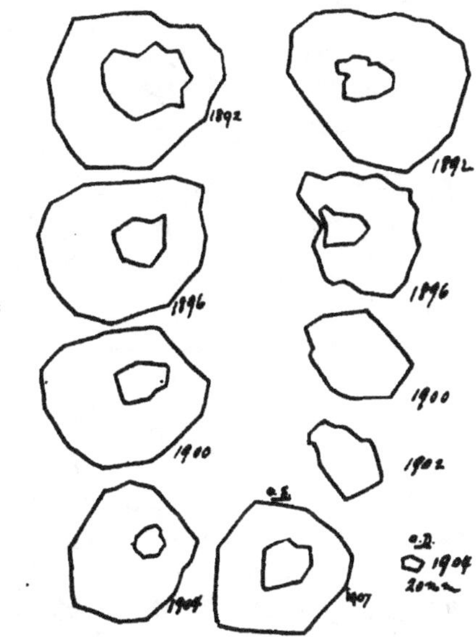

Fig. 1.—Fields of Case 2: 10 mm. white and red.

Case 3.—*History.*—Male, aged 72 years. Under observation thirteen years. When first seen, optic nerves hyperemic; central excavations; anterior chambers shallow.

O. D. V. + S. 0.75 D. ⊂ + C. 0.50 D. ax. 170° = 5/5

O. S. V. + S. 1 D. ⊂ + C. 0.75 D. ax. 10° = 5/5

Seen at intervals of one or two years. Nine years after first observation excavation in left eye found to have extended below to the edge of the disc, and to be distinctly undermined. Sclera resistant. Venous pulse. Anterior chamber shallow in both eyes. Vision and field of vision normal in both eyes. Eserin, gr. 1/10, gtt. ii, O. S., b. d., gtt. ii, O. D. u. d., ordered, and has been continued uninterruptedly and in stronger doses during the past four years. The excavation in the left eye has deepened and extended, and during the past year that in the right eye has also assumed a glaucomatous type. Tension is perceptibly elevated in both eyes and the anterior chambers are shallow.

O. D. + S. 0.75 D. ⊂ + C. 0.50 D. ax. 170° = 5/5
O. S. + C. 0.62 D. ax. 175° = 5/5

The fields are normal.

Remarks.—The glaucomatous excavations formed while patient was under observation, the degenerative process in the nerves being preceded by a stage of hyperemia. Though the excavations have extended and the tension has become more elevated, vision and fields have remained normal.

CASE 4.—*History.*—Male, aged 51 years. Under observation thirteen years. At time of first observation, both optic nerves hyperemic, especially the left.

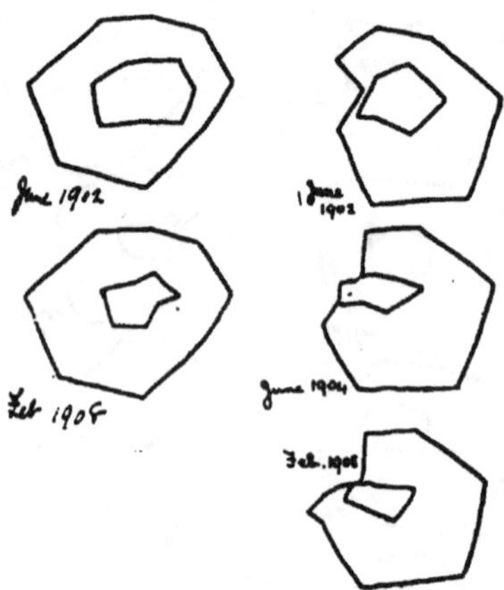

Fig. 2.—Fields of Case 1: 10 mm. white and red.

O. D. + S. 0.50 D. ⊂ + C. 0.75 D. ax. 90° = 5/5
O. S. + S. 0.50 D. ⊂ + C. 1 D. ax. 70° = 5/5

Fields of vision normal. Left-sided neuralgia at times, with some pain in corresponding eye. Seen at intervals of one or two years. Eight years after first observation excavations in each eye noted as being suspicious, and eserin, gr. 1/12, gtt. ii. u. d., prescribed. Two years later excavations more pronounced, especially in O. D. Vision and field of vision normal in each eye. Eserin, gr. ½, gtt. ii. b. d. At present time quite a deep glaucomatous excavation in O. D., extending to scleral ring externally. The excavation in O. S. has also become glaucomatous, being more extended but not so deep as in the fellow eye. Sclera rigid in each eye. Pilocarpin, gr. i. gtt. ii. b. d.

O. D. + S. 0.25 D. ⊂ + C. 0.75 D. ax. 100° = 5/5
O. S. + S. 0.25 D. ⊂ + C. 0.62 D. ax. 65° = 5/5

Some contraction of O. S. field to nasal side.

Remarks.—Development of the disease while under observation. Miotics have maintained normal vision, but excavations have become glaucomatous.

CASE 5.—*History.*—Female, aged 58 years. Unuer observation twelve years. At first examination in 1896:

O. D. + S. 1.75 D. ⊃ + C. 0.75 D. ax. 100° = 5/5
O. S. + S. 1.25 D. ⊃ + C. 0.50 D. ax. 60° = 5/5

Both optic nerves hyperemic, with central excavations.

Patient seen at intervals of one or two years for change of glasses and minor symptoms. Eight years after first observation, both optic nerves were noted as being pale and "luminous" and the excavations were deep and undermined above, this being the more pronounced in the right eye. The anterior chambers were shallow and the sclera rigid. Vision and fields normal. Eserin, gr. 1/6, gtt. ii, t. i. d. The strength of

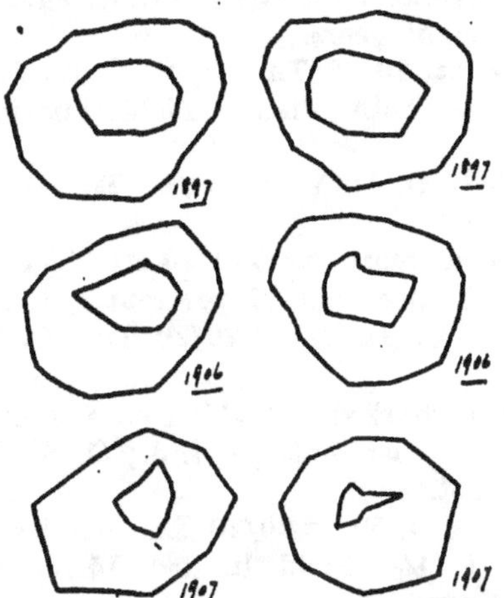

Fig. 3.—Fields of Case 6: 10 mm. white and red.

the miotics has been gradually increased, the pupils being maintained at pin-point contraction, but the excavations have gradually extended until they are now pronouncedly glaucomatous. Vision and fields normal in each eye.

O. D. + S. 2 D. ⊃ + C. 1.25 D. ax. 120° = 5/5
O. S. + S. 1.37 D. ⊃ + C. 0.50 D. ax. 40° = 5/5

Remarks.—Development of glaucoma cups while under observation. Stage of hyperemia of the nerve preceding the atrophic process. Maintenance of full visual acuity and extent of visual fields with miotics.

CASE 6.—(Reported in 1906).—*History.*—Female, aged 73 years. Under observation eleven years. Gradually failing vision in each eye for some months at time of first consultation. Gouty. Suffers from nasal catarrh. Both optic nerves hyperemic, with large temporal excavations. Sclera rigid. Anterior chambers shallow. Fields of vision normal.

O. D. V. + S. 1.75 D. ⊂ + C. 0.50 D. ax. 30° = 5/5
O. S. V. + S. 1.25 D. ⊂ + C. 0.75 D. ax. 60° = 5/5

Eserin, gr. 1/10 to fl. oz. i, gtt. ii, b. d., the strength being gradually increased until at the end of eleven years a solution of gr. ii to fl. oz. i is employed. The patient has been seen at intervals of six months, and, though the nerves have become somewhat atrophic and large shallow glaucomatous cups have developed in each eye, the anterior chambers shallower and tension increased, central vision and the fields of vision have remained normal (Fig. 3).

O. D. V. + S. 1.75 D. ⊂ + C. 1 D. ax. 45° = 5/5
O. S. V. + S. 2.5 D. = 5/5

Remarks.—Glaucoma developed under observation, despite use of miotics, but vision and visual field have remained normal.

CASE 7 (Dr. Weeks).—*History.*—Male, aged 61 years. Under observation eight years.

O. D. V. = 20/20 Tn. O. S. V. = 20/20 Tn.

Slight cupping both discs. Fields normal. Prescribed glasses.

Nov. 26, 1906: O. D. V. = 20/20 Tn. O. S. V. = 20/20. T. + ½.

Cupping of disc more marked. Left field slightly limited nasally. Advised pilocarpin (1 per cent.), t. i. d., left eye.

Jan. 2, 1907: O. D. V. = 20/20 Tn. O. S. V. = 20/20. T. + ½.

Cupping more marked. Fields more reduced. Advised: O. S. V., eserin (½ per cent.), t. i. d.; O. S. V., pilocarpin (1 per cent.) at night.

September 2: O. D. V. = 20/20 Tn. Field normal. O. S. V. = 20/20. T. + ½. Field limited 15 degrees nasal side. Treatment continued.

Remarks.—Full central vision and but slight loss in visual field during eight years under observation.

CASE 8.—*History.*—Male, aged 59 years. Under observation eight years. When first seen, large shallow excavations in each eye; nerves gray. Tn. Heavy user of tobacco. Fields of vision normal.

O. D. + S. 1.5 D. ⊂ + C. 0.50 D. ax. 180° = 5/5
O. S. + S. 0.75 D. ⊂ + C. 0.50 D. ax. 175° = 5/5

Tobacco prohibited. Eserin, gr. 1/20, gtt. x, in each eye, u. d. Strychnia. Seen at intervals of one or two years. Third year after first observation marked glaucomatous excavations in outer parts of both nerves. T. elevated. Pupils large. Fields and vision normal. Eserin, gr. ½ to fl. oz. i, gtt. ii, in each eye twice daily. Eserin continued in increasing strengths until 1901, when patient died of heart disease. Shortly before death fields normal in each eye.

O. D. + S. 2.25 D. ⊂ + C. 1.25 D. ax. 180° = 5/5
O. S. + S. 2 D. ⊂ + C. 1 D. ax. 170° = 5/5

(A year ago I successfully operated on the son of this patient for a subacute attack of glaucoma in one eye.)

Remarks.—Glaucoma developed while under observation, though the miotics which were employed maintained normal vision and fields of vision.

CASE 9.—*History.*—Female, aged 68. Under observation seven years. Gouty. Has always suffered from head pain. At time of first consultation nerves gray; shallow physiologic excavations, that in the left eye with undermined edges. Sclera rigid. Fields normal.

O. D. + S. 0.75 D. ⊃ + C. 0.50 D. ax. 50° = 5/5

O. S. + S. 0.75 D. ⊃ + C. 0.25 D. ax. 120° = 5/5

Second observation, a year later, when excavation in O. S. was found to be deeper and more glaucomatous in type.

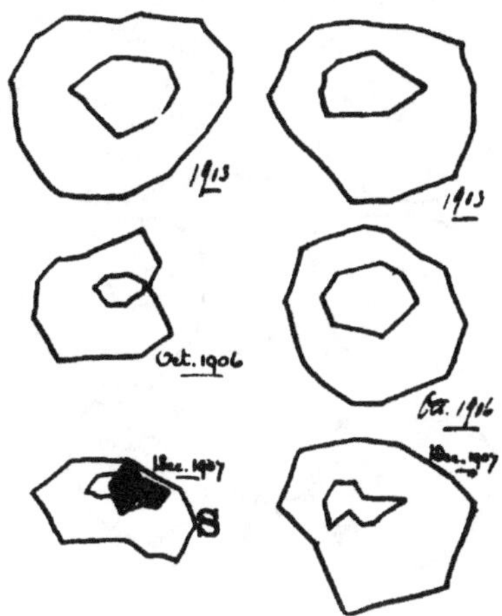

Fig. 4.—Fields of Case 9: 10 mm. white and red; S, absolute scotoma for 10 mm. white.

Head pain had persisted despite use of glasses, but there was no obscuration of vision in either eye. Vision and field still normal.

The patient then passed from observation for four years, although she had been warned of the necessity of frequent observations of the left eye and told of its glaucomatous nature. At the visit, four years later, complaint of failing vision in O. S. for a year or more was made and also of a continuance of the head pain. Examination showed a deep typical glaucomatous cup in the left eye and a shallow glaucomatous one in the right (Fig. 4). O. S. T. + 2, O. D. T. + 1. Both nerves quite gray and walls of retinal vessels thickened. Pilocarpin, gr. i to fl. oz. i, t. i. d. with strychnia and nitroglycerin.

O. D. V. + S. 1.5 D. ⊃ + C. 0.50 D. ax. 30° = 5/5

O. S. V. — C. 0.50 D. ax. 30° = 5/7½

The patient has been seen frequently during the past two years, the miotic being increased in dose, so that the pupil has been kept at maximum contraction (Fig. 4). Now using a solution of gr. iii to fl. oz i of pilocarpin.

O. D. V. + S. 1.25 D. ⌒ + C. 0.50 D. ax. 20° = 5/5

O. S. V. = 5/40 eccentric.

O. D. field still normal for form and color.

Remarks.—Glaucoma cups slowly developed in both eyes during five years of interrupted observation and without treatment, so that O. S. V. became much compromised both centrally and peripherally. During the two years miotics have been employed, disease has been arrested in the right eye, though a slow progression has occurred in the left.

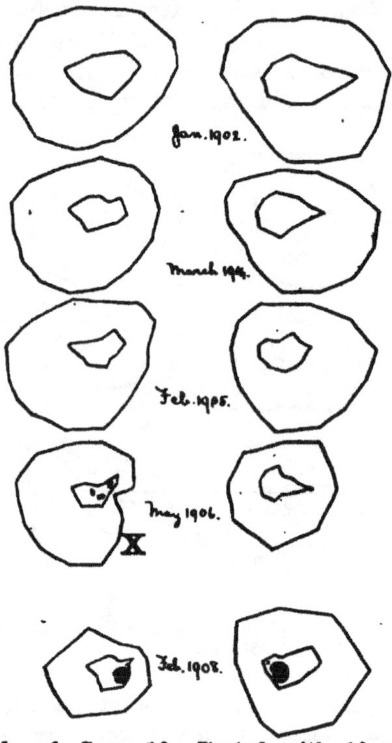

Fig. 5.—Fields of Case 10: Tested with 10 mm. white and red; X, relative scotoma for 10 mm. red. Fields of 1907 remain practically as in 1906. In February, 1908, tested with 10 mm., white and red; absolute scotoma for 10 mm. red.

Case 10.—*History.*—Female, aged 71 years. Under observation six years. At time of first consultation, vision said to have failed in each eye during the six months previous. Both nerves hyperemic, with large excavations becoming undermined to nasal side. Venous pulse. Anterior chambers shallow. Sclera rigid. Fields normal.

O. D. V. + S. 2.5 D. ⌒ + C. 0.25 D. ax. 145° = 5/5

O. S. V. + S. 2.5 D. ⌒ + C. 0.25 D. ax. 160° = 5/5

Eserin, gr. 1/10 to fl. oz. i, gtt. ii, in each eye, b. d. Seen at intervals of six months and strength of eserin gradually increased. At end of two years cups had assumed a typical glaucomatous appearance and tension was appreciably elevated in each eye. Central vision still normal, but form fields somewhat compromised concentrically, that for red being decidedly restricted. Eserin, gr. ½, gtt. ii, b. d.

At end of six years, moderately deep glaucoma cups, anterior chambers quite shallow (Fig. 5). Tension elevated.

O. D. V. + S. 0.25 D. ⊃ + C. 0.62 D. ax. 30° = 5/5

O. S. V. + S. 1.25 ⊃ + C. 0.37 D. ax. 30° = 5/5

Using pilocarpin, gr. i, gtt. ii, b. d.

Remarks.—Glaucoma developed under observation. Retention of normal central vision, but loss in visual fields during six years of observation under continuous use of miotics.

Case 11 (Dr. de Schweinitz).—*History.*—Male, aged 71 years. Under observation six years. Right eye removed for sarcoma of chorioid March 31, 1898. Corrected vision of the left eye at that time — 1.75, axis 75, 6/5, with a suggestive cup, but not typical. Three years later no return of sarcoma and apparently no increase in the size of the cup, vision 6/6. One and one-half years later, with corrected vision, O. D. + .50 ⊃ — 1.50 axis 75, 6/6; cup now distinctly and typically glaucomatous, no pulse, no tension, contraction of nasal field and characteristic ring scotoma. Operation suggested but declined. Persistent use of miotics. Two years later no return of sarcoma, vision 6/9 O. S. Increase in size of scotoma and greater contraction of visual field. Operation declined. Four years later patient (himself not seen) is reported by an intelligent relative to be practically blind, having always declined any operative interference, believing that his case was in the hands of God.

Remarks.—Miotics failed to control glaucomatous process, blindness ensuing.

Case 12.—*History.*—Female, aged 61 years. Under observation six years. At time of first observation there had been a dimness of vision in the left eye for two weeks, associated with symptoms of a mild attack of subacute glaucoma. The anterior chambers in both eyes were shallow; O. S. pupil was somewhat more dilated than that of O. D.

O. D. V. + S. 1.75 D. ⊃ + C. 0.25 D. ax. 110° = 5/5

O. S. V. + S. 2 D. ⊃ + C. 0.75 D. ax. 110° = 5/5

No pathologic excavation in O. D., but in O. S. commencing glaucoma cup to nasal side. Retinal veins full and pulsating.

Pilocarpin and eserin have been maintained without interruption in each eye ever since. The right eye has remained normal, and the left eye has suffered no further glaucomatous attacks, though the progress of the disease is evidenced by an increase in the extent of the excavation, so that it now embraces nearly the entire head of the nerve, and the field is somewhat cut nasally (Fig. 6). There has been a persistent tendency to conjunctival irritation, which has been successfully combated, from time to time, by local applications of argyrol and astringents. Now using pilocarpin, gr. ii, gtt. i, O. D., u. d.; O. S., gtt. ii, O. S., t. i. d.

O. D. + S. 2.75 D. = 5/5

O. S. + S. 2.25 D. ⊃ + C. 0.25 D. ax. 105° = 5/5

Remarks.—Disease held in check six years by miotics.

CASE 13 (Mr. E. T. Collins, *Clin. Jour.*, March 1, 1905).—*History.*—Female, aged 79 years. Under observation five and one-half years. Left eye lost from consequences of operation of iridectomy performed for relief of glaucoma. Symptoms of glaucoma in right eye at that time, held in check by regular and continuous use of pilocarpin.

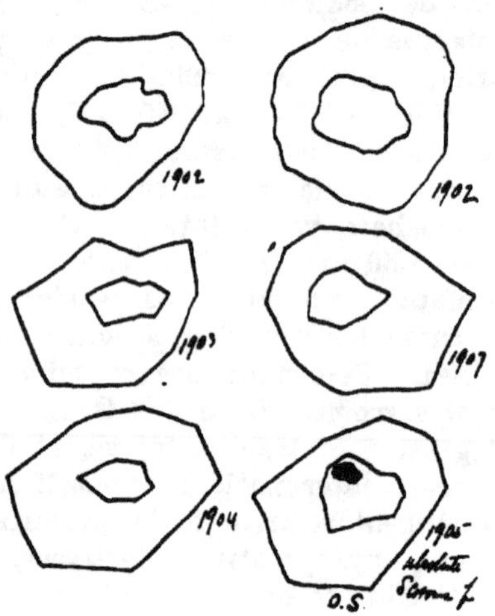

Fig. 6.—Fields of Case 12: 10 mm. white and red.

CASE 14 (Dr. Cheney).—*History.*—Female, aged 66 years. Under observation five years. When first seen (September, 1901) was using a strong eserin solution in each eye. No cupping of disc, but an unusual degree of venous pulsation. Halos and smoky vision at times. Both fields were normal.

O. D. V. — S. 0.25 D. ⊃ + C. 0.75 D. ax. 70° = 18/30

O. S. V. — S. 0.25 D. ⊃ + C. 0.75 D. ax. 120° = 18/30

Pilocarpin, ¼ per cent., t. i. d., increasing shortly afterward to 1 per cent. solution. One year later, corrected vision, O. D. 18/20, O. S. 18/15. Tension slightly +. Six months later, no contraction of fields, pupils very small, occasional halo of short duration.

When last seen (September, 1906) she reported that sight was about the same and she came simply for a change in her near glasses. There was a well-marked glaucomatous cup. The pupils were very small and the field of the left eye was considerably contracted at the lower inner segment. The tension was perhaps a little increased, but not greater than in many normal eyes.

O. D. V. — .50 ⌢ + .75 C. ax. 90° = 20/30
O. S. V. — .50 ⌢ + .75 C. ax. 105° = 20/40

Remarks.—Disease held in check by miotics while under observation five years.

Case 15 (Mr. E. T. Collins, *Clin. Jour.*, March 1, 1905). —*History.*—Male, under observation three years. Eserin (gr. i to fl. oz. i), cocain (gr. v to fl. oz. i), into each eye daily. Vision and field of vision have remained normal.

Case 16 (Dr. Weeks).—*History.*—Female, aged 70 years. Under observation two years. O. D. V. = 20/30. T. +. Field slightly reduced on nasal side. O. S. V. = L. P. T. + 1.

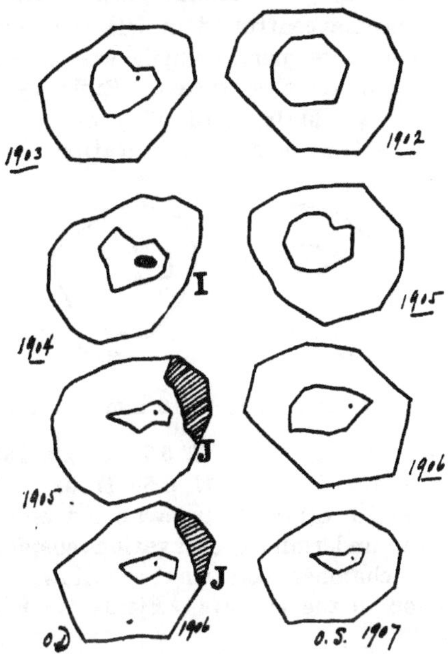

Fig. 7.—Fields of Case 17: 10 mm. white and red; I, relative scotoma for 10 mm. red; J, in shaded area 10 mm. white seen with difficulty.

Advised eserin solution (½ per cent.), b. i. d., in both eyes. October 26: O. D. V. = 20/30. T. + ½. Fields slightly more reduced. O. S. V. ———. T. + 1. Eye quiet.

Advised eserin (1/3 per cent.), b. i. d., in both eyes.

Jan. 17, 1906: O. D. V. = 20/30 +. T. + ½. Field same. O. S. V. ———. Eye quiet.

Nov. 13, 1907: Conditions same as at last visit.

Remarks.—Vision and field maintained practically the same. during the two years under observation.

Case 17.—*History.*—Female, aged 55 years. Under observation two and one-half years. At time of first observation dimness in left eye of six weeks' standing. Gouty. Mother had glaucoma. Both optic nerves gray; central excavation in the right eye and a forming glaucomatous one in the temporal half of the left nerve; sclera rigid, especially in O. S.; both anterior chambers shallow (Fig. 7).

O. D. V. + S. 0.50 D. ⊃ + C. 0.37 D. ax. 110° = 5/5.
O. S. V. + S. 0.50 D. ⊃ + C. 0.37 D. ax. 70° = 5/5.

Pilocarpin, gr. ss to fl. oz. i, gtt. ii, in left eye, q. d.; in right eye, b. d. Seen at intervals of six months, dose of pilocarpin being gradually increased, until now (two and one-half years after first observation) using pilocarpin, gr. ii, in left eye, q. d.; in right eye, b. d. O. S. excavation somewhat deeper, but that in O. D. still physiologic.

O. D. + S. 0.37 D. ⊃ + C. 0.50 D. ax. 150° = 5/5.
O. S. + S. 0.37 D. ⊃ + C. 0.37 D. ax. 45° = 5/5.

Remarks.—Glaucoma controlled in left eye, despite the considerable involvement of nerve which was present when the patient first came under observation. Right eye still normal.

Case 18.—*History.*—Male, aged 57 years. Under observation two years. At time of first consultation:

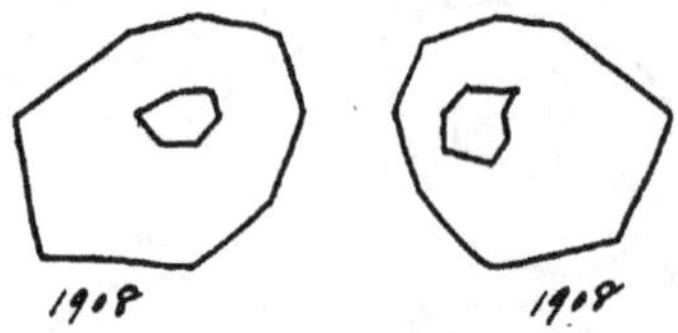

Fig. 8.—Fields of Case 19: 10 mm. white and red.

O. D. V. — S. 2.25 D. ⊃ — C. 0.75 D. ax. 180° = 5/5.
O. S. V. — S. 4.5 D. ⊃ — C. 0.50 D. ax. 60° = 5/9.

Localized traumatic cataract, from an old blow, in left eye. In the right eye, undermined excavation suspicious of glaucoma. Anterior chamber somewhat shallow. Sclera rigid. Central excavation in the left eye. Fields of vision normal in each eye.

After six months, excavation appears more extended and deeper. Pilocarpin (gr. 1/5, gtt. ii, b. d.) was prescribed. Three months later, gr. ½, gtt. ii, O. D., b. d. Field of vision and central vision normal. One year after observation, glaucomatous cup fairly well pronounced in the right eye, that in the left still physiologic. Pilocarpin, gr. i, gtt. ii, O. D., b. d.; gtt. i, O. S., b. d. Field of vision normal in each eye.

O. D. — S. 2.25 D. ⊃ — C. 0.62 D. ax. 155° = 5/5.
O. S. as at first examination.

Remarks.—Glaucoma cup developed under observation. Normal visual acuity and field of vision maintained despite steady progress of excavation.

Case 19.—*History.*—Female, aged 63 years. Under observation eighteen months. At time of first consultation, right eye just recovering from an iridectomy which had been done by another surgeon on account of acute glaucoma. Shallow excavation in head of optic nerve, but eye quiet and no glaucomatous symptoms. Left eye free from glaucoma, save for a doubtful excavation to outer side of nerve. Anterior chamber in each eye shallow. Tn. Fields of vision normal in each eye. Gouty subject.

O. D. V. + S. 1.5 D. ⊃ + C. 1.75 D. ax. 160° = 5/5.

O. S. V. + S. 2.5 D. ⊃ + C. 0.62 D. ax. 90° = 5/5.

Pilocarpin, gr. ½, gtt. ii, in each eye b. d., prescribed. Seen at intervals of every three or four months since. No glaucomatous symptoms in either eye, but excavation seems to be spreading and becoming deeper in the left eye. Now using pilocarpin, gr. i, gtt. ii, in each eye, b. d. (Fig. 8).

Remarks.—Despite glaucomatous outbreak in right eye, no glaucomatous symptoms have appeared in either eye, though a pathological excavation is forming in the left eye, even while the pupil is maintained at pin-point contraction.

MODERATELY ADVANCED CASES.

CASE 20.—*History.*—Female, aged 79 years. Under observation fifteen years. At time of first observation complained of occipito-frontal pains radiating into the eyes, worse on the left side. Six months previous she had had several attacks of sudden failure of vision in the left eye, which had lasted for a few minutes. During these periods of visual obscuration, the defect began in the temporal field. Both nerves were hyperemic, central excavation in the right eye becoming undermined down and out. Excavation in the left eye shallow but typically glaucomatous. Anterior chambers shallow. Scleræ rigid, especially in O. S. (Fig. 9).

O. D. V. + C. 0.25 D. ax. 180° = 5/5.

O. S. V. + S. 0.25 D. = 5/7½.

Eserin, gr. 1/20 to fl. oz. i, gtt. ii, O², b. d., prescribed.

One year later: O. D. V. = 5/5; O. S. V. = 5/7½. T. higher in O. S.

Two years later: O. D. V. = 5/5; O. S. V. = 5/7½.

Eserin, gr. ¼ to fl. oz. i, gtt. ii, O², b. d. Excavation in O. D. now typically glaucomatous as well as that in O. S.

One year later (1896): O. D. V. = 5/5, O. S. V. 5/7½. O. S. T. + 1, O. D. Tn. Eserin, gr. ½ to fl. oz. i, gtt. ii, b. d. Patient not seen for three years, eserin being employed, though irregularly, during the interval.

O. D. V. + C. 0.25 D. ax. 180° = 5/5; O. S. V. = 5/15.

Discs quite gray. Excavations of pure glaucomatous type. T. + 1 in O. S. elevated in O. D. Eserin, gr. i, gtt. ii, in each eye, q. d. Now seen regularly at intervals of six months until present time, seven years later.

At end of two years, vision had deteriorated in O. S. to 3/60, and at the end of another year to 1/60, at which it still remains.

1901: O. D. V. + C. 0.25 D. ax. 70 = 5/5.
1902: O. D. V. — S. 0.25 D. ⌒ — C. 0.50 D. ax. 120 = 5/5.
1903: O. D. V. — S. 0.50 D. ⌒ — C. 0.75 D. ax. 145 = 5/5.
1905: O. D. V. — S. 1 D. ⌒ — C. 1.25 D. ax. 145 = 5/5.
1906: O. D. V. — S. 2 D. ⌒ — C. 1.25 D. ax. 145 = 5/5.
1907: O. D. V. — S. 1.25 D. ⌒ — C. 1.25 D. ax. 145 = 5/5.

Now using pilocarpin, gr. vi to fl. oz. i, 2 drops in each eye, q. d., pupils being kept at pin-point contraction.

Remarks.—Glaucoma held in abeyance in O. D. for sixteen years, in O. S. five or six years, by miotics. It is probable that a more favorable result would have been gained in O. S.

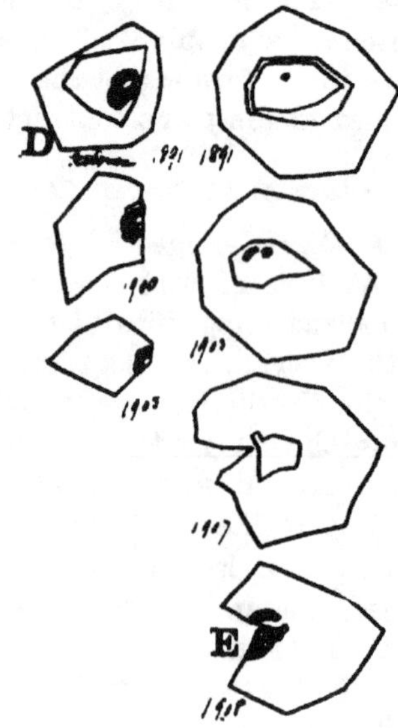

Fig. 9.—Fields of Case 20: 10 mm. white and red; D, absolute scotoma; E, absolute scotoma for 10 mm. white.

had an interval of several years not elapsed during which the miotics were used irregularly. At times, during the course of the disease, subacute symptoms arose which were promptly made to disappear by stronger doses of pilocarpin.

Case 21 (Bjerrum, *Centralb. f. prakt. Augenh.*, August, 1907.) Under observation twelve years. This author cites the case of a woman 85 years of age, whom he had treated with miotics for twelve years. The same vision, i. e., 5/9, and the same characteristic field of vision (a nasal scotoma defect with a paracentral scotoma under the fixation point to the blind spot being maintained as long as the case was under observation). Tn. A 2 per cent. solution of pilocarpin was employed, t. i. d.

CASE 22.—Female, aged 66 years. Under observation ten years. At time of first observation, sight said to have failed rapidly during year previous. Anterior chambers shallow; pupils small (i. e., pupils eccentric, irides reactionless, occasioned by anomalous formation in irides). Deep glaucomatous excavations. Venous pulse. T + 1 in each eye. (Fig. 10).

O. D. V. + S. 1 D. ○ — C. 6 D. ax. 100° = 5/15.
O. S. V. + S. 8 D. ○ — C. 2 D. ax. 90° = 5/22.

Eserin gr. ½ to fl. oz. gtt. ii, in each eye, b. d. Seen at intervals of six months or a year over a period of ten years., when patient passed from observation. Miotics gradually increased in strength, until pilocarpin, gr. ii to fl. oz. i, employed in each eye, b. d. Three years after time of first observation, retinal hemorrhages occurred in each eye which dimmed central vision for some months, but when last seen

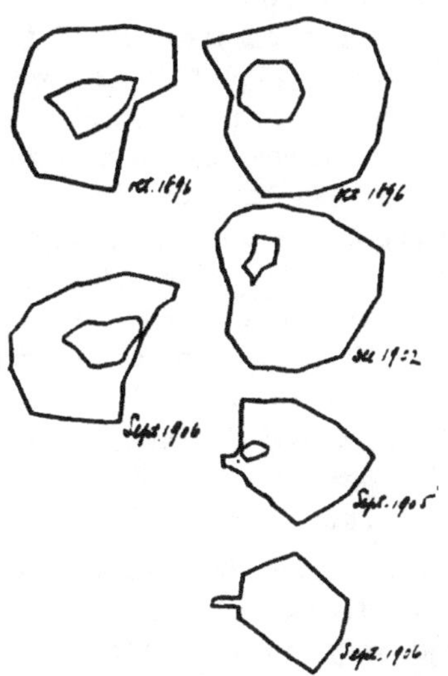

Fig. 10.—Fields of Case 22: 10 mm. white and red.

O. D. + S. 1.5 D. ○ — C. 8 D. ax. 100° = 5/18.
O. S. — S. 8.5 D. ○ — C. 4 D. ax. 70° = 5/18.

Remarks.—Miotics controlled the disease the ten years the patient was under observation, despite its quite advanced character and the degeneration of the retinal vessels as evidenced by retinal hemorrnages.

CASE 23.—(Dr. de Schweinitz. Reported 1899.) *Patient.*—Aged 50 years. Under observation ten years. Cornea anesthetic; anterior chamber shallow, deep cup, O. D. T. + 2. O. D. + S. 2 D. ○ + C. 0.60 D. ax. 15° = 5/7½.

Field: Concentric contraction, later loss of nasal half, final complete loss. Miotics and strychnin employed.

Remarks.—The vision of glaucomatous eye did not fail for two years, when it was 6/15. Two years later eye was blind.

Case 24.—(Dr. Cheney.) Male, aged 55 years. Under observation seven years. Seen July 4, 1899. A gradual failure of sight had been noticed in the right eye for at least five years, and it is probable that the disease had existed for a considerably longer period. There had been no pain, redness or other symptoms, and he had neglected to consult an oculist until this time. The tension was increased, the chamber a little narrow, the pupil of moderate size, and the disc deeply cupped. There was an arterial but no venous pulse. Vision = fingers at 20 cm. The left eye was normal in every respect, and the first suggestion of glaucoma was nearly three years later, when he reported some blurring of vision and an occasional halo about the light. The tension was not increased, but there was a slight cupping of the disc over the outer half and the vision had fallen off from 20/15 to 20/20 minus. A weak pilocarpin solution (¼ of 1 per cent.) was prescribed, and he has used this myotic constantly up to the present time. There is an occasional period of blurring for a day or two and the tension has been at times above normal. The strength of pilocarpin has been gradually increased, and for the last six months he has used a 1½ per cent. solution four times a day. There is now a cup of moderate depth over the outer two-thirds of the disc, but the central vision and field have continued perfectly normal.

Remarks.—Glaucoma held in check by miotics for the five years during which patient was under observation.

Case 25.—(Dr. Ayres.) *Patient.*—Aged 54 years; chronic glaucoma both eyes. Under observation seven years.

1900: O. D. V. = 1. O. S. V. = 0.6. Tn. + 1. Right field normal; left field very much contracted. Weak eserin prescribed.

1903: O. D. V. = 1. Tn. O. S. v. = motions of hand outward. Tn. + 1. O. S. nerve blanched and excavated. Operation declined.

1904: O. D. V. = 1. Tn. +. O. S. V. = shadows. Eserin.

1905: O. D. V. = 1. Tn. + 1. O. S. V. = 0.

1906: O. D. V. = 1. Tn. + 1. O. S. V. = 0.

1907: O. D. V. = 15/20. Tn. + 1. Field vision more contracted.

Still uses eserin. Operation refused.

Remarks.—Vision in O. D. maintained at normal for seven years under weak eserin.

Case 26.—(Dr. Hansell.) Male, aged 59 years. Under observation seven years. At time of first observation nerve white and completely cupped; pupils dilated; tension normal.

O. D. + S. 0.25 D. ⌢ + C. 0.50 D. ax. 90° = 5/4.

O. S. + C. 0.50 D. ax. 90° = 5/4.

Fields: White field unaffected. Color field concentrically contracted. Eserin, gr. ½ to fl. oz. i.

Two months later, left field limited to 70 degrees, right to 80 degrees, temporal side.

Three years later, O^2V. with correction = 5/5. Discs white and fields slightly smaller.

Three years later, O^2V. with correction = 5/7½. Cupping much deeper. O. D. T. + ½; O. S. T. normal.

One year later, O^2V. with correction = 5/5 partly. No ocular symptoms.

Remarks.—Patient under observation seven years, and using eserin, gr. ½ to fl. oz. i, continuously, glaucoma being held completely in check by the drug.

Case 27 (Dr. de Schweinitz, reported 1899).—Female, aged 72 years. Under observation five years.

O. D. lenticular opacity; complete cup.

O. D. + S. 3 D. = 6/12.

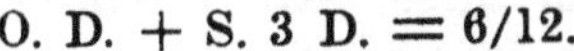

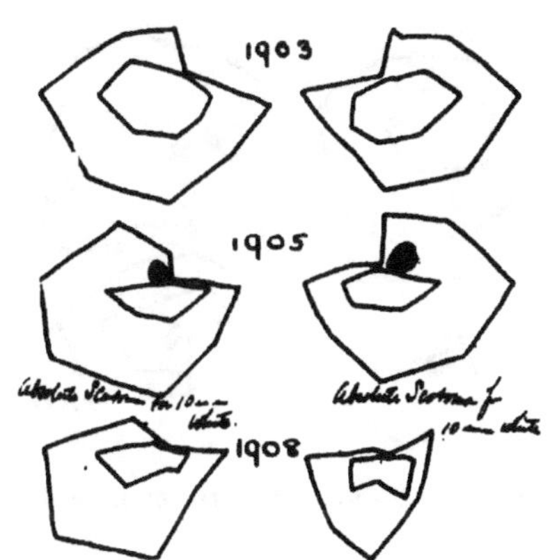

Fig. 11.—Fields of Case 30: 10 mm. white and red.

Complete loss of upper half, moderate contraction of remaining half. Eserin. After five years, hand movements only.

Remarks.—Miotics apparently powerless to control course of disease, though influence of cataract in reducing vision not noted.

Case 28 (Dr. de Schweinitz).—Patient, aged 72 years. Under observation eight years.

O. D., anterior chamber normal; complete cup; venous pulse; halo, T. +.

O. D. + S. 1.5 D. ⌒ + C. 0.50 D. ax. 90° = 6/12

Field: contraction moderate, chiefly nasal side, later scotoma. Miotics. Strychnin. Bichlorid of mercury.

At the end of eight years, V. = 4/60.

Remarks.—Lowering of vision, due partly to development of lenticular opacity, eye becoming myopic, miotics controlling the disease in a measure only.

Case 29 (Dr. de Schweinitz).—Patient, aged 75 years. Under observation six years.

O. S. shallow anterior chamber, almost complete cup, broad halo T. +.

O. D. V. + S. 0.50 D. ⊂ + C. 0.50 D. ax. 165° = 6/5

Field.—Slight concentric contraction. Miotics and strychnia. O. D. V. at end of six years, 6/9.

Remarks.—Vision preserved and apparently never any rise of tension or visual disabilities with this eye after six years.

Case 30.—Female. Under observation five years. When first observed aged 65. History of failing sight for two years. Rheumatic. Large glaucomatous excavations in each eye, more pronounced in the left eye. T. + in each eye (Fig. 11).

O. D. V. + S. 0.50 D. = 5/5 partly

O. S. V. + S. 0.50 D. ⊂ + C. 0.50 D. ax. 145° = 5/5 ptly

Eserin, gr. 1/10, gtt. ii, in each eye, b. d., increasing in three months to gr. ½. Not seen for three years, eserin being continued with interruptions during that period.

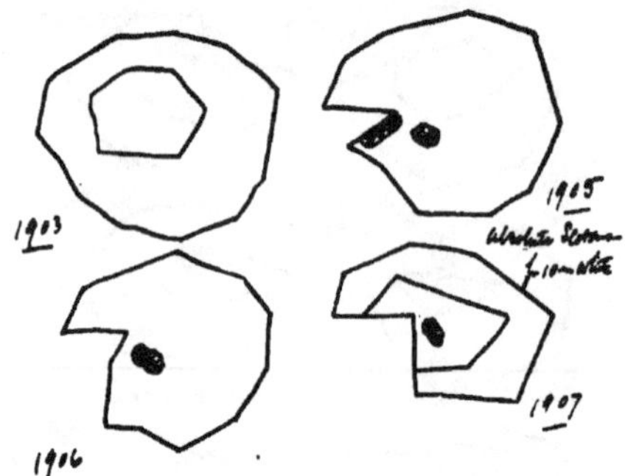

Fig. 12.—Fields of Case 32: 10 mm. white and red.

O. D. V. + S. 0.50 D. = 5/22

O. S. V. + S. 0.75 D. ax. 150° = 5/5 partly

Remains of old hemorrhages in right eye. Tension elevated in each eye. Eserin, gr. i, gtt. ii, in each eye, q. d.

O. D. V. + S. 0.50 D. = 5/15

O. S. V. + C. 0.75 D. ax. 150° = 5/6

Remarks.—Eserin held disease in check five years, vision in right eye being lowered chiefly through hemorrhages in macular region.

Case 31 (E. T. Collins, *Clin. Jour.*, March 1, 1905).—Female, aged 66. Under observation five years.

At time of first observation there was glaucomatous cupping of both nerves. Slight fulness of tension in the left eye, but none in the right. O. D. V. = 6/6. O. S. V. = 6/12. Fields of vision normal. Eserin prescribed. Seen at intervals of two years, eserin being employed continuously. Five years after first observation O. D. V. = 6/9. O. S. V. = 6/12. Fields of vision normal.

CASE 32.—Male, aged 64. Under observation five years. Poor vision in right eye for some years past, following dynamite explosion. Vision of left eye totally lost at that time. O. D. V. worse past six months. Halos at times. Large glaucomatous excavation in right eye; anterior chamber shallow; pupil large; cornea maculated in pupillary area; T. +. Left eye phthisis bulbi.

O. D. — S. 1 D. ⊃ — C. 1.5 D. ax. 180° = 5/9

Eserin, gr. ¼ to fl. oz. i, gtt. ii, O. D., t. i. d.

Seen at intervals of six months, miotics being increased from time to time. Now using pilocarpin, gr. iii to fl. oz. i, gtt. iii, t. i. d., and eserin, gr. i. to fl. oz. i, gtt. ii, at night. During the five years of treatment vision has practically held its own (Fig. 12).

O. D. V. + S. 0.75 D. ⊃ — C. 4 D. ax. 160° = 5/12 ptly

Remarks.—Central vision maintained for five years, despite some loss of field in an eye far advanced in glaucoma and the seat of a central corneal scar, the left eye being blind with phthisis bulbi.

CASE 33 (Dr. de Schweinitz).—Female, aged 72 years. Under observation five years.

O. S. complete cup, halo, lenticular opacity. O. D. + S. 3 D. = 6/15.

Complete loss of upper and inner quadrant, contraction of remaining portion. Eserin. At end of five years V. = 6/9.

Remarks.—Improvement in central vision after five years, though field became considerably contracted.

CASE 34 (Dr. de Schweinitz).—Female, aged 60 years. Under observation four years. Chronic rheumatism and arteriosclerosis; typical glaucoma cups — 2. Corrected vision O. D. — 6/12, O. S. 6/10. Operation not advised owing to general condition. Persistent and careful use of pilocarpin with internal administration of strychnia and antirheumatics. First examined May 12, 1904. One and one-half years later original vision preserved, but visual fields distinctly contracted, especially on the left side, which at that time and originally was only a small field on the temporal side. In the next six months (exact date not known) vision of O. D. suddenly disappeared; left eye continued unchanged. At the present time, or four years after the original examination, O. D. without 1 p.; left eye practically unchanged in vision, possibly a little less accurate, 6/12. Within the last few months occasional attacks of halo vision and slight rise of tension, always controlled by increased use of pilocarpin. Operation declined or, rather, forbidden by family physician.

Remarks.—Miotics failed to control glaucomatous process in right eye, but maintained vision and fields in the left for the four years patient was under observation.

CASE 35 (Dr. de Schweinitz).—W. E. H., male, aged 74 years. Under observation four years. First examined July 21,

1903. Corrected vision O. D. + 2 ⊂ + .75 C. axis 30, 6/6, O. S. + 1.50, 6/15. Moderate cup, each side, smaller on the right and not quite typical; left eye typical loss of nasal field. Right eye slight concentric contraction; no rise of tension. Operation always declined. Persistent use, except when conjunctival symptoms forbade, of miotics. Patient not seen for two years, then vision of O. D. still 6/6, left eye absolutely blind; patient unable to tell when this loss of sight occurred. Again two years later V. of O. D. 6/6, no change in O. S. No increased contraction of visual field. Cup in this eye, however, never typically glaucomatous, although distinctly pathologic.

Remarks.—Vision and field maintained in the right eye, but no power to check glaucomatous process in the left eye.

Case 36 (Dr. Ayres).—Patient, aged 55 years. Under observation four years. At time of first observation, glaucoma cups in both eyes, discs pale. Tension somewhat elevated. O. D. V. = .06, O. S. V. = .02. Weak eserin. One year later condition much the same. Iridectomy refused. Weak eserin continued. Three years later O. D. V. = .07, O. S. very amblyopic. Tension + 1 in each eye. (Iridectomy performed at this time, but result of operation marred by onset of albuminuric retinitis.)

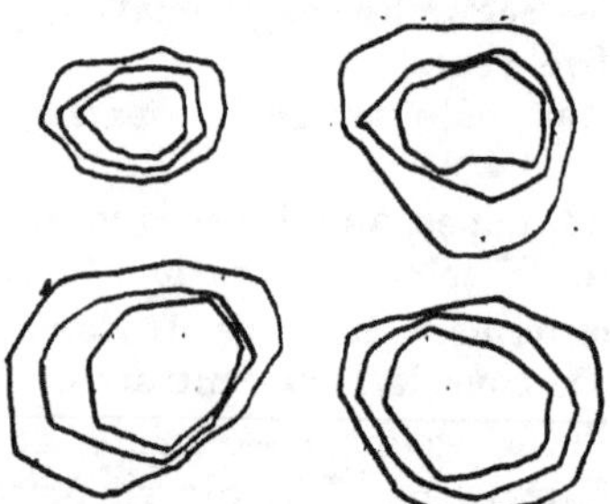

Fig. 13.—Fields of Case 37: 10 mm. white, red and green.

Remarks.—Eserin employed apparently very weak, not perhaps in sufficient strength to obtain very small pupils.

Case 37 (Dr. Holmes).—A middle-aged male. Under observation four years. When first seen (October, 1903):

O. D. V. + S. 1.25 D. = 20/20. T. + ½. Halos at times.
O. S. V. emmetropic 20/20

Fields concentrically contracted, especially in left eye, in which there was some loss of nasal field (Fig. 13). Eserin, gr. i to fl. oz. i. Three months later eserin discontinued for a time, glaucomatous symptoms having disappeared. Miotic resumed, however, in a few weeks, as halos reappeared. One year later, vision in each eye still 20/20. One year later vision 20/20 in each eye and field of vision normal. No halos as long as miotic is employed. One year later, four years after first observation, vision 20/15 in each eye and fields normal. One per cent. solution of eserin in olive oil employed daily.

Remarks.—Glaucomatous symptoms held in check by eserin during the four years of observation.

Case 38 (Dr. de Schweinitz).—Male, aged 69 years. Under observation four years.

O. D. sluggish pupil; complete glaucoma cup.

O. D. + S. 1 D. ⊃ + C. 0.75 D. ax. 15° = 6/22

Field, contractions general, with re-entering angles. Miotics.

Remarks.—After four years of treatment, gradual contraction of field and increase of scotoma. Slow progress of the disease in spite of miotics.

Case 39 (Dr. Veasey).—A young colored woman. O. D. V. began to fail after an attack of typhoid fever when 16 years of age, becoming blind at the end of three years. At time of examination right eye found to be blind with a deep glaucoma cup; eye emmetropic. The left eye appeared to be normal, and there was a small physiologic cup.

Three years later, seventeen years after the appearance of glaucoma in O. D., the left eye became glaucomatous, the cup being undermined and tension slightly elevated. Miotics were faithfully employed and strychnia and nitroglycerin adminis-

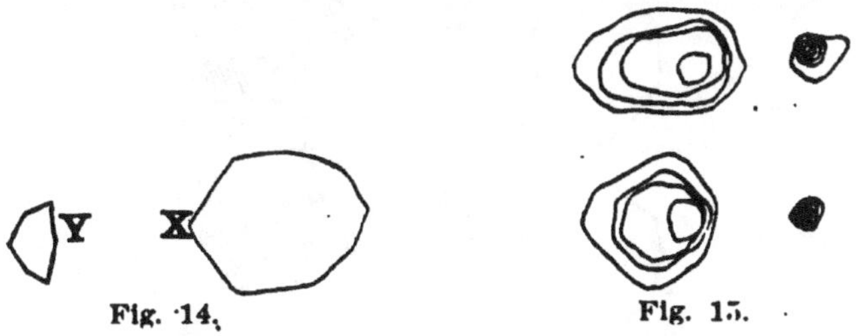

Fig. 14. Fig. 15.

Fig. 14.—Fields of Case 39: Y, obj. 2 mm. square; X, obj. 1 cm. square. Fig. 15.—Fields of Case 40: 10 mm. white, blue, red and green.

tered internally, but the cup became larger and the field smaller. Iridectomy was advised but declined, and, although the treatment has been persistently carried out, at this time, ten months after the eye became affected, but a small amount of eccentric vision remains (Fig. 14).

Remarks.—This case appears to be an atypical form of chronic glaucoma, induced, perhaps, by some disease within the eye, and is of value as indicating the inability of miotics to control its course.

Case 40 (Dr. Callan).—Male, aged 73 years. Under observation three years. At time of first observation deep glaucomatous excavations in both eyes, the entire nead of the right nerve being involved. Halos at times; no pulsation in vessels. Iridectomy refused. Miotics employed, keeping pupils at pinpoint contraction. Under close observation three years, central vision being well maintained (Fig. 15) i. e., O. S. V. = 20/40, O. D. V. = 10/200. Three years later O. D. V. = 20/30; O. S. V. = 20/30.

Remarks.—Well-developed stage of disease held in check in both eyes over a period of three years by miotics.

CASE 41.—Male, aged 51 years. Under observation three years. At time of first consultation vision in right eye had been misty six months. Halos at times. Rheumatic history. Had been under ophthalmic care, but no drops had been employed. There was a large glaucomatous excavation in right eye, with a shallower but also a characteristic excavation in the left. Tension markedly elevated in both eyes. Anterior chambers shallow.

O. D. V. + C. 1 + D. ax. 20° = 5/15

O. S. V. + S. 0.25 D. ⌒ + C. 0.50 D. ax. 180° = 5/5

Eserin, gr. ½ to fl. oz. i, gtt. ii, in each eye, at night; gr. ¼, gtt. iii, t. i. d.

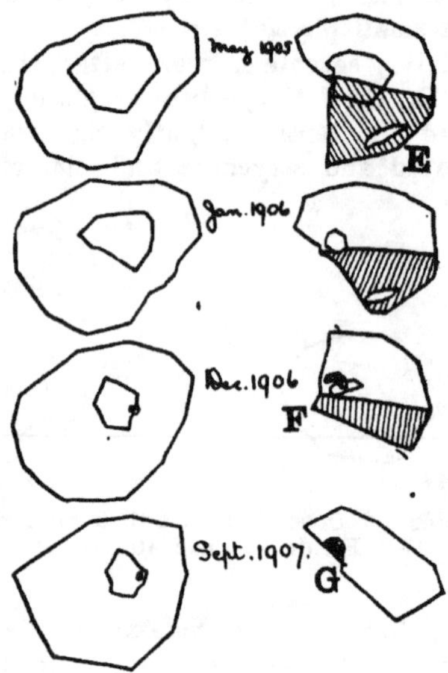

Fig. 16.—Fields of Case 41: 10 mm. white and red; E, white and red seen dimly in shaded area; F, absolute scotoma; G, absolute scotoma.

Patient has been seen at intervals of every three or six months since, at which times stronger miotics were found necessary to control the appearance of halos and to prevent loss of vision in the right eye. At end of three years

O. D. V. + S. 0.25 D. ⌒ + C. 0.50 D. ax. 10° = 5/22

O. S. V. + S. 0.50 D. ⌒ + C. 0.62 D. ax. 170° = 5/5

The glaucomatous excavations are deeper and more pronounced (Fig. 16). Halos have disappeared and there are no subjective symptoms.

Remarks.—The miotics have controlled the glaucoma, notwithstanding the somewhat advanced stage of the disease when the patient came under treatment and the tendency which the disease manifested to assume a subacute type.

CASE 42 (Dr. de Schweinitz).—Female, aged 65 years. Under observation two years. Corrected vision O. D. 6/9, O. S. 6/15; refraction hyperopic astigmatism, the astigmatism against the rule. Typical glaucoma cups; no rise of tension ever demonstrable; characteristic contraction of visual fields from nasal side, with marked contraction of preserved field on the left side; no scotomas. Persistent use of pilocarpin and internal administration of strychnia for two years, with practical preservation of the vision already recorded, possibly a little less accurate in the left or poorer eye, which is now about 6/20. No change in the visual field. Marked arteriosclerosis in retinal vessels.

Remarks.—Vision and fields maintained for the two years under observation.

CASE 43 (Dr. C. A. Wood).—Male, aged 72 years. Under observation two years. At time of first examination complained of a misty sensation with fatigue on use of eyes.

O. D. V. with correction = 20/100
O. S. V. with correction = 20/200

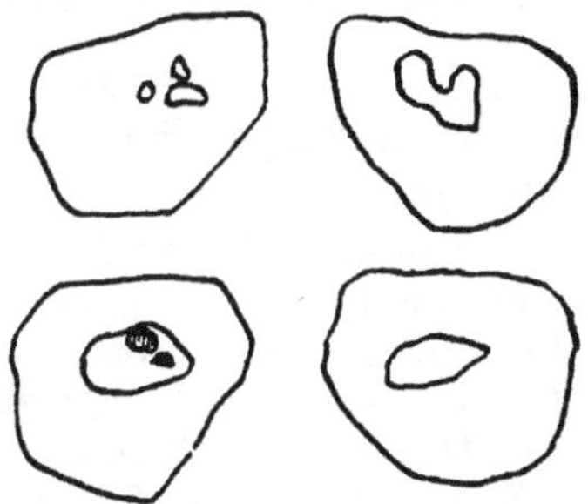

Fig. 17.—Fields of Case 43: 5 mm. white and red. W, scotoma (eccentric) white called red; relative central scotoma for red.

Tension and pupillary motions normal. Anterior chamber shallow. Glaucomatous excavations in each eye. Pulsation of retinal arteries produced by experimental instillation of homatropin. Massage of eyeball with ½ per cent. solution of eserin and eserin, ½ per cent., in oily mixture, t. i. d., and gently rubbed in each time. Seen at intervals of every few months and treatment maintained two years, O. D. V. improving to 20/70 and O. S. V. = 20/100 (Fig. 17).

Remarks.—Arrest of glaucomatous process, with improvement of central vision and enlargement of visual fields.

CASE 44 (Dr. Ayres).—Female, aged 68 years. Under observation two years; 1906, chronic glaucoma in both eyes. Deep excavations. T. + ? + S. 3 D. in each eye. O. D. V. = 15/20. O. S. V. + S. 3 D. ⊃ + C. .05 ax. 180° = 15/30. Field of vision slightly contracted. Pain in eyes frequent; rheumatic; thickened finger joints. Ordered eserin, ¼ gr. to fl. oz. ½, two or three times a week, and 15 grains of salicylate of sodium each day.

Remarks (1908).—Has used weak eserin nearly two years, and vision remains the same. Tension is barely + ? Continues the salicylate of sodium. Operations not recommended.

CASE. 45 (Dr. Weeks).—Male, aged 56 years. Under observation two years. First seen Nov. 30, 1905.

O. D. V. = 8/200. T. + ½. Marked cupping.

O. S. V. = 20/20. T. + —. Slight cupping.

Fields normal. Pilocarpin b. i. d. January 22: Halos recently; had neglected to use pilocarpin. O. S. V. = 20/20 +. Continue treatment.

April 5: O. D. V. = 8/200; O. S. V. = 20/20. Fields the same.

November 24: O. D. V. = 6/200. T. + ½. Some reduction in color field. O. S. V. = 20/20. T. +. Eserin (¼ per cent.). O. D. b. i. d.; O. S. u. i. d. at night. Extract of jaborandi continued.

Jan. 12, 1907: O. D. T. + O. S. T. +. Field slightly reduced. Is losing ground slowly. Eserin (¾ per cent.) b. i. d. Pilocarpin at noon. O. D. V. = 10/200. O. S. V. = 20/20.

March 21, 1907: O. S. field slightly larger. T. + on. Continue treatment.

Remarks.—Disease controlled by miotics during the two years patient under observation, despite a very advanced stage of the disease in one eye.

CASE 46 (Dr. Ayres).—Female, aged 65 years. Under observation one year; 1906, chronic glaucoma in both eyes. Deep excavation in each eye, most pronounced in O. D. O. D. T. + 1 ? O. S. T. T.n. O. D. pupil sluggish, O. S. responsive. O. D. V. = 15/100. O. D. + S. 1.5 D. = 15/20. O. S. V. = 15/100. O. D. + S. 1.75 D. = 15/15. O. D. field contracted all around, but especially the nasal side and in. Notch in field at ax. 110 degrees contracted to 20 degrees. O. S. field contracted slightly all around. Weak eserin and salicylate of sodium prescribed.

1907: O. D. T. + 1. Field contracted. V. = 15/20. With correction, O. S. V. = 15/20 Tn. Iridectomy in both eyes. Tension normal afterwards.

Remarks.—Vision maintained without change for one year by miotics, despite cutting of visual fields.

CASE 47 (Dr. Weeks).—Male, aged 52 years. Under observation one year.

O. D. V. = 20/20. T. +. Slight cupping of disc. Field normal.
O. S. V. = 20/20. T. +. Slight cupping of disc. Field normal.

Has seen halos for more than ten years—attacks of blurred blindness. Advised pilocarpin (1 per cent.) at night.

January 31: No "mist" or "fog." Advised eserin (1/3 per cent.) at night; pilocarpin (1 per cent.) mornings.

October 3: Slight halos occasionally. Slight aching at times. O. D. V. = 20/20 Tn. Continue treatment. O. S. V. = 20/20.

December 27: O. D. Tn. V. = 20/20; O. S. Tn. V. = 20/20; fields normal; no halos. Pupils small.

Remarks.—Central and peripheral vision maintained, with control of halos by miotics during the year under observation.

ADVANCED CASES.

CASE 48 (Reported 1906).—Male, aged 66 years. Under observation fifteen years. At time of first consultation O. D. blind from subacute glaucoma, and O. S. vision much reduced from same cause, the glaucoma having supervened on an attack of grippe three years previously. Tension in both eyes equaled + 2. The anterior chambers were very shallow, the scleral vessels were dilated and engorged and the nerves were deeply excavated.

O. D. V. hand movements in temporal field.

O. S. V. + S. 0.25 D. ⊂ + C. 0.50 D. ax. 180° = 5/5

Eserin, gr. ½ to fl. oz. i, gtt. ii, O², q. d. as an initial dose. In a few weeks, using gr. i to the ounce, and a similar increase was made each month until in four months a gr. iv. to the ounce solution was employed. At the end of six months pilocarpin in twice the strength was substituted for the eserin, and during the past fifteen years the miotic has been employed three or four times daily. For thirteen years there was full central visual acuity, though a study of the fields will show (Fig. 18) that as the years went by the field of vision became more and more contracted and the paracentral scotoma became steadily larger. Two years ago, after an attack of dysentery, there were several recurring attacks of blindness in the left eye which persisted from five to ten minutes. Central vision sank after this to 5/7½ and so remained for about a year, when other attacks of blindness supervened, vision finally failing to re-establish itself. The eyes were acutely inflamed for a time after this and the acute glaucoma which supervened was controlled with great difficulty by miotics and cocain.

Remarks.—Full central vision maintained in typically glaucomatous eye with field cut almost to fixation for fourteen years by miotics.

CASE 49.—Female, aged 85 years. Under observation three years. At time of first observation: O. D. + S. 1 D. = 5/15. O. S. + S. 2 D. ⊂ + C. 1 D. ax. 180° = 5/7½. Deep glaucomatous excav. in each eye, embracing entire head of nerves. Senile changes in chorioid and some spiculæ in lenses. T. elevated in each eye (Fig. 19). Eserin, gr. ¼, gtt. ii, in each eye, b. d. Seen at intervals of about four months, and eserin increased in strength; now using gr. 2½, gtt. ii, O², q. d.

At end of one year O. D. V. had failed to 1/60; O. S. V. + S. 1 D. = 5/15. Tension is decidedly elevated in both eyes. Lenses hazy, the reduction in vision being probably occasioned quite as much by the cataracts as by the glaucomatous process.

Remarks.—**Despite the great age of the patient and the advanced character of the glaucoma, vision maintained three years.**

CASE 50 (Dr. de Schweinitz).—Female, aged 48 years. Under observation two years. O. D. pupil dilated and fixed. Cornea anesthetic. Deep cup. T. + 2.

O. D. + S. 1.75 D. $\supset$ + C. 0.50 D. ax. 165° = 6/9

Fields.—**Great contraction, only a small patch remaining on temporal side, with partial scotoma. Eserin. Vision after two years 6/12.**

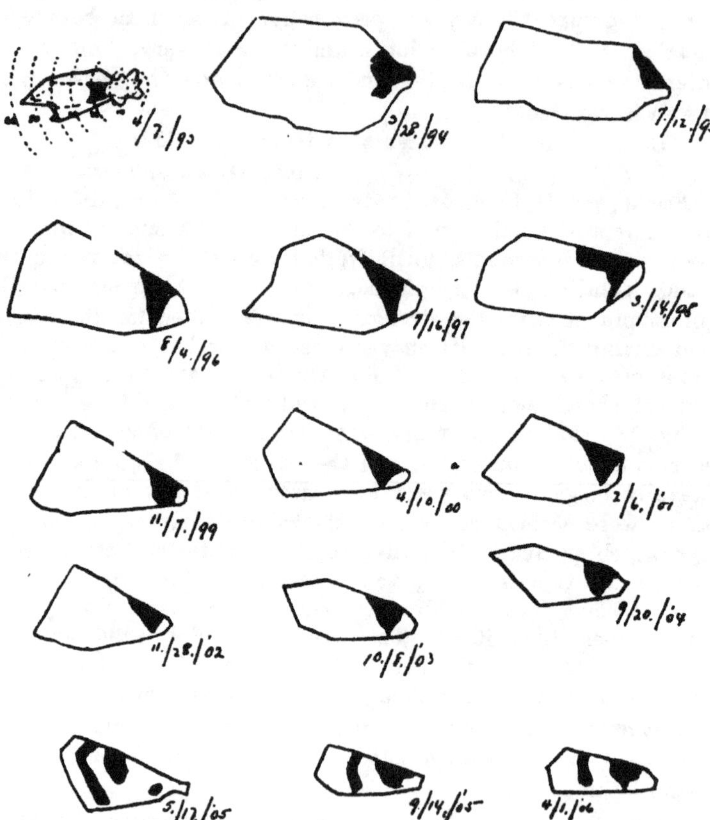

Fig. 18.—Fields of Case 48: The fields of vision in the left eye show gradual peripheral restriction and the extension of scotoma.

Remarks.—Disease held in check two years, despite its advanced type.

CASE 51 (Dr. C. A. Wood).—Female, aged 46 years. Under observation two years. Dimness of vision for one year, preceded by ten years of asthenopia, before first consultation. Pupils had been widely dilated for one month before; photophobia, occipital headache had been complained of and halos had been observed. Large glaucomatous excavation in each eye with pulsating retinal arteries and veins. The anterior chambers were shallow and the pupils semi-dilated and sluggish (Fig. 20).

O. D. T. + 1; O. S. T. + 2. Both cornea were slightly hazy.

O. D. V. = 20/40. O. S. V. = finger counting at three inches eccentrically.

Pilocarpin, gr.: 1/20 to fl. oz. i, t. i. d. Massage with eserin ointment, t. i. d.; a 5 per cent. solution of dionin preceding

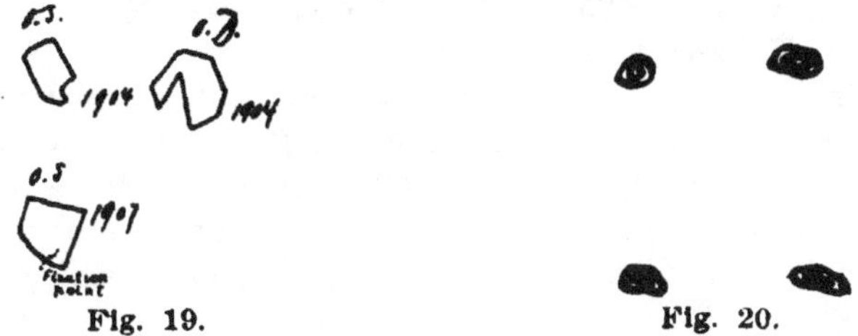

Fig. 19. Fig. 20.

Fig. 19.—Fields of Case 49: In 1907 it was impossible to outline field of O. D. for white, though the patient could apparently see the fixation point; 10 mm. white. Fig. 20.—Fields of Case 51: 5 mm. white and red.

the eserin. At the end of one week O. D. V. improved to 20/30.

The patient has been under observation every few weeks for the past two years; central vision has been retained and there has been no further contraction of the fields.

Remarks.—Vision held in abeyance for the two years under observation, notwithstanding the advanced stage at which treatment was inaugurated.

CASE 52 (Dr. C. A. Wood).—Male, aged 60 years. Under observation two years. Vision failing five years before Dr. Wood first saw him. Iridectomy had been performed on the right eye three years before, notwithstanding which blindness gradually ensued. O. S. V. = 20/200. Dionin and massage with eserin improved vision to 20/70. Both discs deeply ex-

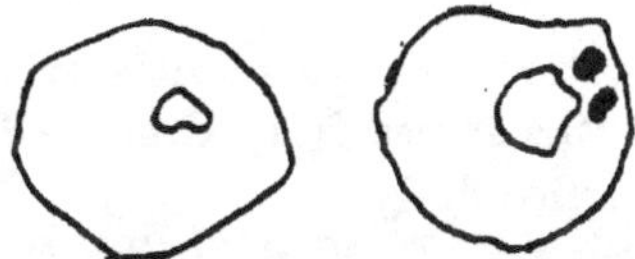

Fig. 21.—Fields of Case 52: 5 mm. white and red.

cavated and pallid. Anterior chambers are shallow and tension full. Has been under constant observation during the past two years and the miotic treatment has been continued uninterruptedly.

Remarks.—Central vision improved and no loss in peripheral field in a very advanced case, after two years of treatment, in which vision in one eye had deteriorated following iridectomy (Fig. 21).

Case 53.—Female, aged 65 years. Under observation two years. At time of consultation all the signs of advanced chronic glaucoma in each eye, the anterior chamber being very shallow, tension + 1 or more, and large excavations in each eye, that in the left embracing the entire head of the nerve, that in the right the outer 4/5 of it. Vision had been failing for ten years and for a year or more had been using eserin (gr. ¼ to fl. oz. i) once or twice a week. Subject of advanced arterial sclerosis.

O. D. V. + S. 2.75 D. ⊃ + C. 0.37 D. ax. 90° = 5/5

O. S. V. hand movements at ½ m.

Pilocarpin, gr. ½, gtt. ii, in each eye, t. i. d., increased in one week to gr. i, q. d., and to gr. 2, gtt. ii, O², t. i. d., and eserin, gr. 2, gtt. ii, O², at night by the end of three months. Seen at intervals of three months, and assurance obtained that miotic was being employed faithfully, maintaining pupils

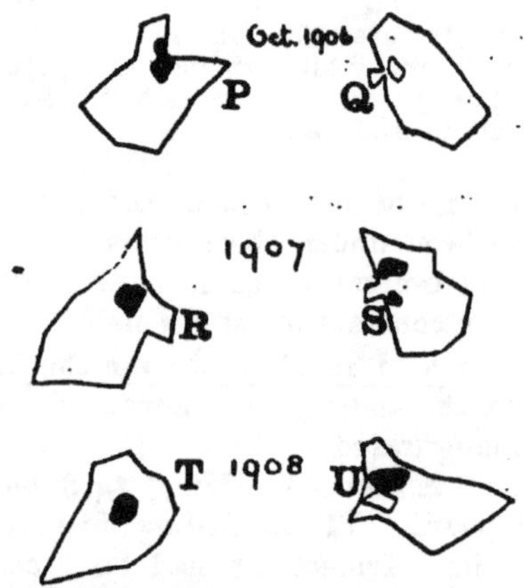

Fig. 22.—Fields of Case 53: P, absolute scotoma for 20 mm. white; Q, 10 mm. white and red; R, absolute scotoma for 20 mm. white; S, absolute scotoma for 10 mm. white; T, absolute scotoma for 15 mm. white; U, absolute scotoma for 10 mm. white.

at pin-point contraction. Conjunctivitis arising at times from the use of the miotic successfully combated with argyrol, 25 per cent., once or twice daily.

At end of two years O. D. V. + S. 2.5 D. = 5/5. Anterior chamber in each eye very shallow and both nerves deeply and completely cupped (Fig. 22).

Remarks.—O. D. vision normal, and the fields but little contracted after two years, the disease having steadily progressed under weak eserin, being controlled only by strengths of the drug sufficient to maintain the pupils at pin-point contraction.

Case 54.—Female, aged 74 years. Under observation eighteen months. Poor health. Advanced vascular degeneration, vision in the left eye failing five years, in the right three years. Had never used miotics, though under the care of an eye specialist for five years. At time of first consultation:

O. D. + S. 0.50 D. ⊂ + C. 0.50 D. ax. 180° = 5/7½

O. S. V. faint light perception only.

Deep glaucomatous cups in each eye (Fig. 23). T. + 1 or more, pupils 2/3 dilated. Pilocarpin at once ordered, gr. ½, gtt. ii, in each eye, t. i. d., rapidly increasing at end of two months to gr. 2, gtt. ii, in each eye, q. d. Has been seen at intervals of three months, and despite the advanced degree of cupping of the nerve and the cutting of the field. O. D. V.

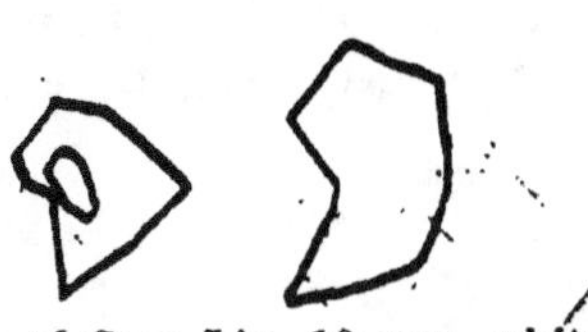

Fig. 23.—Fields of Case 54: 10 mm. white and red.

+ C. 0.62 D. ax. 180° = 5/6. The field has been but slightly more cut than at the first observation.

Remarks.—This case represents the power of miotics to retain vision for a long period even under the most desperate conditions, vision being maintained for eighteen months in an individual of very advanced years and great debility, the field of vision being greatly contracted and vision rapidly deteriorating.

CASES SUBJECTED TO BOTH MIOTICS AND IRIDECTOMY.

Case 55 (Dr. de Schweinitz).—Male, aged 69 years. Under observation nine years. First examined Dec. 5, 1894. Typical chronic glaucoma, with deep cups. No demonstrable increase of tension. Corrected vision: O. D. 6/12, O. S. 6/6; moderate contraction of each field, paracentral scotoma in right. Persistent use of eserin, alternating with pilocarpin. Operation advised and declined. One year later O. D. 6/60, O. S. 6/5. Operation still declined. Ten months later O. D. 2/50, O. S. 6/5. Operation still declined, miotic treatment continued. Two years later O. D. counts fingers, O. S. 6/6. One year later O. D. 1 p., O. S. 6/6. Field gradually contracting and Bjerrum's scotoma beginning to appear. One year later same conditions. One year later same conditions, except O. S. 6/6?. Practically no change for two years, except increase in the size of the scotoma of the left eye and reduction of vision to 6/7.5. Iridectomy now accepted. Performed first on the right or nearly blind eye with perfect operative result, and one month later on the left eye, or eye with a vision of 6/7.5. Corrected vision after operation 6/6. Six months later corrected vision 6/9. Seven months later 6/12; some increase in the scotoma and contraction of the visual field. Patient not seen since last named date, namely, April 8, 1903. Patient had rheumatism and was a sufferer from persistent attacks of hay fever.

Remarks.—Gradual loss of vision in right eye following use of miotics for eight years. For three years vision and field conserved in left eye, but at end of that time gradual diminution, falling from 6/6 to 6/7½. Paracentral scotoma. Iridectomy. Improvement in vision and field about six months, then gradual loss in both central and peripheral vision.

CASE 56 (Dr. Hansell).—Male, aged 50 years. Under observation eight years. At time of first observation O. D. V. = 5/5; O. S. V. — S. 0.25 D. ⌒ — C. 0.75 D. ax. 90° = 5/5. Tension normal. O. S. nerve slightly cupped below.

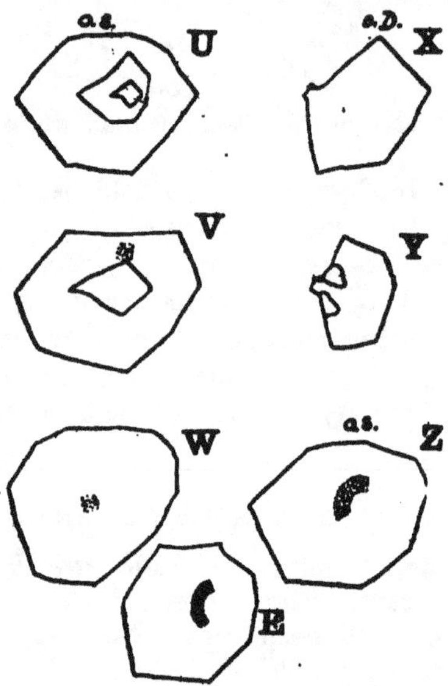

Fig. 24.—Fields of Case 57: U, obj. 1 cm. square; field for white and green; X, obj. 1 cm. square; V, obj. 0.5 cm. square; field for white and green. In the scotoma white appeared gray; W, obj. 1 cm. square; scotoma forred and green, white appeared grayish; Z, obj. 0.5 cm. square; scotoma for red and green, white was grayish; E, obj. 1 cm. square; absolute and relative scotoma.

Four years later both discs slightly cupped and pale. O. D. V. = 5/5; O. S. V. = 5/7½. Fields limited on nasal side. Eserin, gr. ½ to fl. oz. i; strychnia. One year later, fields for white and colors limited to nasal side. Shallow glaucomatous cups. Nerves white. Eserin, gr. i to fl. oz. i. One year later O. D. V. = 5/5, O. S. V. = 5/22. Left field limited upward, inward and downward. Nerves white and cups pronounced.

Iridectomy performed on both eyes with an interval between. Two months later O. D. V. = 5/5, O. S. V. = 5/60. Fields more contracted. Has had several attacks of blurred vision in O. S.

Remarks.—Despite the continuous use of eserin through eight years, loss of vision steadily progressed. Iridectomy also powerless to check glaucomatous process.

CASE 57 (Dr. Veasey).—Patient aged 60 years. Under observation eight years. At time of first observation typical glaucoma cup in O. D. and a probable commencing cup in O. S. O. D. V. + S. 1.75 D. = 5/7½. O. S. V. + S. 2 D. = 5/4.

Iridectomy performed on O. D. one month later, O. D. V. + C. 3 D. ax. 15° = 5/7½.

Eserin and pilocarpin continuously and faithfully employed in O. S., but at end of two years, while central vision remained good, the field became more contracted (Fig. 24). The field in O. D. has decreased but little since the iridectomy, vision equaling 6/9. Iridectomy advised on the left eye, but refused. Six years after first observation O. D. V. = 6/12, O. S. V. = 6/9. Anterior chamber of left eye was shallower, but tension normal. One month after operation there was somewhat less contraction of the field and scotoma was somewhat smaller than before the iridectomy was performed. One year ago, eight years after first observation, O. D. V. = 6/12; O. S. V. = 6/12.

Remarks.—This case is of interest, inasmuch as it shows relatively that iridectomy and miotics have about equal influence in controlling the course of chronic glaucoma, the degenerative process advancing about *pari passu* in each eye.

CASE 58 (Dr. Ellett).—Female, aged 42 years. Under observation six years. At time of first observation there was a history of chronic simple glaucoma in the left eye for five years. Vision 20/60. Iridectomy. Now, six years after operation, field is not more contracted than when the case first came under observation, though central vision is not so good. When first seen O. D. V. normal, but anterior chamber shallow and tension sometimes elevated. Halos at times. Eserin prescribed, but used only regularly when halos are seen. Despite this irregular use of miotics, central vision is still perfect and field normal.

Remarks.—This illustrates the power of both miotics and iridectomy in checking the progress of the disease, both means having successfully combated the glaucomatous process for a period of six years.

CASE 59 (Dr. Weeks).—Male, aged 72 years. Under observation three years. First seen Jan. 13, 1903.

O. D. V. = 20/40 +. T. +. Anterior chamber slightly shallow.

O. S. V. = L. P. T. + 2. Cupping of disc 1 1/3 mm.

Prescribed pilocarpin, 1 per cent., O. D., u. i. d.; O. S., b. i. d. Right field very slightly contracted.

Oct. 5, 1903: O. D. V. = 20/20. T. +. Field normal. O. S. V. = L. P. T. + ½.

May 23, 1905: O. D. V. = 20/20 —. (Pilocarpin, b. i. d.) Field of right eye more reduced, especially for colors.

Jan. 17, 1906: O. D. V. = 20/30. T. + ½. O. S. V. = L. P. T. + 1. Slight glaucomatous attack yesterday, affecting both eyes.

May 4: O. D. V. = 20/30. T. + ¼. The disease is slowly progressing and operation is advised.

May 9: Broad iridectomy in right eye.

June 7, 1906: O. D. V. = 20/20.

July 5: + 20/30 +. Field for form almost normal. Field for colors slightly larger.

September 10: O. D. V. = 20/30 +. Field as on July 5.

November 26: O. D. V. = 20/30 +. Patient died in December, 1906.

***Remarks.*—Disease controlled for three years by miotics. Field then gradually contracting, iridectomy done with restoration of field to normal until patient died six months later.**

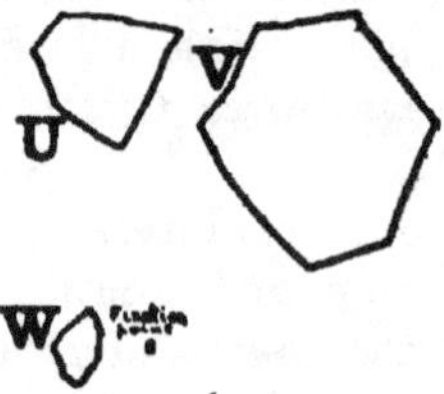

Fig. 25.—Fields of Case 61: U, obj. 2 cm.; V, obj. 1 cm.; W, obj. 2 cm. square.

One eye blind from glaucoma when patient came under treatment.

CASE 60 (Dr. de Schweinitz).—Female, aged 55 years. Under observation two years. O. D. pupil moderately dilated; hazy cornea; typical glaucoma cup; full veins. T. + 2. Has V. = 6/45.

Field—Contracted above and on nasal side. Eserin; later iridectomy. + C. 2 D. ax. 180° = 6/15.

Remarks.—Iridectomy was performed when visual acuity had been raised to 6/12 by eserin, showing efficacy of miotics.

CASE 61 (Dr. Veasey).—Male, aged 65 years. Under observation two years. At time of examination, typical chronic simple glaucoma in each eye. Vision said to have been failing for four years (Fig. 25). O. D. V. = 5/27; O. S. V. = 3/160; O. D. Tn., O. S. T. + 1. Solutions of eserin alternated with pilocarpin were employed constantly. Two years later, fields were greatly contracted in both eyes.

Iridectomy O. D., but without avail, vision deteriorating. Miotics continued in O. S., but total blindness ensued in two years.

Remarks.—This case, well advanced in glaucoma when it came under treatment, shows the inability of either iridectomy or miotics to control the progress of the disease.

Case 62 (Dr. Weeks).—Female, aged 76 years. Under observation one year.

O. D. V. = 20/40 —. T. + ½. Field reduced 20° on nasal side.

O. S. V. = 20/30 —. T. + ½. Field reduced 15° on nasal side.

Pilocarpin (1 per cent.), O. D., t. i. d.; O. S., u. i. d.

September 4: O. D. V. = 20/40. T. + 1; O. S. V. = 20/70. T. + ½. Pilocarpin not used this morning. Pilocarpin (1 per cent.) O. D. every three hours; O. S., t. i. d. Fields contracting a little slowly.

September 8: Fields more contracted. Advised operation. Eserin (½ per cent.) O. D. every three hours; O. S. t. i. d. Much "mist."

September 25: O. D. V. = 20/50. T. + ¾. Myopia increasing. O. S. V. = 20/40 +. T. + ¾. Fields more reduced.

October 2: Double iridectomy.

October 17: O. D. V. = 20/70 Tn.; O. S. V. = 30/100 Tn.

October 24: O. D. V. = 20/50
O. S. V. = 20/70

Both eyes 20/40.

Patient was seen almost weekly, and conditions remained about the same up to July 26, 1907, when there was a slight improvement in the sight and no reduction in the fields. Eserin (1/3 per cent.) had been used two or three times daily.

Nov. 8, 1907: O. D. T. +; O. S. T. +. Pupils small, vision the same.

Remarks.—Miotics employed two months; failing to control the glaucoma, iridectomies were performed, which seemed to check the course of the disease the remaining ten months patient was under observation.

MEMORANDA

[APPENDIX.]

REPORT OF THE COMMITTEE ON LEGISLATION CONCERNING OPTICIANS.

At the last annual meeting of this Section the following resolution was unanimously adopted:

WHEREAS, Opticians in various states have endeavored to obtain by legislation the right to practice what is usually called optometry; and,

WHEREAS, The proper fitting of glasses means in most cases really the practice of medicine, and physicians, realizing this, have often strenuously urged that such a right should be granted only to persons who take the course of study and pass the examinations already defined by the statutes; and,

WHEREAS, The members of the Section on Ophthalmology of the American Medical Association, in common with other physicians, would be glad to cooperate with opticians in obtaining for them legislation which is fair and safe; therefore, be it

Resolved, That a committee of three be appointed, two of these being ophthalmologists named by the chairman of this section, and one a physician named by the president of the Association. It shall be the duty of that committee to collect facts concerning the claims of the opticians to any recognition, and if these facts show that any legislation is needed, then to report to this section some plan in which we might all cooperate because of its justice to the opticians, to physicians, and above all, because it is the safest and best for the public.

The stenographer omitted to forward this resolution early enough for publication with the rest of the minutes, but as it had been duly recorded and formed a well-known part of the proceedings of our section, the chairman accordingly appointed two members, and at the request of the President of the Association, Dr. George M. Sternberg, U. S. Army, consented to act as the third member.

As the resolution constituting this committee instructed it to collect facts concerning the claim of opticians to recognition, therefore the first step was to prepare a series of questions on the subject. A rough proof of these questions was first sent to the secretaries of about sixty-five state and national societies of opticians with a request for comments or suggestions. The object of this was to obtain information and to draw out in advance any adverse criticisms on these questions. The answers which came from opticians showed the wisdom of this plan. A few stated the claims of the opticians to legal recognition clearly and with apparent honesty, and the data were specially valuable in showing what had been accomplished in that direction or what was proposed. Most of these correspondents, however, were rather resentful and suspicious of any interference. In spite of considerable provocation in the form of "open letters" to this committee, and otherwise, care was taken to avoid discussion in any form.

After deciding on the form of the questions, they were sent to members of this section, of the American Ophthalmological Society, and to a few other ophthalmologists of good standing who were not members of either organization. It seemed desirable thus to gather information from as many different sources as possible. As each member of the section is already familiar with these questions they need not be repeated here, but the more important points will be referred to later in this report.

As bills for the recognition of optometry had been introduced into the legislatures in different states during the early part of last winter, therefore, in the latter part of January, a brief note was issued to those who had already replied to the first letter. This note simply gave the names of those interested in the subject, thus placing them in communication with each other, if desired. Also the names were given of physicians who had been suggested for chairman of a committee on the subject in the various state medical societies.

That letter from this committee was not in any way advisory, and certainly we did not venture to interfere with the legislation in any state, having quite enough to do otherwise.

It is well to make this explanation as one or two letters which came soon after the issue of that list, indicated that perhaps its object had not been understood.

For the sake of clearness it is desirable thus to refer to the resolution which called this committee into existence, and to show briefly its plan of study.

Having done this we should understand clearly what is meant by the terms optician and optometrist, and then ask, as the resolution provides, what claims they make to recognition. After that we can ask ourselves whether this section or any other body of physicians should take action at all in the premises, and if so what that should be.

To avoid misunderstandings it is worth while to define the meaning of terms used. The word "optician" means, as the dictionaries say, not only "one skilled in optics," but also one who simply "sells glasses." By optometrist we will understand not only those who are permitted by law to sell glasses, but also those who have formally combined, and under this name, are endeavoring to obtain a legal status.

As the term "optometrist" has a legal status, and as it is more specific than optician, we gain in clearness by using it in a restricted sense. But the term optician or optometrist does not describe a body of men who, like those of most similar occupations have about the same amount of training to fit them for their work, or who are held by custom or tradition to a certain line of conduct. To select a few of any type as samples is manifestly unjust. But this diversity of acquirement and of character is so great that when we consider any claims for legal recognition we should remember that what applies to one group may not hold good at all for the others.

With this understanding of terms we can ask what the claims of the optometrists are to recognition. Although these have been often published, it is desirable, if only in fairness, to repeat them here distinctly, and in as strong terms as possible, even though it must be briefly. These claims are:

First.—The existence already of a very considerable body of optometrists organized partly for the purpose of obtaining legal recognition. According to one of their trade journals, *The Keystone*, October, 1907, their organizations in the United States are as follows: National, four; interstate, two; state, forty-one; and local societies, twenty-two. It is difficult to obtain the total number registered. But it is stated that in New York alone the societies of optometrists include at least 1,200 to 1,400 members. The American Association of Opticians contained at last accounts, over 5,000 members, and the number was constantly increasing.

Second.—In a considerable number of states and territories laws have been already passed legalizing optometry, for example, in Arizona, California, Idaho, Indiana, Minnesota, Montana, New Mexico, North Dakota, Oregon, Tennessee, Utah, Nebraska. Strenuous efforts are also being made to obtain similar recognition in an increasing number of states, and apparently with increasing success. During the last winter, bills have been introduced in legislatures of New York, Massachusetts, Maine and a number of other states, and in several of these the efforts have been more or less successful.

It is desirable for our purpose at this point to obtain some idea at least in what this legislation consists. The laws enacted show a remarkable degree of similarity in the following points:

(A) They usually define optometry about as follows: "The employment of subjective or objective methods or means to determine the accommodative and refractive state of the eye and the scope of its functions in general."

(B) According to all the laws passed or bills presented the governor (in New York, the Board of Regents) is empowered to appoint a board of examiners in optometry. In most of the states this board is selected entirely from optometrists. In Indiana there must be at least one oculist on the board, and in Ohio two. In none of the laws or bills is there any specification of standards of excellence. The board thus composed entirely or almost entirely of opticians can admit to the practice of optometry any one whom they wish.

(C) According to all laws passed or bills presented all persons who have practiced optometry for a time varying from two to five years may receive the certificate of this board of optometry on the payment of a nominal fee.

Accompanying is a tabular statement of these facts concerning optometry as they could be ascertained by the committee:

Third.—It is claimed, usually with much emphasis, that there is a desire on the part of the optometrist to raise their standard of excellence.

Fourth.—It is claimed that the optometry laws which have been passed or the bills which have been presented to regulate optometry would give protection to the public, because the optometrist who had a state certificate would be considered by

TABLE OF REGULATIONS IN VARIOUS STATES CONCERNING OPTOMETRY.

STATE.	When Bill Was Presented.	By Whom Appointed.	Number in Board.	Number of Optometrists.	Others on Board.	Certificate Because in the Business at the Time.	Certificate Because of Experience of Years.	Amount of Fee for Certificate
Arizona	1907	Governor	3	3		Yes		$5.00
California	1907	Governor	8	8		Yes		5.00
Indiana	1907	Governor	5	4	1 oculist		3 years	5.00
Massachusetts	1907	Governor	5	5			2 years	5.00
Minnesota	1901	Governor	5	5		Yes		3.00
Montana	1907	Governor	5	5		Yes		5.00
Nebraska	1906	Governor	3	3			2 years	5.00
New York	1908	*	5	5			2 years	5.00
North Dakota	1905	Governor	5	5		Yes		3.00
Ohio	1908	Governor	5	3	2 oculists		2 years	5.00
Oregon	1907	Governor	3	3		Yes		5.00
Rhode Island	1908	Governor	3	3			2 years	5.00
Tennessee	1907	Governor	3	3		Yes		1.00
Utah	1907	Governor	3	2	1 oculist	Yes		3.00

* Appointed by state Board of Regents.

the public as competent, in contradistinction from the optician who does not hold a state certificate and is therefor incompetent.

Fifth.—That the average doctor of medicine knows but little about the fitting of glasses, and though he was taught to do this during his college course, has either forgotten how or he is so much engaged with other branches of the practice of medicine that he does not care to do this work.

Sixth.—The fitting of glasses by optometrists is convenient and economical for the public.

Seventh.—It is a physical impossibility for the few ophthalmologists to provide glasses for all who need them, among fifty odd million inhabitants in the United States.

Eighth.—It is practically impossible to prohibit entirely by law the sale of glasses by opticians.

Ninth.—It is unnecessary to prohibit entirely the sale of glasses by opticians to the public because in many cases glasses from opticians do no harm, but on the contrary they do afford distinct relief from discomfort. The evidence for this statement is too abundant to be denied.

The validity of each of these claims will be considered later.

The foregoing includes the principal claims which the opticians usually make to legal recognition. The question before this committee is, shall any action be taken in the matter, and if so, what?

Four plans of procedure suggest themselves:

First.—To do nothing. There are excellent reasons for such an attitude. Discussions like this are not scientific and the whole subject smacks so much of trade unionism as to be distasteful to us all. One of the most honored members of this section simply said, "I hate such discussions."

Besides, they are unprofitable. Although opticians may fit many of our patients with glasses, we know that often those same glassses, or diseases of the eyes, incipient or advanced, which pass undetected, ultimately increase the total amount of our work. Considered from the financial standpoint the ophthalmologist is often the better off because of such competition.

As for the public, the efforts in its behalf are seldom appreciated, and if it really wishes to be cheated by the incompetent optometrist, some might say, why not let them both alone?

But many practitioners have decided convictions on the subject, and if we are to express any opinions as individuals it is becoming to consider the facts together, to formulate and express an opinion collectively.

Moreover, it is a proud tradition of the American Medical Association that when public health is threatened in any way that association has always been ready to speak—and in no uncertain tone. It therefore does not seem proper for this section to remain mute and apathetic concerning a subject which is also important, as we shall see, to the public health. Instead, we ought to examine these claims of the optometrists to legal recognition. If they are just claims we should admit that frankly and promptly. If they are not, we should know exactly why. Or in case they are unjust, and if in spite of that, one sort of such legislation is inevitable, as seems probable, then we should have some substitute to propose which is better than the laws thus far made.

If, in the second place, any action is to be taken or even any opinion is to be expressed concerning laws already enacted or proposed, we should ask whether the claims made by the optometrists, as already cited, are valid. Let us consider them in the order in which they have been given to see if it is possible to accord with these views:

First.—The simple existence of a body of men organized for a special purpose, does not prove that their object is worthy. If so, there might be equal reason for the legal recognition of the anarchists or any similar body.

Second.—The fact that legislation favorable to such an organization has been enacted does not prove that the law is a good one.

Third.—The claim that legislation is desired by the opticians in order to raise the standard of excellence among them shows a laudable ambition. But it is impossible, in any case, to prove that a certain motive does or does not exist. That is indicated only by the action, and if a higher standard is the object aimed at, then no objection ought to be made to having this standard still higher—such, for example, as is now required by the three years' course in pharmacy or dentistry. This higher standard will be dealt with later.

Fourth.—It is claimed that the optometry law would be a protection to the public by the creation of a class of men who have a certificate showing their proficiency, as compared with those who do not possess such a certificate. This claim would be valid were it not that each law enacted and also each law proposed, so far as can be ascertained, permits all persons who have practiced optometry for a certain few years also to receive this certificate of the board of optometry by paying for it a nominal fee. In other words, the public are no more protected with such legislation than without it. We should bear in mind, too, that such a certificate has a certain trade value. The state thereby certifies that that man is qualified to do that work—and it is proposed that the state shall certify to that simply on the payment of a fee. The very natural inference is that many opticians, at least, desire an optometry law because the certificate which they could so easily obtain declares their proficiency.

Fifth.—As for the claim that the Doctor of Medicine knows little or nothing about the fitting of glasses, or frequently that he does not care for such practice, that is true. It is generally conceded that the course of study in the average medical school might be changed so as to give more time to the study of ophthalmology. That, however, needs no additional legislation, and improvements in this respect are constantly being made. Moreover, if a doctor does not wish to fit glasses he can not be compelled to do so.

Sixth.—The claim that the fitting of glasses by optometrists is convenient and economical for the public means but little. It is also true that all drugs, including poisons, might be sold conveniently and economically by any person at any store with greater convenience and economy to the public. Nevertheless, the law provides that they shall be sold by qualified persons only, and if, as we shall see, the fitting of glasses is the practice of medicine, then we may point out that permission to practice medicine has thus far been given by law to physicians only.

Seventh.—We must admit the claim that it is a physical impossibility for the few ophthalmologists in this country to provide glasses for all who need them.

Eighth.—We must also admit that it is practically impossible to prohibit entirely by law the sale of glasses by opticians to the public. If a man who is a presbyope of one or two diopters has lost his glasses, and wishes to sign his name or attend to some business transaction, he will pay the optician for those glasses. It is not probable that any law would be or could be made to prohibit this transaction on the ground that it was sufficiently dangerous to public health or public morals.

Ninth.—The claim must also be admitted that the glasses prescribed by opticians may do no harm, and frequently do relieve a certain amount of considerable discomfort.

But the facts warrant us in going still further. They show that the opticians or optometrists, or both, not only practice medicine but do so frequently to the detriment of the patient. It requires no elaboration to show that the fitting of glasses is, in most cases, the practice of medicine. Glasses can and do affect the eyes as much as applying drops to them.

But it is a general impression among laymen and among doctors also that this effect of glasses on the eyes of patients or on other organs of their bodies is, after all, very slight, and that opticians could not do very much harm under any circumstance—that it has been unduly imagined by the eye doctors.

This point appeared of sufficient importance to this committee to warrant some investigation.

It was mainly to collect data concerning this aspect of the subject that the questions already referred to were prepared and issued, though it was not expected that many of the busy practitioners could review their case records in order to answer all these questions.

The number of replies received to the circular letter sent out by this committee was 204. Of these, 26 were fragmentary or indefinite, leaving 178 quite complete. These contain a very considerable amount of interesting information and valuable detail. It would, however, form too voluminous a report to give the experience or opinions in detail. Moreover, that would be only to obscure the other objects of this report, and also give the impression, probably, that the ophthalmologists were anxious to prove a case against the opticians. It seems better, therefore, to state only the more prominent facts, and in as few words as possible.

An examination of these replies shows the following:

First.—It is the opinion of every practitioner, without exception, that not every person should be allowed to sell any kind of glasses to any person who wishes to buy them.

Second.—Nearly every ophthalmologist without exception has seen numerous cases in which an optician, failing to recognize the underlying disease, gave glasses to improve the vision or to relieve the discomfort complained of, and the patient, relying only on those glasses to do this, was thereby caused:

(A) Unnecessary suffering: (a) In headaches directly or indirectly from the eye or from imbalance of ocular muscles; (b) in headaches from diseases of the stomach, kidneys, or other parts of the body, or from anemia or general diseases; (c) in nervous diseases. In this connection it is not meant that the glasses prescribed by physicians all give immediate relief. Far from it. It is meant, however, that unnecessary suffering has been found to have been produced under such circumstances, which was relieved by other glasses or by other treatment.

(B) A distinct majority of physicians who replied to our circular letter had not only seen unnecessary suffering following the use of glasses which had been prescribed by opticians, but had also seen cases in which such opticians had overlooked or neglected pathologic conditions of the eyes, which were apparently present, with a resulting partial or total loss of vision, because of the continued diplopia, or iritis, glaucoma, chorioiditis, or retinitis with or without neuritis.

(C) A much less number of physicians observed under similar circumstances not only the unnecessary suffering or imperfect vision, but the entire loss of an eye from glaucoma or malignant diseases of the chorioid or retina.

(D) A few of these correspondents reported also cases in which failure to recognize an albuminuric retinitis in the early stage, and the consequent delay in instituting the proper treatment had resulted fatally, when such a result could probably have been retarded or possibly prevented. With this additional medical testimony as to the sins of commission and omission which are committed in the effort to practice medicine by those not qualified to do so, the case appears still stronger against legislation such as has been already enacted for the recognition for optometry.

A third plan of procedure which we might adopt would be to oppose all such legislation because it is unfair to physicians, as the fitting of glasses is really the practicing of medicine; and as physicians are required to pass certain examinations before they are permitted to practice, therefore it is unfair to them to allow opticians to prescribe glasses. That seems self-evident. But no ophthalmologist wishes to plead his own case in that way. Nor is it necessary. With his training as a physician he has no fear of small competition, though he still sees the injustice done to him by legislators. For, although other physicians or committees of medical societies have again and again shown to legislators the injustice to physicians of the present optometry laws, that was counted simply as jealousy and the law usually passed just the same. It therefore seems in questionable taste, and is usually useless to object to optometry laws on the ground that they are unfair to physicians.

For the sake of clearness it is desirable to review our study of the subject to this point. We have found:

First.—That in order to define the condition to ourselves, and to act in harmony and in accordance with the traditions of this Association concerning public health, it is desirable to agree on some statement in regard to legislation concerning optometry.

Second.—When we examine the laws which have been passed or which have been proposed concerning optometry, we find that we can not endorse the legislation in that form. Among other reasons, because no standard of excellence is established. Almost any one can obtain the certificate to practice optometry.

Third.—At the same time we are forced to admit that it is physically impossible for ophthalmologists in this country to provide with glasses all who require them. It is practically impossible to prohibit their sale, and sometimes at least the glasses obtained from opticians do no harm, but do afford distinct relief from discomfort.

In view of these facts, there seems to be only one rational solution of the question: That is, to pass laws regulating their sale.

The committee appreciated that it is very difficult to decide under just what circumstance they may or may not be sold. Nor is it probable that any recommendation would meet unanimous approval. Apparently, however, the permission to sell glasses might be given in cases where the ametropia does not exceed one or two diopters or the vision fall below a certain fraction. Although it is well-known that our worst cases of so-called asthenopia are those with a low degree of ametropia, still those are not the persons who are ordinarily in danger of losing their sight.

The exact degree of imperfection of the eyes, or the imperfection of vision, or both of these factors together, which should be a reason for deterring an optician from selling glasses without a prescription are all details to be decided on by medical men in each state. The standards proposed would depend on the personal opinion of different ophthalmologists, or necessary local conditions, especially in sparsely settled states. The essential point on which this committee desires to lay stress is that some restriction in the sale of glasses is desirable. The problem is not unlike the problem concerning the sale of liquor. Experience shows that restriction is the most practical plan.

But if the dispensing of glasses is to be limited, then who would be allowed to prescribe for or furnish glasses to persons whose eyes are in a more or less dangerous condition—for example, those who have high degree of ametropia or diseasesd condition of the interior of the globe? Apparently, that should be under the direction of a doctor of medicine, or at least be done by some person better qualified than those who have thus far been recognized by law as optometrists.

In reality, that is just the practice at present with the better class of opticians. They furnish glasses for presbyopia and low degree of ametropia, the doubtful or dangerous cases they refer, when they can, to some one who is better qualified to judge of such conditions. That arrangement seems to work satisfactorily. It is not easy to formulate into some statute what is now the ordinary practice in this respect, but that again is rather a question of detail, to be determined by local conditions in each state.

But we have already admitted that it is physically impossible for the opthalmologists in this country to provide glasses for all who require them. Experience shows that laws have been passed admitting optometrists to prescribe glasses for all conditions, and that the number of these optometrists is constantly increasing and probably will increase still more.

In view of such facts the only rational plan seems to be to use whatever influence we have, to assist in creating a body of these men whom we can respect as being competent, and above all, who are not dangerous to the community.

The plan for this would be as follows:

First.—If a board of examiners in optometry is to be created, it should not be appointed from any optical society, but that board should include physicians, as is the case in one or two states already.

Second.—The standard of examinations should be such as presupposes a good preliminary education and a course of at least three years special study as is demanded for dentists or pharmacists. It is true that both of those departments began at first with low standards, and medicine began ages ago with a standard lower still. But modern conditions demand that if any one now wishes to practice medicine or surgery even in part, he should possess a corresponding part of what is the common fund of modern knowledge. Moreover, this can be easily done if a few of the many schools of optometry will simply raise their standards.

Third.—The schools of optometry should be those in which the students are taught the higher mathematics and physiologic optics thoroughly, the anatomy and physiology of the eye, a certain portion of its pathology, especially that which related to ametropia, together with the art of making lenses and fitting glasses. The certificate of such a school would command confidence and respect, and could easily lead to the certificate or diploma of the board of optometry.

This committee is well aware that many opthalmologists and other physicians will at once protest against any plan to assist the optician in obtaining legislation, which means almost the creation of a department as distinct from ophthalmology as pharmacy is from medicine, and dentistry from other branches of surgery. But we must all learn that laws are not made by physicians but by legislators, and, ultimately, by the people whom those legislators represent. Whether those laws are right or wrong, they exist, and other laws of like character are rapidly increasing.

The question is whether we will attempt opposition to legislation in which we are constantly defeated (although such legislation is grossly unfair to those who have been required to pass examinations) or on the other hand, whether we abandon all discussion in which our own interests are in any way concerned and then unite in advocating restriction in the sale of glasses and also a standard for the opticians which is worthy of the best among them and of every one with whom they have to deal.

It is a question whether, in spite of opposition, laws shall be made which constantly increase the number of incompetent opticians or whether those laws shall confer a few certificates on those who are really competent. It is a question whether the medical profession must in this respect follow ignominiously the uneducated public, or by advocating a high standard of efficiency, that the profession, in fact this section, may lead in a distinct advance in ophthalmic science and in giving comfort and safety to a considerable number of the afflicted public.

As one of the principal objects of this inquiry is to find if possible a few fundamental principles which will serve as a basis for uniform opinion or for action, if necessary, on the part of the members of this section in their relation to legislation concerning optometry, this committee offers the following preamble and resolutions. If the section approves them they may assist somewhat toward clearer thought or more intelligent action on this question. If the conclusions are not approved, the section may suggest from the data something better:

Whereas, The ophthalmologist constantly sees cases in which the use of glasses furnished by opticians has produced unnecesary discomfort, suffering, or more or less injury to the eyes, and

Whereas, He also sees cases in which the failing vision was due to some disease of the eyes or even to a disease of organs in other parts of the body, and this abnormal condition having been naturally overlooked by the optician who furnished glasses for that failing vision, the patient delayed the proper treatment for the original disease, thereby suffering more or less loss of vision of the eye, and in some cases loss of life, and

Whereas, The collective experience of ophthalmologists in different parts of the country indicates that the frequency and importance of such errors is much greater than is generally supposed, and

Whereas, The number of ophthalmologists in certain parts of this country is not sufficient to give suitable attention to all persons whose eyes require careful examination and accuracy in the prescribing of glasses, therefore, be it

Resolved, That it is the sense of this Section that the well-being of the public requires that the sale of glasses should be restricted by law, especially for those whose vision falls below a certain standard of excellence which has been agreed on by medical experts.

Resolved, That in the states where legislators consider that the conditions demand the recognition of optometrists, the lawmakers should be impressed with the fact that legislation for that purpose which has thus far been enacted, is imperfect and inadequate, especially because no standard of excellence is specified for optometrists, as the Board of Examiners can grant a certificate by the payment of a nominal fee.

Resolved, That when any Board of Optometry is to be created, its standard of excellence should be defined by the act creating it, and this standard should be as high as possible from the first. The examination for a certificate or diploma should presuppose, at least, a high school education, with a subsequent course of three years in studies relating to what is therein defined as optometry.

Resolved, That the previous practice of optometry for a certain number of years should not, on the payment of a fee, enable an applicant to obtain the certificate of the Board, but the high standard of excellence established from the first should be maintained without favors to any individuals or groups of persons.

Lucien Howe.
George M. Sternberg.
William H. Wilder.

CPSIA information can be obtained
at www.ICGtesting.com
Printed in the USA
LVHW08*1616110818
586684LV00009B/180/P

9 780260 115348